# Advanced Practice and Leadership in Radiology Nursing

Kathleen A. Gross
Editor

# Advanced Practice and Leadership in Radiology Nursing

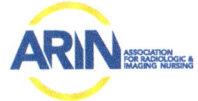

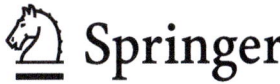

*Editor*
Kathleen A. Gross, MSN, BS, RN-BC, CRN
Owings Mills, MD
USA

ISBN 978-3-030-32678-4    ISBN 978-3-030-32679-1  (eBook)
https://doi.org/10.1007/978-3-030-32679-1

© Springer Nature Switzerland AG 2020, corrected publication 2020
This work is subject to copyright. All rights are reserved by the Publisher, whether the whole or part of the material is concerned, specifically the rights of translation, reprinting, reuse of illustrations, recitation, broadcasting, reproduction on microfilms or in any other physical way, and transmission or information storage and retrieval, electronic adaptation, computer software, or by similar or dissimilar methodology now known or hereafter developed.
The use of general descriptive names, registered names, trademarks, service marks, etc. in this publication does not imply, even in the absence of a specific statement, that such names are exempt from the relevant protective laws and regulations and therefore free for general use.
The publisher, the authors, and the editors are safe to assume that the advice and information in this book are believed to be true and accurate at the date of publication. Neither the publisher nor the authors or the editors give a warranty, expressed or implied, with respect to the material contained herein or for any errors or omissions that may have been made. The publisher remains neutral with regard to jurisdictional claims in published maps and institutional affiliations.

This Springer imprint is published by the registered company Springer Nature Switzerland AG
The registered company address is: Gewerbestrasse 11, 6330 Cham, Switzerland

*To my husband, Richard J. Gross, MD, and sons, David and Jonathan, who have taught me much about life and professional dedication through their own work. Also, to Abigail, Whitney, and Evan who give me cause to laugh and remind me of balance in living.*

# Foreword 1

Evidence-based practice (EBP) is widely considered the foundation of quality health care practice. EBP is no longer just a buzzword but a requirement that clinical practice is based on scientific evidence. As health care professionals, we have a duty to be concerned that we are achieving the best patient outcomes from our interventions and that those interventions, protocols, and policies are based on scientific evidence and best practices.

It was these very concerns that led to the development of the Johns Hopkins Nursing EBP Model and Guidelines that has driven nursing practice across all specialties at the Johns Hopkins Medical Institutions for the last 15 years. The JHNEBP Model defines EBP as a problem-solving approach to clinical decision-making within a health care organization that integrates the best available scientific evidence with the best available experiential (patient and practitioner) evidence, considers internal and external influences on practice, and encourages critical thinking in the judicious application of such evidence to care of the individual patient, patient population, or system [1].

The goals of EBP are to assure the highest quality of care by using evidence to promote optimal outcomes and to create a culture of critical thinking, ongoing learning, and a spirit of inquiry for clinical decision-making. The benefits of implementing the latest clinical evidence in practice are overwhelming for providers and make sense for so many reasons. Evidence-based interventions are more likely to produce positive results and hence improve patient outcomes. They very often eliminate ineffective practices that have become obsolete but are used by clinicians because "that is the way we have always done it." Instead, using EBPs can differentiate your practice and your organization as a high quality provider, and consumers are looking for those providers. The current focus on value-based reimbursement demands that providers use EBP as the Medicare program and many state quality improvement agencies are incorporating EBPs into their reimbursement mechanisms. And, they are making the data public that support those differentiated reimbursement methods.

What does this mean for radiology nursing? First, this book makes an important contribution by presenting a strong evidence base for radiology nursing practice. The focus on clinical effectiveness, efficiency, cost-effectiveness, safety, and quality is evident throughout. Radiology nursing involves critical skills in assessment and monitoring. The availability and use of evidence-based checklists and assessment tools to measure a variety of patient outcomes have become essential to quality care. In addition, accepted scientific evidence used in general nursing practice, such as turning schedules to prevent the development of pressure sores, requires the radiology nurse to use the evidence and their assessment skills to determine their patient's needs based on the individual's risk for skin breakdown. There are many topics relevant to radiology nursing that need to be addressed. What about safe injection of contrast media or extravasation of contrast media? What is the latest evidence, the strength of that evidence, and how will you use it in your practice? Finally, radiology nursing deals with advanced technology and the ongoing acquisition of new technology that requires the development of and dissemination of new scientific knowledge to accompany the new practice. This creates many challenges to develop and maintain an EBP when health care delivery is constantly and rapidly changing. However, the opportunities to contribute in your specialty abound! Be that change leader who questions practice, discusses concerns with other members of the team, and is an early adopter who searches for evidence that will contribute to the delivery of better health care and improve patient outcomes.

Kathleen M. White, PhD, RN, NEA-BC, FAAN
Johns Hopkins School of Nursing
Baltimore, MD, USA

## Reference

1. Dang D, Dearholt S. The Johns Hopkins Nursing evidence-based practice model and guidelines. 3rd ed. Indianapolis, IN: Sigma Theta Tau International; 2017.

# Foreword 2

It is a privilege to be able to introduce this new book which is specifically designed to meet the needs of the advanced practice provider and manager in the radiology setting and will be a useful resource to any nurse regardless of area or location of practice. It is a first of its kind in the radiology nursing literature. Historical and current influences have molded today's practice in radiology. Radiology is synonymous with change, and practitioners in this environment need to be open to new technology, procedures, and outside influences on all the modalities as radiology is constantly evolving and advancing. This book will enable the nurse to be informed.

This book is divided into sections that include roles, clinical issues, safety topics, topics of importance to the patient, and professional topics that are essential to the changing imaging environment. The breath of the authors' knowledge and abilities is a very positive aspect of this book; readers will learn from experts in their respective areas as relevant information is presented that will influence the nursing process. The emphasis on topics in addition to the clinical practice topics, including the patient's perspective and professional and system concerns, makes this book unique as a source for information.

The editor of this text has shown professional nursing leadership through advancing the literature for radiology professionals. With the knowledge and skills discussed in this book, the practitioner and manager will be better able to lead a highly functional and cohesive team and cope with changes that occur. Nurses can then be the change agents that are needed to improve quality radiology nursing care to all patients in a variety of settings.

Christine Keough, BSN, RN, CRN  
University of Rochester Medical Center  
Rochester, NY, USA

# Preface

No nursing specialty has piqued my interest as much as radiology nursing because of its relative newness as a nursing specialty and evolving nature but mostly because of the demands it places on the nurse. It is *very* challenging to be a radiology nurse. I once said that working in radiology was like "practicing in a sea of contrast media: the environment is fluid, the situations can be 'sticky,' and all actions and reactions are highly visible" [1].

Radiology nurses do not have the advantage of a specific academic career path for radiology nursing but use combined education and past experiences such as critical care and emergency or peri-anesthesia nursing to guide quality patient care. The nurse must be very curious and able to absorb new information quickly. Continuous on-the-job learning is an important part of working in the radiology department. This factor is highly variable based on the setting and mentor, if one is available. In addition to the nuances of all the procedure-related care, radiology nurses need to learn the language of radiology, understand principles of radiation safety, understand the chemistry and physiological effects of the contrast media or isotopes that are used, and be aware of new occupational hazards, all largely foreign to nurses prior to entry into the department. Conceptually, the radiology department is organized and run differently than traditional hospital departments where nurses have past experience. Radiology nurses interact with patients of all ages who have a vast array of problems for which they need diagnostic tests or interventions in a variety of imaging modalities.

A developing nursing specialty faces many growing pains, not the least of which is the development of a specialized knowledge base and available literature resources. Radiology nursing is further challenged by the rapid growth in imaging and introduction of new diagnostic imaging examinations and therapeutic procedures which the nurse needs to understand to be able to provide safe and effective patient care. The nurse's critical thinking skills are constantly challenged. Although the radiology nurse's practice may be very autonomous, being *a member of the team* is also an important aspect of being a radiology nurse. The two features are not mutually exclusive. Good communication skills and interdisciplinary collaboration are important attributes for the nurse working as part of the skilled radiology team. Involvement in coordination of care, whether within a hospital system or with outside agencies, is increasingly needed as patient acuity is higher. This is not likely to change. Radiology nurses also function as educators, researchers, and resources to others in and outside the department.

Radiology nursing is also affected by challenges that face all specialties in health care. Regulatory influences change, cybersecurity threats to patient care and welfare take place, new legal and ethical issues arise and healthcare insurance companies exert power on patient care. Radiology nurses do impact patient care outcomes and the ability to demonstrate that is essential to the influence nurses can have on quality. Radiology nurses are leaders in the department and can bring about positive changes by role modeling and *proactive* leadership. Radiology nurses are in an excellent position to be spokespeople for services offered within the radiology department and to promote new less invasive procedures to providers in many medical specialties. Engaging in research to demonstrate better outcomes is another role which the nurse can fulfill.

The nursing advanced practice provider and radiology nurse manager need a text which addresses topics of unique interest to them. The expert authors who have written in this text speak to this audience, as well as, to all radiology nurses, even those who might just be starting in the radiology department. Reading many chapters will make the reader feel as if a colleague is speaking with them about issues or concerns. Other chapters are more tutorial in nature, laying out new information. Areas where radiology nursing needs some work are discussed candidly. It is important that we can look critically at our specialty and identify needs and opportunities for change and growth. The book is divided into five sections as place markers to aid the reader.

*Section I* addresses the roles of the advanced practice provider and also the nurse manager.

*Section II* assists the provider in understanding best practices in clinical care.

*Section III* focuses on topics related to patient safety in the imaging modalities.

*Section IV* adds the dimension of the patient experience, whether it be understanding how literacy impacts outcomes, the process of consents or communications, or guiding children and young people in radiology.

*Section V* focuses on professional issues of interest to nursing and also highlights future horizons in radiology that will impact nursing and radiology.

I wish to thank all the authors who have persevered to complete the work needed to produce a chapter in this first edition. It is no easy task as it takes much time and genuine hard work to write for publication. Early on I placed my trust in each of the authors. While there is no paper on the cutting floor our computers house many revised versions of the chapters. Each author, regardless of their discipline, was given the freedom to approach the topic in a way they deemed most appropriate. I am sure that all would agree it is difficult to say with finality, "The chapter is complete*." There is always one more piece of information authors and editors wish to add as a publication progresses but I assure the readers all have tried their best to provide a current, concise, and informative chapter with emphasis on associated society standards where applicable.

My goal was to provide a text that was not only informative to improve patient care but also inspirational to radiology nurses, regardless of role. We are the gatekeepers and advocates for patients in radiology. We can help avert problems, triage adverse events of all types, and provide follow-up as needed.

We assess and monitor during procedures. We communicate with other providers and staff. We provide 1:1 care for the patient and share in the patient's *lived* experience. We are often there when "news" is delivered and provide emotional support for the patient and significant other. We greet and discharge patients leaving a first and last impression of radiology on their minds. Radiology nurses can and do make an incredible difference in patient care and experience in the radiology department and need to be recognized for their value.

My hope is that radiology nurses and leaders will also share this text with related professionals who care for radiology patients, e.g., the intensive care nurse, the peri-anesthesia nurse, the emergency nurse, the medical surgical nurse, the pediatric nurse, and others as dissemination of knowledge will only serve to enhance the nursing profession as a whole and improve patient care. We need to practice in collaboration not in silos.

Radiology nursing is dynamic; this theme should be foremost in our thoughts. Radiology nurses can be creative and innovative in so many ways. That is part of the essence and pure joy in being a radiology nurse.

*Editor's note: Careful editing of the information was carried out but the professional is advised to always question, if needed, as new information is constantly forthcoming as knowledge expands.

Owings Mills, Maryland      Kathleen A. Gross, MSN, BS, RN-BC, CRN
October 10, 2019

## Reference

1. Gross KA. Core curriculum for radiologic and imaging nursing. 3rd ed. Association for Radiologic and Imaging Nursing; 2014.

# Acknowledgments

I want to send a special thanks to all, including the Springer staff, who supported me during the task of planning, preparing, and bringing this project to the finish line. There are too many to mention by name, but I especially want to thank my spouse, Richard J. Gross, MD, who understood the long days and discipline that I would need to complete this book.

I also want to thank Dina A. Krenzischek, PhD, RN, CPAN, FAAN, FASPAN, and Sharon L. Kozachik, PhD, RN, FAAN, for their encouragement and professional advice throughout the course of this project and at other times in my career.

# Contents

**Section I  Radiology Roles**

1. **Advanced Practice Providers**.................................. 3
   Randi L. Collinson

2. **Role of the Clinical Nurse Specialist in Radiology**........... 15
   Sharon L. Lehmann

3. **Radiology Nurse Manager**..................................... 25
   Valerie Aarne Grossman and Alexandra Penzias

**Section II  Clinical Patient Care Topics**

4. **X-Ray Interpretation**......................................... 41
   Michael Bowen and Tina Sankhla

5. **Point-of-Care Laboratory Testing in Radiology**................ 53
   Kent B. Lewandrowski

6. **Pre- and Post-Procedure Nursing Care**......................... 59
   Patricia Tuck and Dina A. Krenzischek

7. **Procedural Sedation and Analgesia in Radiology**............... 77
   Michael J. Long and Lois Elaine Stewart

8. **Positioning the Patient for Procedures**....................... 91
   Lois Elaine Stewart and Michael J. Long

9. **Transradial Arterial Access**................................. 105
   Paula Dixon

**Section III  Safety in Radiology**

10. **Contrast Reactions**......................................... 119
    Alexandra Penzias and Gloria M. Salazar

11. **Infection Prevention in Radiology**.......................... 129
    Caroline McDaniel, Sandra L. Schwaner, and Costi D. Sifri

12. **Radiation Safety Considerations in Interventional Fluoroscopy**........................................................ 141
    Michael C. Talmadge

| 13 | Waste Anesthetic Gases (WAGs): Minimizing Health Risks and Increasing Awareness .......................... 149 |
|---|---|
| | John E. Moenning Jr., Dina A. Krenzischek, and James D. McGlothlin |

| 14 | Medical Laser Safety ...................................... 161 |
|---|---|
| | Vangie Dennis |

| 15 | Minimally Invasive Image-Guided Procedures .............. 173 |
|---|---|
| | Margaret M. Doherty-Simor |

| 16 | MR Safety Essentials for Nurses ........................... 183 |
|---|---|
| | Maureen N. Hood |

| 17 | Alarm Fatigue .......................................... 199 |
|---|---|
| | Stacey Trotman |

| 18 | Patient Falls in Radiology................................. 205 |
|---|---|
| | Greg Laukhuf |

| 19 | Adverse Events ......................................... 213 |
|---|---|
| | Shawna M. Butler |

### Section IV  The Patient in Radiology

| 20 | Legal and Ethical Considerations for Radiology Procedural Consent....................................... 225 |
|---|---|
| | Adrienne N. Dixon and Meghan Stepanek |

| 21 | Telephone Communications............................... 235 |
|---|---|
| | Mary Elizabeth Greenberg and Carol Rutenberg |

| 22 | Health Literacy ......................................... 245 |
|---|---|
| | Beth Ann Hackett |

| 23 | The Patient Experience in Radiology ....................... 253 |
|---|---|
| | Sanne H. Henninger |

| 24 | Children and Young People in Radiology.................... 263 |
|---|---|
| | Joan Turner |

| 25 | Forensic Patients in the Healthcare Setting .................. 273 |
|---|---|
| | Debra S. Holbrook |

### Section V  Professional Topics

| 26 | Cybersecurity: Cyberspace Wars—The Unseen Enemy........ 285 |
|---|---|
| | Thomas Hough and Kathleen A. Gross |

| 27 | Nursing Research and Outcomes........................... 291 |
|---|---|
| | Kathleen Shuey and Marygrace Hernandez-Leveille |

| 28 | Interprofessional Education and Collaboration............... 301 |
|---|---|
| | Wendy Manetti |

| 29 | Social Media ........................................... 313 |
|---|---|
| | Saad A. Ranginwala |

| 30 | **Response to Violence**............................... 319 |
|---|---|
|   | Jeffrey Strickler |
| 31 | **Current Trends in Radiology**............................ 329 |
|   | Thomas Hough and Joseph Marion |

**Correction to: Advanced Practice Providers** ..................... C1

## About the Editor

**Kathleen A. Gross, MSN, BS, RN-BC, CRN** is the Editor-in-Chief of the *Journal of Radiology Nursing (JRN)*, which publishes works relevant to all imaging modalities across the life span. Kathleen's experience includes working as a clinical radiology nurse in interventional radiology for 21 years. She taught nursing students and radiology technology students. She also served as an adjunct faculty for a university nursing program.

She served in a national capacity as secretary, president-elect, president, and past president of the Association for Radiologic and Imaging Nursing (ARIN).

Kathleen has served on the American College of Radiology's (ACR's) Safety Committee and is currently on the ACR Commission on Patient and Family-Centered Care Education Committee. Kathleen has held committee appointments with the Society of Interventional Radiology (SIR), serving since 2006 as a committee member of the Safety Committee as well as SIR's Standards Committee. Her knowledge and skills contributed to her work as one of the founding members of the Peripheral Arterial Disease (PAD) Coalition; she served on the PAD coordinating committee and nominating committee. She is a member of the Committee on Publication Ethics (COPE) and the International Academy of Nursing Editors.

Professional contributions as a nurse leader are evidenced by her numerous publications. She has authored and coauthored articles specific to radiology and/or radiology nursing in peer-reviewed journals and written columns, editorials, and book chapters. She edited the *Core Curriculum for Radiologic and Imaging Nursing, 3rd edition.*

Kathleen was instrumental in the development of the first radiologic nursing certification examination and served on the Radiologic Nursing Certification Board. Kathleen is the recipient of the *Johns Hopkins School of Nursing Dean's Award for Outstanding Nurse Leader* 2018, the 2018 Maryland Nurses Association *Outstanding Pathfinder Award* (for excellence and creative leadership in nursing), and the *Albert Nelson Marquis Lifetime Award*, 2018. She is a member of Sigma Theta Tau International.

# Contributors

**Michael Bowen, ANP, RN** Department of Radiology, Emory Healthcare, Atlanta, GA, USA

**Shawna M. Butler, DNP, JD, RN, CPHRM** Massachusetts General Hospital, Boston, MA, USA

University of Massachusetts, Boston, MA, USA

**Randi L. Collinson, MSN, CRNP, RN** Department of Neurointerventional Radiology and Neurosurgery Department, Hospital University of Pennsylvania, Philadelphia, PA, USA

**Vangie Dennis, MSN, RN, CNOR, CMLSO** WellStar Atlanta Medical Center, Atlanta, GA, USA

**Adrienne N. Dixon, JD, MS, PA-C** Legal Department, The Johns Hopkins Health System Corporation, Baltimore, MD, USA

**Paula Dixon, MSN, RN, CCRN, CEN** Department of Cardiology, Medical University of South Carolina, Charleston, SC, USA

**Margaret M. Doherty-Simor, MSN, RN** The Interventional Initiative, Oakland, CA, USA

**Mary Elizabeth Greenberg, PhD, RN-BC, C-TNP** School of Nursing, Northern Arizona University, Tucson, AZ, USA

**Kathleen A. Gross, MSN, BS, RN-BC, CRN** Owings Mills, MD, USA

**Valerie Aarne Grossman, MALS, BSN, RN** Department of Radiology, Highland Hospital (An affiliate of the University of Rochester), Rochester, NY, USA

**Beth Ann Hackett, DNP, APRN, CRN** Midstate Radiology Associates, LLC, Meriden, CT, USA

**Sanne H. Henninger, Ed.D, MSW, LCSW** Duke Health—Private Diagnostic Clinic, PLLC, Durham, NC, USA

**Marygrace Hernandez-Leveille, PhD, RN, ACNP-BC** UT Southwestern Office of Advanced Practice Providers, Dallas, TX, USA

UT Southwestern Medical Center, Dallas, TX, USA

**Debra S. Holbrook, MSN,RN,SANE-A,FNEA/P,DR-AFN,FAAN** Mercy Medical Center, Baltimore, MD, USA

**Maureen N. Hood, PhD, RN, RT (R)(MR), FSMRT, FAHA** Department of Radiology & Radiological Sciences, Uniformed Services University of the Health Sciences, Edward Hébert School of Medicine, Bethesda, MD, USA

**Thomas Hough, CMC** True North Consulting & Associates Inc., Mississauga, ON, Canada

**Dina A. Krenzischek, PhD,RN,MAS,CPAN,CFRE,FAAN,FASPAN** Patient Care Service, Mercy Medical Center, Baltimore, MD, USA

**Greg Laukhuf, ND, RN-BC, CRN, NE-BC** Department of Radiology, University Hospitals Cleveland Medical Center, Cleveland, OH, USA

**Sharon L. Lehmann, MS, APRN, CNS, CRN** Department of Interventional Radiology, University of Minnesota Physicians, Minneapolis, MN, USA

**Kent B. Lewandrowski, MD** Division of Clinical Laboratories and Molecular Medicine, Department of Pathology, Massachusetts General Hospital, Boston, MA, USA

Harvard Medical School, Boston, MA, USA

**Michael J. Long, DNP, CRNA** Community Health Network Anesthesia, Indianapolis, IN, USA

**Wendy Manetti, PhD, CRNP** Department of Nursing, University of Scranton, Scranton, PA, USA

**Joseph Marion, MBA, BA** Healthcare Integration Strategies, LLC, Waukesha, WI, USA

**Caroline McDaniel, MSN, RN, CWON** University of Virginia Health System, Charlottesville, VA, USA

**James D. McGlothlin, PhD, MPH, CPE, FAIHA** Emeritus Purdue University, West Lafayette, IN, USA

**John E. Moenning Jr, DDS, MSD** Indiana Oral & Maxillofacial Surgery Associates, Fishers, IN, USA

**Alexandra Penzias, DNP, MEd, APRN, ACNS-BC** Cooley Dickinson Hospital, Northampton, MA, USA

**Saad A. Ranginwala, MD** Department of Medical Imaging, Ann and Robert H. Lurie Children's Hospital of Chicago, Chicago, IL, USA

**Carol Rutenberg, MNSc, RN-BC, C-TNP** Telephone Triage Consulting, Inc., Hot Springs, AR, USA

**Gloria M. Salazar, MD** Department of Radiology, Massachusetts General Hospital, Boston, MA, USA

**Tina Sankhla, MD** Department of Radiology, Emory Healthcare, Atlanta, GA, USA

**Sandra L. Schwaner, MSN, RN, ACNP-BC** Department of Interventional Radiology, University of Virginia Health System, Charlottesville, VA, USA

**Kathleen Shuey, RN, ACNS-BC, AOCN** Department of Nursing, Baylor University Medical Center, Dallas, TX, USA

**Costi D. Sifri, MD** Division of Infectious Diseases and International Health, Department of Medicine, University of Virginia Health System, Charlottesville, VA, USA

**Meghan Stepanek, Esq, MPH** Legal Department, The Johns Hopkins Health System Corporation, Baltimore, MD, USA

**Lois Elaine Stewart, PhD, CRNA** Community Health Network Anesthesia, Indianapolis, IN, USA

**Jeffrey Strickler, DHA, RN, NEA-BC** UNC Health, University of North Carolina Health Care, Cary, NC, USA

**Michael C. Talmadge, DABR, CHP** Radiation Oncology, Massachusetts General Hospital (MGH)/Newton Wellesley Hospital, Newton, MA, USA

**Stacey Trotman, DNP, RN, CMSRN, RN-BC, NE-BC** Department of Nursing and Critical Care Unit, Mercy Medical Center, Baltimore, MD, USA

**Patricia Tuck, MSN, RN, NE-BC** Interventional Radiology Department, Mercy Medical Center, Baltimore, MD, USA

**Joan Turner, PhD, CCLS** Child and Youth Study Department, Mount Saint Vincent University, Halifax, Nova Scotia, Canada

# Section I
# Radiology Roles

# Advanced Practice Providers

Randi L. Collinson

## 1.1 Introduction

In the field of radiology, technology has aided the growth of radiology departments to become one of the largest departments within the medical arena. Radiology offers a plethora of services and revolutionary procedures to assist with patient diagnosis and innovative treatments. As the field of radiology continued to develop and grow so did the need for multiple medical professionals to form the radiology team of today. The focus of this chapter is to discuss the role of the advanced practice provider (APP) in radiology primarily addressing the nurse practitioner (NP) and physician assistant (PA) role in the realm of interventional radiology.

## 1.2 Discovering the Diagnostic X-Ray

In the late 1800s, Wilhelm Rontgen, a German engineer and physicist, produced and detected radiation which became known as X-rays. The first machines that produced X-rays were used by professional photographers for the curious public to see their own boney structures. In the early 1900s, X-ray equipment became an additional medical tool, purchased by physicians, to assist in diagnosing and treating illness. Quickly a need for additional professionals to manage, maintain, and perform the radiologic images was recognized. Many of the first X-ray assistants were nurses since they were already professionally trained and educated. In the years that followed, perfecting X-ray techniques, developing positioning guidelines, and educating radiology specific professionals became the goal in radiology. The role and profession was organized to form the professional known as a radiologic technologist who then replaced the first nurses in radiology [1].

In the years that followed, radiology developed from a service dependent on referrals to a true clinical practice. As the clinical practice continued to emerge into the radiology service of today, it became evident there was an overwhelming need to incorporate several other medical professionals to the radiology team. The significance of nurses and advanced practice professionals, along with several other medical professionals, has shown to provide an advantage to the radiology department and the patients they serve.

### 1.2.1 Radiology Infancy

Radiology departments in the early 1960s consisted mainly of radiologic technologists (RTs),

---

The original version of this chapter was revised. The correction to this chapter can be found at https://doi.org/10.1007/978-3-030-32679-1_32

R. L. Collinson, MSN, CRNP, RN (✉)
Department of Neurointerventional Radiology and Neurosurgery Department,
Hospital University of Pennsylvania,
Philadelphia, PA, USA

certified to assist radiologists with noninvasive and minimally invasive procedures. Some of the noninvasive imaging would include X-rays of body parts, with minimal to no introduction of a contrast media. The minimally invasive imaging procedures would include entering the skin or body cavity with a needle, tube, or catheter with minimal to no damage to those structures, while imaging the specific body parts with some form of radiation [2] (see Chap. 15).

### 1.2.2 CT and MRI Influences

Radiology advancement in the early 1970s was related to the development of the *first* computerized axial tomography (CAT) scanners or CT scanners, as they are called today, for medical imaging. This expanded the radiologist's ability to visualize abnormal and normal conditions, including soft tissue via cross section views aided by the computer, allowing a more accurate plan to diagnose and treat the patient. Similarly, the magnetic resonance imaging (MRI) scanners which were being used in the field of science were now being transitioned to medicine. This newer imaging modality was considered safer since there was no radiation exposure to the patient while providing an additional noninvasive imaging tool to aid radiologists with diagnosing and planning for patient treatment [3, 4].

### 1.2.3 Interventional Radiology Expansion

While these newer imaging modalities were on the rise, advancement continued evolving within the radiology area. A vascular radiologist, Dr. Charles Dotter, began experimenting and discovering the potential treatment use of catheters within the intravascular anatomy. This became known as minimally invasive procedures which led to additional treatment possibilities. The radiologist could perform a specific treatment within the blood vessel, at the site of the problem with the use of fluoroscopy to guide the procedure while providing a quicker recovery for the patient [5, 6].

The development of this section of radiology historically known as "Special Procedures" has come to be known as "Interventional Radiology" or IR. This development led to the formation of what is now called the Society of Interventional Radiology (SIR) in the late 1980s. The SIR then established specific IR training, which was then approved for medical education and incorporated into accredited programs. The IR departments encompass board-certified radiologists specializing in minimally invasive treatment which include subspecialties of Interventional Cardiology, Interventional Radiology, and Neuro Interventional Radiology [5, 6].

Today in the IR department, there are many more minimally invasive procedures. These procedures are performed on a daily elective and emergent basis with the use of catheters, guide wires, balloons, occlusive materials, implantable devices, and medications.

The procedures vary from ballooning an area with stenosis, implanting a stent to assist with vessel patency, creating dialysis access, placing a percutaneous drainage tube, ablating tumors, and embolizing tumors prior to surgical tumor removal just to name a few. In addition to vascular treatments there are special spinal procedures performed to assist with pain alleviation or diagnosis. Even though the procedures that are performed are minimally invasive and considered safe, there is always a risk of complications with any procedure; pre, during, and post procedure [7]. As the procedures performed by the radiologists, known as interventionalists, became more involved and more complicated, the need for nurses and more recently advanced practice professionals was evident.

## 1.3 Evolution of Radiology Nursing

The radiology nursing role began to evolve in the late 1940s when a nurse visionary, named Charlotte Louise Goodwin, RN, joined the radiology team at The Johns Hopkins Hospital in Baltimore, Maryland. She went on to become the director of radiology nursing at Johns Hopkins with a goal to provide recognition, education, and information to the nursing profession. She conducted a national survey by reaching out to other nursing professionals within the radiology field of medicine in 1979 with a surprising positive response. This response was the motivation she needed to present her goals to the Johns Hopkins radiology team and the Radiological Society of North America (RSNA) to obtain recognition, support, and time for the radiology nursing professionals at the RSNA meeting in Chicago, Illinois, November 1981. Thus, the first meeting was held to create the American Radiologic Nurses Association (ARNA) in November 1981 which continued to evolve and focus attention with recognition on nursing in the field of radiology on a national scale [8].

### 1.3.1 Professional Responsibilities Advance in Radiology

As stated above, nurses were hired in radiology as early as the 1940s for patient care management, which then continued to develop into administering conscious sedation during procedures along with short-term recovery of the patient. The nursing responsibilities expanded to include a pre-procedure assessment, history and physical, pretesting review prior to proposed procedure, along with discussion of any abnormal findings with the performing physician. As the nursing responsibilities for providing conscious sedation developed, the required credentialing began to emerge, with many radiology departments requiring nurses to obtain critical care certification and/or advanced cardiac life support with conscious sedation certification [9].

The registered nurse's role in the radiology department has continued to evolve with nurses managing every aspect of the radiology department (see Chap. 3). Nursing coverage may be present in any area that could or may involve intravenous injection, which predominately includes IR, CT, MRI, diagnostic radiology, and nuclear medicine (NM) areas but may also include virtually all modalities. Depending on the size of the department there may also be a designated team of nurses who travel throughout the radiology department medically managing any issues that may develop [9].

### 1.3.2 Recognition as a Specialty

Radiology nursing was recognized by the American Nurses Association as a nursing specialty in 1991 [10]. The organization for radiology nurses is now known as the Association for Radiologic & Imaging Nursing (ARIN), which transitioned from The American Radiologic Nurses Association in September 2007. The ARIN's goal is to promote quality patient care while providing radiology nursing professionals with support and continuing education within the radiology environment [11]. *The Scope & Standards of Practice—Radiologic & Imaging Nursing* was first published by the American Nurses Association (ANA), with the second edition copublished in 2014 by the ARIN and the ANA. The association's official journal, *Journal of Radiology Nursing* (formerly *Images*), continues to provide current evidence-based information for professional radiology nurses within the many aspects of radiology [12–14].

## 1.4 Development of the Advanced Practice Roles in the USA

From 1940 to 1960s the nursing profession developed such a severe shortage resulting in a government solution by signing into law the Nurse Training Act of 1964. This act was developed to provide federal funding to colleges throughout the country to encourage the nursing professions into advanced educational nursing degrees. This federal assistance resulted in the development of several advanced educational programs for nurses, which expanded their knowledge base along with the development of requirements of advanced certification in certain specialized areas [15].

The nurse anesthetist role was developed in the late 1800s, to assist the physicians with anesthetic patient care with the first nurse to administer anesthesia in 1861. The first trained nurse anesthetist to assist with performing patient anesthesia was Sister Mary Bernard employed at a hospital in Erie, Pennsylvania, in 1877 [16].

The clinical nurse specialist (CNS) role was established in the 1950s influenced by the need in the field of psychiatry. Professor Hildegard Peplau at Rutgers University established the first master's program to provide additional assistance in the area of mental health. Then the CNS role continued to evolve into specialty areas of today, as experts in evidence-based practice providing assistance and education for the medical team [17] (see Chap. 2).

Following World War II, an acute shortage of physicians was noted in the United States compared with the growing population and demanding health care needs. As early as 1961, an article was published by Dr. Charles Hudson regarding the concept of using physician extenders to address the growing shortage of primary care providers. Thus, the physician assistant (PA) role was established in the early 1960s while the nurse practitioner (NP) role was conceived in 1965 by a nurse and physician in Colorado to assist with this national physician shortage [16, 17].

### 1.4.1 Education for the Nurse Practitioner

The current requirements to apply to become a NP in the United States (US) include prerequisites of a current nursing license, preferable 1–2 years of nursing experience and a bachelor's degree preferably in nursing science. Additional requirements are a completion of advanced education at a nationally recognized school and accredited curriculum with a completion of certification in the specific designated specialty areas of education. The specialty areas that are accepted in 2019 are patient population focused and include Family/Individual Across the Lifespan, Pediatric (acute or primary), Neonatal, Women's Health and Psychiatric/Mental Health. Upon completion of the advanced education of the Masters in Nursing Science program and passing the national certification exam, practicing as an NP in that specialty is awarded on a state level, with variable state regulations [18]. In an attempt to remedy the varied state level requirements, the National Council of State Boards of Nursing (NCSBN) created an APRN Consensus Model to move to uniform state laws which has been slowly adopted with legislation in some states [19]. Since 2004, The American Association of Colleges of Nursing (AACN) has been recommending to require the standard for entry level NP to become a Doctor of Nursing Practice (DNP) by 2015 but as of 2019 this is not a requirement to practice [20].

### 1.4.2 Education for the Physician's Assistant

The current preferred requirements to apply to practice in the USA as a PA include prerequisites of some type of medical experience as a nurse, paramedic, or emergency medical technician. The training for the PA curriculum requires completion at an approved, accredited physician assistant program with many offering a Bachelor of Science in PA studies or a Master of Science in PA studies with some opportunity to specialize in subspecialties, completion of clinical supervised training, and completion of PA national certification exam. This completion allows the PA to practice in any state in the USA after completing each state regulatory requirement [21].

## 1.5 Need for Advanced Practice Providers

In a survey from 2000 to 2001 performed by the SIR it was reported by interventional radiologists that 65% conducted preprocedure visits, with only 53% performing post procedure follow-up visits. In the same survey, while 84% had admitting privileges only 75% utilized them with 70% mainly accepting direct referrals [22]. Thus, revealing the interventional practices that would prosper would need to expand into a full clinical service by including advanced practice providers to the radiology team. As a clinical service the interventional radiology sections must provide alternative patient treatment options with current and future patient management. In a literature review published in 2018, evidence supported positive benefits of advanced practice providers in reducing patient waiting times, decreased workload on physicians, cost-effectiveness, and job satisfaction [23].

The advanced practitioner is an ideal addition to the radiology team by assisting with patient clinic consultations, performing specific percutaneous procedures, along with continued patient management in the hospital setting and with the continued outpatient follow-up responsibilities.

### 1.5.1 Types of Advanced Practice Provider Roles in Radiology

The term "Advanced Practice Providers" (APP) is used to describe a medical professional with advanced academic and clinical education in a specific specialty or general medicine that allows them to diagnose and manage common or chronic illnesses. The APP is required to obtain advanced certifications and may work in collaboration or independently as per their state requirements. APPs incorporate certain areas of education and expertise, which include the nurse practitioner (NP), the nurse anesthetist (NA), the clinical nurse specialist (CNS), and the physician's assistant (PA). The APPs best suited for the interventional roles are mainly the NPs, CNSs, and the PAs [24].

In 1999, the first NPs were hired into the IR team at the University of New Mexico, having completed a 6-month radiology training program providing additional education and final credentialing on completion [25]. An article located on the American Academy of Physician's Assistant website, noted a PA, scheduled his own rotation with the IR team while in PA school, and began employment in 1999 for Mecklenburg Radiology Associates, located in Charlotte, North Carolina [26].

In some radiology departments another role was being developed and recognized by the American College of Radiology (ACR), the American Registry of Radiologic Technologists (ARRT), and the American Society of Radiologic Technologists (ASRT) in early 2002 [27]. The role was an advanced role for the radiologic technologist referred to as a radiology assistant (RA) and radiology practitioner assistant (RPA). The RPA role is considered *mid-level provider* working *under the supervision of a radiologist* with additional education. The RPA acts as a radiologist "extender" and can perform specific radiologic procedures under direct radiologist supervision. The RPA typically receives Bachelors of Science degree upon completion of approved curriculum and obtains certification.

The RA is considered an *advanced level* radiologic technologist who can lead in patient management, patient assessment and perform exams and procedures with image evaluation but not final written reporting. The RA curriculum requires a baccalaureate degree with 1 year full-time clinical experience, preceptorship of 18–21 months, and certification [28].

The RA is certified by the Certifying Board for Radiology Practitioner Assistants (CBRPA) and registered by the American Registry of Radiologic Technologists (ARRT) following the completion of the advanced curriculum. The RA/RPA work with the radiologist's supervision, and guidance as delineated in the Joint Policy Statement of the American College of Radiology (ACR) and the American Society of Radiologic Technologists (ASRT). As of today there are 31 states in the USA that recognize or license the RA/RPA [27, 28].

## 1.6 Advanced Practice Providers Billing for Services

Non-physician advanced practitioners in the United States employed by interventional radiology can obtain history and physical exams, deliver clinical care and participate with radiology physicians in forming a clinical assessment and plan. After credentialing and appropriate training the non-physician practitioners can perform minor interventional procedures that otherwise would require the radiologist to perform as guided by the regulations of each state. The NP and PA practitioners are recognized by Centers of Medicare & Medicaid Services (CMS) as qualified health providers that acquire their own national provider identification number which allows billing under their own identification numbers for services provided [29].

The most recent changes by Centers of Medicare & Medicaid Services (CMS) were allowing the RAs the ability to perform diagnostic testing under "direct supervision" rather than "personal supervision" starting in January 2019. The CMS define *personal supervision* requiring the physician to be in the room while the test is being performed in comparison to *direct supervision* in the office which requires the physician to be present in the office suite, immediately available to provide guidance and assistance throughout the procedure. The next step is in progress with the Medicare Access to Radiology Care Act (MARCA) which was introduced into the US Congress in March 2019 and would allow RAs to be recognized as non-physician providers. This allows the RAs to become another autonomous integral member of the radiology team while continuing to contribute to interventional department productivity allowing reduction of some of the burden for the physicians [30–32].

Table 1.1 depicts the nurse practitioner, the physician assistant, and the registered radiology assistant/extender (advanced provider) roles with consideration to similarities, differences, educational requirements, and independent allowable billing status.

### 1.6.1 Medicare Reimbursement for Advanced Practice Professionals

In 1948, the American Nurses Association (ANA) was instrumental in presenting outcome data to prove how quality, cost-effective care provided by advanced practice nurses (APNs) should be

**Table 1.1** Provider comparison chart

| Medical Professionals | Nurse Practitioner | Physician Assistant | Radiology Assistant/Radiology Extenders |
|---|---|---|---|
| Degree required | Masters or Doctorate of Nursing | Masters of Medicine | Majority bachelors prepared |
| Model of studies | Nursing model | Medicine model | Radiology/medicine model |
| Study model focus | Holistic approach with patient focus | Disease approach with diagnosis/treatment | Patient assessment/management approach |
| Training required | RN license, 400–1000 h studies | 2000 h studies | RT license, additional Radiology MD preceptorship |
| Available curriculum | College classes or online/clinical training | College classes/clinical training | College/clinical based training with MD |
| Areas of study | Multiple age/gender/mental health focused | Diagnostic/treatment for all areas of life span | Radiology/procedural focused |
| Pre requisite | Bachelor's in Nursing | Bachelor's in Medicine | Certified radiologic technologist |
| Practice authority | Independent, reduced and restricted authority | Physician collaboration | State regulated practice |
| Advanced professional associations | American Association of Nurse Practitioners | American Academy of Physician Assistants | American Society of Radiologic Technologists |
| USA national total | 270,000+ (estimated) | 123,000+ | RA's—392/RPE's 640+ |
| Recertification | 100 h CE's + 1000 h every 5 years, no exam | 100 h CE's every 2 years, exam every 10 years | 12 h CE's yearly, qualifications required every 10 years |
| Radiology training | No | No | Yes |
| Providers recognized by CMS | Yes | Yes | No |
| Transferring skills to other practice | Yes | Yes | No |

Source: From refs. [18, 20, 21, 28, 29, 32, 36, 37, 49–60]

eligible for Medicare reimbursement. The value of this data was not truly recognized until the 1990s due to the barriers that existed.

There were several barriers to granting direct reimbursement to APNs. One of the barriers was due to opposition of organized medicine questioning the quality of the APN services with no physician supervision or control. Another barrier was noted when health care cost continued to increase with an inability to demonstrate APN contribution to cost containment. Still another barrier to APN direct reimbursement was the absence of consumer demand for APN services due to the lack of consumer education regarding available APN services.

The benefits to granting direct reimbursement to the APNs included, providing community recognition as an independent professional, allowing autonomy or enhancing employment revenue and enabling APNs with independent practice and patient management. By direct reimbursement to APNs additional data collection and research would provide valuable information of cost-effectiveness, patient outcomes and services provided.

In 1989, the US Congress enacted a law to recognize APNs as direct providers of services to residents of nursing home facilities. The government focus at this time was to provide comprehensive care to populations residing in nursing home facilities and rural areas [33]. Direct reimbursement by Medicare in 1990 for APRNs was limited to only professionals working in countryside areas and skilled nursing facilities. Expansion of Medicare reimbursement for clinical nurse specialists and nurse practitioners, including nurse anesthetists and nurse midwives, started in the late 1990s. The reimbursement for the APN professionals allows 85% of the physician reimbursement and continues to be a complicated process which incorporates state and federal level regulatory factors [34].

The Institute of Medicine (IOM) reported recommendations regarding the future of advanced practice nursing in 2011, stating the barriers of advanced practice nursing should be removed to allow the communities more access to cost effective health care. The U.S. Department of Health and Human services is continually refining the plan to meet health care needs of the American population. The impact of nurse practitioners on health outcomes of Medicare and Medicaid patients has been evaluated and determined to be equivalent to or above expected care when compared to physicians [35].

## 1.7 NP/PA Education in Radiology

In any advanced practice role the education and information provided while in training is at a rigorous and demanding pace to meet the curriculum schedule. While the basic classes must be met to form the framework for appropriate diagnosis and treatment, a lack of radiologic education is definitely evident when considering the NP and PA curriculum. This is evident in a small study of almost 700 NPs graduating from 2006 to 2011 which was related to clinical preparedness and practice transition. The study revealed the NPs rated X-ray interpretation as lowest on the scale of preparedness and competence [36]. While yet another study of approximately 900 NPs surveyed reported an NP program curriculum with a dedicated clinical rotation for education and training in diagnostic imaging and testing would be overwhelmingly beneficial. In addition, the NPs surveyed revealed they would welcome the opportunity for continuing education in radiological imaging and testing [37].

As an advanced practitioner in the medical field, the responsibilities of the role are guided by the professional practice in that specific area of expertise. The advanced practice provider in the radiology realm can be a key professional asset to the radiology team while providing individual patient care.

## 1.8 Patient Care

Starting with the clinic visit the provider will review the medical history, medications, and allergies with the patient while simultaneously developing a relationship with each patient. This first visit will assist the team in forming and establishing a trusting relationship of communication between the patient, the practitioner, and the treating physician. While coordinating all the aspects of preparing the patient for a procedure, the provider will be responsible for any information and education the patient and family will require which assists in decreasing anxiety and clarifying expectations. The relationship that is formed will assist in determining the need for any emotional or spiritual support prior to, during, and post procedure. The advanced practitioner is the continuous connection and the key link to optimize patient care and management [38].

Many interventional radiologists today specialize in certain procedures that are treatment focused which require the APP to provide specialized care for each patient. As the APP role continues to evolve in the radiology field, each radiology service, from the specific specialties, such as neuroradiology to the interventional radiology focus, to chemoembolization focused to vascular access focused, the responsibilities for the APP can vary immensely.

### 1.8.1 Advanced Practice Provider Responsibilities

Many of the general responsibilities of the APP are listed below which can include specialty-specific responsibilities along with procedural responsibilities and can vary with each specific practice and state regulations [39, 40] (Table 1.2).

### 1.9 Recent Advanced Professional Growth in the USA

With the use of data collection from the National Provider Identifier (NPI), The Centers for Medicare and Medicaid Services (CMS) reported an estimated 106,000 practicing NPs and 70,000 PAs in 2010 [41]. In the year 2017 the NPs employed in the USA grew from 166,280 to 179,650 in 2018 as shown by statistical information provided by the US Bureau of Labor Statistics (USBLS). In just 1 year, the PAs employed in 2017 went from 109,220 to 114,710 in 2018. The RTs employment increased from 201,200 in 2017 to 205,590 in 2018, which does not separate RAs from RTs. As the numbers of these professionals increased, so did the wages, proving that with an advanced educational degree and clinical training, the financial worth of these medical professionals is recognized and compensated. The mean wage provided by the USBLS for NPs in 2018 was $110,030; PAs was $108,430; RNs $75,510; and Radiologic Technologist (RT) was $61,540 [42]. The ASRT performed a small survey in 2008 to determine the mean wages of Radiology

**Table 1.2** Responsibilities of the APP

*Responsibilities that may be required of NP/PA/RA/RPA in radiology*
History and physicals
Preprocedure testing with review and management
Inpatient evaluation and management/outpatient follow-up and management
Communication, consultation with referral to other medical services as needed
Ordering and interpreting labs and imaging studies
Writing prescriptions
Emergency management with appropriate therapies
Clinic visits with management
Admission/discharge orders with follow-up visit established
Patient/family education and resident teaching
Obtaining informed consent
Prescribing conscious sedation (state regulated)
Assisting or performing procedures
Involvement in research/continued data collection of complications and outcomes
Establish and maintain Internal Review Board (IRB) documentation annually
Education and maintenance of continuing education for certain technical staff
*Possible procedure specific responsibilities of PA/NP/RA/RPA*
Lumbar puncture/myelograms
Central vascular access (e.g., port placement, peripheral inserted central venous catheters)
Needle biopsies
Feeding tube exchange
Drainage catheter exchanges and removal
Paracentesis
Thoracentesis
Chest tube placement
Drain exchange/removal
Wound care
Epidural steroid injection
Needle localization

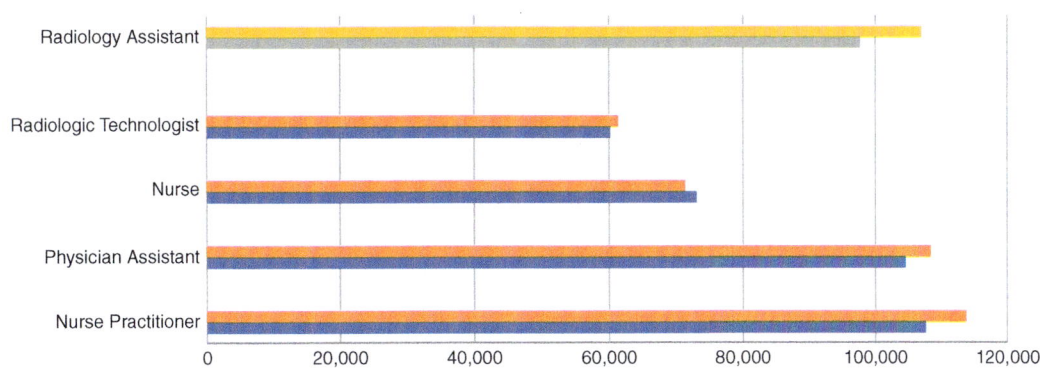

**Fig. 1.1** Medical professionals in the United States. (Source: From refs. [42–44])

| | Nurse Practitioner | Physician Assistant | Nurse | Radiologic Technologist | Radiology Assistant |
|---|---|---|---|---|---|
| 2016 Mean Wages | | | | | 106,777 |
| 2008 Mean Wages | | | | | 97,891 |
| 2018 Mean Wages | 113,930 | 108,430 | 71,730 | 61,540 | |
| 2017 Mean Wages | 107,480 | 104,760 | 73,550 | 60,320 | |

Assistant/Extenders which revealed a mean wage of $97,891 [43]. In 2016 the ASRT again performed a survey to determine wages with results of mean salary for RRA was $106,777 [44]. Thus verifying again, the advanced medical professionals that form the team in radiology continue to develop and enhance the field, while providing additional financial profit with indispensable individual patient care (Table 1.1 and Fig. 1.1).

## 1.10 International Advanced Practice Roles

The nurse practitioner role outside of the USA and around the world differs in the extent of responsibilities they can perform, prescriptive authority granted, and recognition in the country they practice and reside. In 2001 the International Council of Nurses (ICN), a federation of national nurses associations worldwide, confirmed the four common characteristics of nurse practitioners around the world to be, advanced education, required licensure and regulation, authority to prescribe medication/ treatment, and referral to other professionals with common professional functions [45]. A few examples of the advanced practice role and responsibilities in other countries around the world can be located on the web site https://international.aanp.org.

In Canada, the advanced nursing practice (ANP) role incorporates the clinical nurse specialist (CNS) and nurse practitioner (NP). As in the USA, the APN role started in the 1970s, due to the physician shortage, but did not truly expand until 1998, when reforms to the Canadian health care system were developed. A framework developed by several medical professionals became known as PEPPA, which referred to **Participatory, Evidence based, Patient focused, Process and Advanced practice nursing evaluation** [46]. The Canadian Nurse Practitioner Initiative (CNPI) in 2004 guided and assisted in implementing the building of a definitive framework for the ANPs role in the Canadian health care system. The educational requirements of the APN in Canada is similar to the advanced practice nurses in the USA, with the required bachelor's degree in nursing, advanced practice education in nursing, and licensure required for both degrees to practice as an ANP. Since then, the ANP role has continued to evolve to include autonomously prescribing medications including narcotics along with recognizing the NP as a primary care health services provider in March 2017. The Federal Income Tax Act allows the NP to complete the forms required for medical expenses or disability benefits while providing shorter wait times for the patients they care for [47].

In Finland, the advanced roles for nurses are still in the infancy stages. The Finnish Nurses Association reported recommendations for role development for the Finnish Advanced Practice Nurse as recently as 2016. The Finnish Nurses Association has begun to recognize the necessity to their country's health care community of the Advanced Practice Nurse (APN). In Finland the APN roles which are recognized include the Nurse Practitioner and the Clinical Nurse Specialist. The APN and CNS have been developed since the early 2000s. Educational requirements are on a master's level for the APN with prescriptive authority requiring an additional post graduate training. Nursing training in Finland is regulated by national legislation and based on the European Union's Directive which is similar to other European countries.

In the Czech Republic, advanced nursing practitioners (ANPs) have two nursing categories that are recognized, which are: the nurse specialist who is a nurse with a specialization that mainly focuses on chronic diseases and the nurse with a master's degree in a specific clinical discipline. Neither of these roles are autonomous with no prescriptive authority but both have the ability to diagnose, consult, and order testing. The Czech Republic is currently investigating the future role and responsibilities for the ANP while attempting to define the role, develop the educational programs, and provide financial support for the required advanced education [48].

## 1.11 Conclusion

Since the discovery and development of radiologic medicine beginning in the 1800s and the addition of technological advances in the computer age in the 1940s, medicine along with the field of radiology have continued to advance. Radiology began as a referral service but soon realized to continue to provide ideal treatment with optimal patient care, the radiology service would benefit financially and professionally by creating a dedicated clinical service. The radiology clinic was created to provide alternative minimally invasive treatment options for patients while continuing to medically manage the patient on a longer term basis. The clinic with the addition of the advanced practice provider has proven to positively benefit the radiology service. There are a variety of advanced practice providers in radiology departments that are a key member in the clinic who can assist and perform specific procedures, can manage illnesses in the hospital setting, while providing continued outpatient follow-up care for the radiology service. The advantages have proven to increase patient satisfaction with continuity of care, decrease workload for physicians, increase efficiency along with revenue, and provide autonomy with job satisfaction. As health care becomes more progressive regarding the complex diseases and cutting edge treatment options, the advanced practice provider role will continue to be a key element in providing individualized patient care in the radiology arena. APPs may find resources for continuing education and networking through the Society of Interventional Radiology (www.sirweb.org).

## References

1. Asrt.org. ASRT history. 2019. http://www.asrt.org/main/about-asrt/asrt-history. Accessed 28 Feb 2019.
2. Minimally invasive procedure. En.wikipedia.org. 2019 [cited 17 Sept 2018]. https://en.wikipedia.org/wiki/invasive_of_surgical_procedures.
3. Imaginis—The Women's Health & Wellness Resource Network. Imaginis.com. 1991 [cited 17 Sept 2018]. Brief History of CT. http://www.imaginis.com/
4. Bellis M. How magnets and radio waves changed medicine forever. ThoughtCo. 2018 [cited 17 Sept 2018]. https://www.thoughtco.com/magnetic-resonance-imaging-mri-1992133
5. Murphy T, Soares G. The evolution of interventional radiology. Semin Interv Radiol. 2005;22(01):6–9.
6. Lakhan S, Kaplan A, Laird C, Leiter Y. The interventionalism of medicine: interventional radiology, cardiology, and neuroradiology. Int Arch Med. 2009;2(1):27.

7. Sabharwal T, Fotiadis N, Adam A. Modern trends in interventional radiology. Br Med Bull. 2007;81–82(1):167–82.
8. Laukhuf G, Green K, Lehmann S. Behind the images: a history of the Association for Radiologic & Imaging Nursing. Herdon, VA: Association of Radiologic & Imaging Nursing; 2017.
9. What is an Interventional Radiology Nurse? Lifebridgeblogs.org. 2019 [cited 12 Nov 2018]. http://www.lifebridgeblogs.org/2012/06/19/what-is-an-interventional-radiology-nurse/
10. Clark P, McClain I. Interventional radiology nursing. J Radiol Nurs. 2004;23(2):51.
11. Home. The Association for Radiologic & Imaging Nursing. 2019 [cited 17 Nov 2018]. https://www.arinursing.org/
12. Nursing Journal. Journal of Radiology Nursing. Journals. elsevier.com. 2019 [cited 22 Nov 2018]. https://www.journals.elsevier.com/journal-of-radiology-nursing/
13. American Radiological Nurses Association & American Nurses Association. Radiology nursing. Silver Springs, MD: American Nurses Association; 2007.
14. American Nurses Association. Radiologic and imaging nursing. American Nurses Association: Alpharetta, GA; 2014.
15. Yett D. The nursing shortage and the Nurse Training Act of 1964. Ind Labor Relat Rev. 1966;19(2):190.
16. History of Nurse Anesthetists. Nursing in anesthesiology. 2019 [cited 10 Oct 2018]. https://nurseanesthetist57.wordpress.com/history-of-nurse-anesthetists
17. Hamric A, Spross J, Hanson C. Advanced practice nursing E-book. 5th ed. Elsevier Saunders: St. Louis; 2014.
18. Requirements to Become A Nurse Practitioner. NurseJournal.org. 2019 [cited 19 Apr 2019]. https://nursejournal.org/nurse-practitioner/what-to-know-to-become-a-nurse-practitioner/
19. Nurse Practitioner License Requirements: Change is in the Air. Nursinglicensure.org. 2019 [cited 19 Apr 2019]. https://www.nursinglicensure.org/nurse-practitioner-license.html
20. Is a DNP Degree an NP Requirement in 2015 and Beyond? NursePractitionerSchools.com. 2019 [cited 23 Mar 2019]. https://www.nursepractitionerschools.com/faq/dnp-requirement-for-np/
21. Physician's assistant training programs and requirements. Study.com. 2019 [cited 19 Apr 2019]. https://study.com/physician%27s_assistant_training.html
22. Murphy T, Soares G. Tracking changes in the practice of interventional radiology. Semin Interv Radiol. 2005;22(01):15–6.
23. Thom S. Does advanced practice in radiography benefit the healthcare system? A literature review. Radiography. 2018;24(1):84–9.
24. Beach D, Swischuk J, Smouse H. Using midlevel providers in interventional radiology. Semin Interv Radiol. 2006;23(4):329–32.
25. Stowe H. Development of an NP role in interventional radiology. Nurse Pract. 2003;28(8):57–8.
26. Lane S. Ready to intervene—AAPA. AAPA. 2019 [cited 22 Nov 2018]. https://www.aapa.org/news-central/2017/05/ready-to-intervene/
27. History. Asrt.org. 2019 [cited 22 Nov 2018]. https://www.asrt.org/main/careers/radiologist-assistant/ra-history-and-background/history
28. Radsciences.com. 2019 [cited 14 Apr 2019]. http://www.radsciences.com/doc/RPAvsRA10-05.pdf
29. Hawkins C. Rules and regulations relating to roles of nonphysician providers in the radiology practices. Radiographics. 2018;38960:1609–16.
30. Ross J. 10 Things radiologist need to know about radiology extenders. Radiology Business. 2019 [cited 17 Apr 2019]. https://www.radiology-business.com/topics/practice-management/10-things-radiologists-need-know-about-radiology-extenders.
31. About Radiology Physician Extenders. Srpeweb.org. 2109 [cited 14 Apr 2019]. https://www.srpeweb.org/about-radiology-physician - extenders.html
32. Medicare Physician Fee Schedule Final Rule on RAs Supervision Levels. https://www.srpeweb.org/homepage. 2018 [cited 29 Dec 2018]. https://www.srpeweb.org
33. MittelStadt P. Federal reimbursement of advanced practice nurses' services empowers the profession. Nurse Pract. 1993;18(1):43–9.
34. Reimbursement Task Force and APRN Work Group, of WOCN Society National Public Policy Committee, 2011. Reimbursement of advanced practice registered nurse services. J Wound Ostomy Continence Nurs. 2012;39(12):S7–S16.
35. Oliver G, Pennington L, Revelle S, Rantz M. Impact of nurse practitioners on health outcomes of Medicare and Medicaid patients. Nurs Outlook. 2014;62(6):440–7.
36. Hart A, Bowen A. New nurse practitioners' perceptions of preparedness for and transition into practice. J Nurse Pract. 2016;12(8):545–52.
37. Logsdon R, Gleason R. Advanced nurse practitioner educational needs for safe and efficient radiological imaging. Adv Emerg Nurs J. 2015;37(3):233–41.
38. Wempe E. Advanced practice: roles of the advanced practice nurse in the interventional radiology clinic setting. J Radiol Nurs. 2015;34(3):175.
39. Sanders VL, Flanagan J. (2015). Radiology physician extenders: a literature review of the history and current roles of physician extenders in medical imaging. J Allied Health. 2015. [cited 3 Feb 2019];44: 219–224.
40. Taylor K, Sansivero G, Ray C. The role of the nurse practitioner in interventional radiology. J Vasc Interv Radiol. 2012;23(3):347–50.
41. The Number of Nurse Practitioners and Physicians Assistants Practicing Primary Care in the United States l Agency for Healthcare Research & Quality. Ahrq.gov. 2019 [cited 27 Apr 2019].
42. U.S. Bureau of Labor Statistics. Bls.gov. 2019 [cited 19 Apr 2019].
43. Asrt.org. 2019 [cited 28 Apr 2019]. https://www.asrt.org/docs/default-source/research/radextsalandfctn2008.pdf?sfvrsn=4

44. Asrt.org. 2019 [cited 28 Apr 2019]. https://www.asrt.org/docs/default-source/research/radiologic-technologist-wage-and-salary-survey-2016.pdf?sfvrsn=2
45. Cna-aiic.ca. 2019 [cited 10 Feb 2019]. https://www.cna-aiic.ca/-/media/cna/page-content/pdf-fr/fs11_role_nurse_practitioner_march_2002_e.pdf?la=en
46. Bryant-Lukosius D, DiCenso A. A framework for the introduction and evaluation of advanced practice nursing roles. J Adv Nurs. 2004;48(5):530–40.
47. McNamara S, Giguère V, St-Louis L, Boileau J. Development and implementation of the specialized nurse practitioner role: use of the PEPPA framework to achieve success. Nurs Health Sci. 2009;11(3):318–25.
48. Country Specific Practice Profiles—ICN Nurse Practitioner/Advanced Practice Nursing Network. International.aanp.org. 2019 [cited 10 Feb 2019]. https://international.aanp.org/Practice/Profiles
49. Nurse Practitioner vs. Physician Assistant. Nursejournal.org. 2019 [cited 26 Apr 2019]. https://nursejournal.org/nurse-practitioner/np-vs-physician assistants/
50. NP Practice Authority Grows—March 2017 Update. Nurse.org. 2019 [cited 28 Apr 2019]. https://nurse.org/articles/nurse-practitioner-scope-of-practice-expands-mar17/
51. AANP 1 The American Association for Nurse Practitioners. American Association of Nurse Practitioners. 2019 [cited 27 Sept 2018]. https://www.aanp.org/
52. NP Fact Sheet. American Association of Nurse Practitioners. 2019 [cited 27 Sept 2018]. https://www.aanp.org/https://www.aanp.org/about/all-about-nps/np-fact-sheet
53. What is a PA? Learn more about the PA profession—AAPA. AAPA. 2019 [cited 27 Sept 2018]. https://www.aapa.org/what-is-a-pa/
54. Ongoing Requirements. Arrt.org. 2019 [cited 17 Apr 2019]. https://www.arrt.org/earn-arrt-credentials/ongoing-requirements
55. Home—AAPA. AAPA. 2019 [cited 29 Apr 2019]. https://www.aapa.org/
56. Home. Asrt.org.2019 [cited 29 Apr 2019]. https://www.asrt.org/
57. ACR.org Home. Acr.org. 2019 [cited 29 Apr 2019]. https://www.acr.org/
58. Registered Radiologist Assistant. Arrt.org. 2019 [cited 29 Apr 2019]. https://www.arrt.org/earn-arrt-credentials/credential-options/registered-radiologist-assistant
59. Census. Arrt.org. 2019 [cited 30 Apr 2019]. https://www.arrt.org/about/census
60. Society of Radiology Physician Extenders. Srpeweb.org. 2019 [cited 30 Apr 2019]. https://www.srpeweb.org/

# Role of the Clinical Nurse Specialist in Radiology

## 2

Sharon L. Lehmann

## 2.1 Introduction

Clinical Nurse Specialists (CNS) have been educated at the master's degree level since the specialty began in the 1960s, about the same time as the nurse practitioner (NP) programs began. The practice of the CNS is within the domain of nursing and does not usually overlap the domain of medicine, except for the psychiatric CNS, who provides diagnostic counseling and psychiatric services, which sometimes do overlap with the services of treatment provided by physician psychiatrists [1–4]. Many CNSs by virtue of extensive experience and position requirements become proficient at performing comprehensive physical assessments and diagnosing disease states occurring in patients; thus, they may provide medical care, albeit usually under the direction and guidance of a physician.

Table 2.1 provides a historical overview of the CNS in the United States (US) [5–16]. The CNS role was created: (1) to provide direct care to patients with complex disease states or conditions; (2) to improve outcomes by developing the clinical skills and judgements of staff nurses; and (3) to retain nurses who were experts to clinical practice [17]. Psychiatric CNSs became more autonomous, and independent in their practice. As nursing practices expanded such as with cardiology and oncology, the need for expert nurses continued to grow. Typically, the CNS was hospital based, but as the role expanded the CNSs moved into clinics and community settings [4].

In the 1990s, the term "advance practice registered nurse" (APRN) became commonly used in the USA. State nurse practice acts (NPAs) collectively adopted the term to delineate nurse anesthetist (CRNA), nurse midwife (CNM), NP, and CNS. The professional and regulatory influences of the NPAs served to unite the advance practice specialty roles conceptually and legislatively, thereby promoting collaboration and cohesion among APRNs.

In the Statement on Clinical Nurse Specialist Practice and Education, the National Association of Clinical Nurse Specialists (NACNS) defined the CNS as an APRN who manages the care of complex and vulnerable populations, educates and supports nursing and nursing staff, and provides the clinical expertise to facilitate change and innovation in health care systems [18]. Advanced practice nursing is the primary distinguishing feature of CNS practice.

In 2008 the APRN Consensus Model was developed to help take APRN practice to the next level. Over 40 nursing organizations participated to address the inconsistency in APRN regulatory requirements throughout the USA. The result was the Consensus Model for APRN Regulation: Licensure, Accreditation,

S. L. Lehmann, MS, APRN, CNS, CRN (✉)
Department of Interventional Radiology,
University of Minnesota Physicians,
Minneapolis, MN, USA

**Table 2.1** The history of CNS development in the United States (US) following World War II

- The 1946 Mental Health Act was passed into law by President Harry S. Truman. It provided federal research and funds for undergraduate and graduate nursing education; for a time, graduates whose education was supported by federal funds formed the largest cadre of master's-degree prepared nurses in the US [5]
- There was a proliferation of medical, surgical, pediatric and neonatal intensive care units, cardiac surgery, and special needs of physically, mentally and severely ill patients in hospitals
- In 1954 Hildegard Peplau developed the first master's degree program in psychiatric nursing at Rutgers University, New Jersey, USA. Her book, *Interpersonal Relations in Nursing: A Conceptual Frame of Reference for Psychodynamic Nursing,* provided their basic practice for the specialty [6, 7]
- Nurse educator's credit Peplau's work as the driving force for education of the CNS and the development of master's programs, aided in large part by federal funds through the GI bill, and for construction of nursing schools to meet the growing demand and evident need for highly educated nurses
- In 1963, expansion of the US federal government's Professional Nurse Training Act, administered through the Division of Nursing of the Department of Health, Education and Welfare (DHEW), to include CNS education added a major impetus for the development of more master's degree programs to prepare CNSs in all major specialties [8]
- During the 1960s and 1970s CNSs became, the single largest group of nurse experts because there was a shortage of physicians [9]
- The American Nurses Association (ANA) officially recognized the CNS role in the mid 1970's, defining the CNS as an expert practitioner and change agent. The ANA's definition specified a master's degree as a requirement for the CNS (ANA Congress of Nursing Practice, 1974) [10]
- By 1984, National League for Nursing (NLN) had 129 accredited master's degree programs preparing CNSs [11]
- The National Association of Clinical Nurse Specialists (NACNS) was founded in 1995 [12]
- In 1997, The Balanced Budget Act, specifically identified CNS's as eligible for Medicare reimbursement. The law, providing Medicare Part B direct payment to NPs and CNSs regardless of their geographic area practice, allowing both types of APRN's to be paid 85% of the fee paid to physicians for the same services. The law's inclusion and definition of the CNS corrected the previous omission of this group from reimbursement [13]
- In 2010-NACNS published core competencies and criteria for the evaluation of CNS graduate programs and certificates. A new document entitled "*CNS Statement for Clinical Nurse Specialist Practice and Education*" is expected out in the summer of 2019 that will include updated information on core competencies [14]
- In 2004 the Doctorate of Nursing Practice (DNP) degree, was introduced by the American Association of Colleges of Nursing (AACN), aimed at ensuring education preparation for the Advanced Practice Registered Nurse (APRN). In 2015 the DNP would standardize practice entry requirements [15]
- In 2015 NACNS endorsed the DNP as entry into practice for the CNS by 2030. The NACNS Board elected to provide a 15-year transition to the DNP as entry-level for the CNS. The NACNS Board believes that this timeline allows schools, universities and individuals to plan for implementation of the DNP as entry level for CNS practice [16]

Certification, and Education (LACE). The Consensus Model seeks to improve patient access to APRNs, support nurses to work more easily across different states, and enhance the American Nurses Credentialing Center (ANCC) certification process by preserving the highest standards of nursing excellence [19]. Through consistency and clarity of the APRN Consensus Model criteria, APRNs were empowered to work together to improve health care for all [20].

The necessary coordination among licensure, accreditation, certification, and education bodies required by the APRN Consensus Model called for an incremental implementation process. Although the model was completed in 2008, the target date for full implementation of the uniform APRN regulations across the four essential elements for licensure, accreditation, certification, and education was 2015. The National Council of State Boards of Nursing (NCSBN) has a map of the USA with the consensus model implementation status as of April 23, 2018 (see https://www.ncsbn.org) [20].

## 2.2 Educational Preparation for this Role

The NACNS recognizes that there are two routes for completing a clinical doctorate in nursing: post-baccalaureate (i.e., post-BSN) and post-masters. Post-BSN programs must use validated

CNS competencies and education standards to guide the curriculum and ensure that graduates are prepared to practice in the CNS role. NACNS has developed and published nationally vetted CNS competencies [14]. In addition, graduate programs must use the Criteria for the Evaluation of Clinical Nurse Specialist Master's, Practice Doctorate, and Post-Graduate Certificate Educational Programs (2012) for guidance during CNS education program evaluation and/or development. Completion of the CNS specialty didactic and clinical courses in a population of interest, along with completion of the doctorate of nursing practice (DNP) role/practicum hours, will enable graduates to meet or exceed the 1000 clinical hour requirement and to sit for national certification. Post master's of science in nursing (MSN) students who hold current advanced practice certification with verified specialty clinical hours will be required to complete the DNP role/practicum to meet the DNP essentials competencies and the remaining clinical hour requirement [16, 21].

While NACNS supports the DNP as the appropriate degree for future clinical practice as a CNS, the organization supports the right of CNSs who pursued other graduate education to retain their ability to practice within the CNS role without having to obtain the DNP for future practice as an APRN after 2030 [16].

With the APRN Consensus Model CNS education had to shift from an emphasis on role and specialty to a model that includes population and role. CNS programs had to develop curriculums that balanced the requirements for education on population, role and specialty education which is unique to the CNS within the mandated clinical hours [21].

## 2.3 Certification and Licensure

While education, accreditation, and certification are necessary components of an overall approach to preparing an APRN for practice, the licensing boards—governed by state regulations and statutes—are the final arbiters of who is recognized to practice within a given state. Currently, there is no uniform model of regulation of APRNs across the states. Each state independently determines the APRN legal scope of practice, the roles that are recognized, the criteria for entry into advanced practice, and the certification examinations accepted for entry level competence assessment. This has created a significant barrier for APRNs to easily move from state to state and has decreased access to care for patients.

For example, the author graduated in 1995 with an MS in nursing. The author chose to become certified in 1997 although it was not mandated for the author to keep her position. However, having the certification did allow the employer to change the author's position class from nurse clinician to CNS. The author received certification through ANCC by taking the medical surgical nursing examination [19]. This certification has to be renewed every 5 years and has been "relabeled" and the author is now called a CNS certified in Adult Health. The ANCC has now retired this examination but as long as the author keeps renewing she can continue to be certified, otherwise the author will have to find a new examination to take.

The author chose to take the radiology nursing examination which is accredited by the ABSNC [22]. The author chose to take this exam as validation for her practice as a radiology nurse. This examination is not required for the author's position or to keep her state license. Certification showed validation of knowledge.

When certification first became mandatory, many CNSs in the state of Minnesota where the author lives did not have a specialty examination that matched their area of specialty. Nurses were granted waivers for years; however, as certification exams have become available this was no longer an option.

In 2015, statutory barriers were removed in Minnesota for APRN practice. The creation of a formal infrastructure (Minnesota APRN Coalition) was developed to manage financial and communication strategies, provide cohesion among all four roles of APRNs, and encourage engagement of strong legislative authors and bipartisan support, and valuable partnerships among the coalition and external stakeholders.

The Minnesota Board of Nursing was key to the passage of legislation [23].

In 2016, the Minnesota State Board of Nursing issued a license number for the CNS license. Then in 2018 when this author renewed a basic Minnesota registered nurse license, the author also had to pay a given fee for a separate license to practice as a CNS. The author is allowed to practice independently; however, her employer insists that she still have a collaborate practice agreement with a physician.

## 2.4 The Future of the CNS Role

It is believed there are over 72,000 CNSs in the USA. The US Bureau of Labor Statistics has separate classifications for CRNAs, CNMs, and NPs in their standard Occupational Classification listing, so some data is collected when the Bureau does routine surveys. The CNS, however, ends up under the general RN classification, so it is not known how many CNSs are there in the USA [21].

In a US survey of CNSs, conducted by NACNS in 2016, it was found that 3 in 4 clinical nurse specialists specialize in adult health or gerontology, most CNSs work in acute care hospitals that have or are seeking ANCC's Magnet™ Recognition, and more than half have nursing clinical-related responsibility for an entire health system, but only 1 in 5 CNSs are authorized to prescribe medications [24].

As a group, the NACNS survey found that 22% provide direct patient care, 20% teach nurses and staff, 20% consult with nurses, staff, and others, 14% lead evidence-based practice projects, and 12% assist other nurses and staff with direct patient care [24].

### 2.4.1 Title Protection and Prescriptive Authority

Prescriptive authority is a matter of state law in the USA. A 2015 analysis of states, completed by NACNS in collaboration with the NCSBN, indicates that CNSs have independent authority to prescribe in 19 states. The CNS needs a collaborative agreement with a physician to legally prescribe in another 19 states. The total number of states where a CNS may be eligible to prescribe is 38. Although the CNS has the education, competence, skills, and expertise to practice, if she/he moves from one state to another state, it is the nurse practice act of the new state that will determine what the CNS can do [25].

In the state of Minnesota where the author lives and is licensed, many CNSs completed their degrees before prescriptive authority was a part of a degree. As part of the 2016 legislation in Minnesota, CNSs who did not already have prescriptive authority, must practice for 2080 h within the context of a collaborative agreement within a hospital or integrated care setting with a Minnesota-licensed certified NP, certified CNS, or physician who has experience providing care to patients with similar medical problems before she/he can prescribe independently. The CNS in Minnesota can write for controlled substances and a collaborative agreement is not required [26].

### 2.4.2 Reimbursement

One issue highlighted by the NACNS survey findings is reimbursement. CNSs in independent ambulatory care practice, or who have hospital medical board privileges, are able to bill insurance companies directly for their services, rather than through a third party, reducing insurance costs. According to the survey findings, only 6% of CNSs bill directly to a third-party payer, like a private insurance company, Medicare or Medicaid, or an individual patient for the services they provide [24].

Medicare prohibits all APRNs from admitting patients to skilled nursing facilities and certifying for hospice or home care despite the fact that they may serve as the patient's primary care provider. There have been bills placed before the US Congress to amend the Society Security Title XVIII for APRNs to certify for hospice and home care. The Home Health Care Planning Improvement Act (S. 445) to allow APRNs to certify eligibility and make changes to home

## 2.5 The CNS in the Radiology Department

The CNS has a unique APRN role to integrate care across the continuum and through three spheres of influence: patient, nurse, and system. The three spheres are overlapping and interrelated, but each sphere possesses a distinctive focus. In each of the spheres of influence, the primary goal of the CNS is continuous improvement of patient outcomes and nursing care. Key elements of CNS practice are to create environments through mentoring and system changes that empower nurses to develop caring, evidence-based practices to alleviate patient distress, facilitate ethical decision-making, and respond to diversity. The CNS is responsible and accountable for diagnosis and treatment of health/illness states, disease management, health promotion, and prevention of illness and risky behaviors among individuals, families, groups, and communities [21].

To be successful, a CNS must understand and apply the seven competencies (see below) of advanced practice nursing across the three spheres of influence regardless of setting or specialty. Implementing competencies across the three spheres can result in improvement in clinical outcomes, patient safety, patient/family satisfaction, resource allocation, professional nursing staff knowledge and skills, advancement of clinical practice, health care team collaboration, and organizational efficiency [17].

### 2.5.1 Direct Clinical Practice

This core competency is central to and influences all the other competencies. It is important to note that the "3 Ps" that form the core courses in all APRN programs (pathophysiology, pharmacology, and physical assessment) are not separate competences in this understanding, but provide baseline knowledge and skills to support the direct clinical practice competency. Providing regular and consistent direct patient care is essential and has been shown to improve patient outcomes and reduce health care costs when CNSs and other APRNs are directly involved with patient care, including assessing, teaching, counseling, and navigating systems [17].

The author spends the majority of her time in the outpatient clinic setting. My job description can be found in Table 2.2. Below are some examples from the author's practice.

- Evaluate patients for potential biopsies. A consult is sent by the referring service, the chart is reviewed, and the case is presented to the interventional radiologist (IR). The images are reviewed, and the biopsy is either approved or not approved. Most patients are brought into clinic for consultation prior to having the biopsy. They are complex, with multiple health issues and many medications, some of which need to be held for a period of time

**Table 2.2** Sample CNS job description

*Core privileges in adult clinical nurse specialist*
- Perform health histories and physical exams, order and interpret diagnostic tests within protocol guidelines within context of collaborative management
- Care of indwelling vascular catheters, chest tubes, gastrostomy tubes, gastrojejunostomy tubes, cecostomy tubes, sclerotherapy tubes, and abscess drainage tubes
- Discharge patients
- Initial and ongoing assessment of the medical, physical and psychosocial status of patients who are young adult or older
- Initiate admitting starting orders for collaborating physician
- Order and interpret appropriate laboratory studies within protocol guidelines and within context of collaborative management, recording findings
- Order restraints per hospital policy
- Work in specific disease related areas (such as diabetes) assessing and managing symptoms, patient education and assisting with lifestyle changes

*Core privileges in prescriptive core*
- Prescriptive core

*Special request privileges: level II clinical nurse specialist*
- Enteric tube (non-percutaneous) placement and removal

prior to the biopsy, and then the biopsy is scheduled.
- Evaluate patients for venous access when undergoing workup for bone marrow transplant. Some have never had access before, some have had previous venous blood clots and require assessment, and some come with a tunneled central line in place that also must be assessed for adequacy and appropriate placement.
- Evaluate adult cystic fibrosis (CF) population for port-a-cath placement. Some have had multiple intravenous access, previous venous blood clots, and need long-term venous access most frequently for antibiotics.
- Consult with patients who are quite anxious and want more information on gastrostomy tube placement, percutaneous nephrostomy tube placement, etc.
- Follow-up with patients after gastrostomy tube placement, perform button changes once the initial change has occurred and remove gastrostomy tubes when no longer needed.
- Assume responsibility for patients who are referred from outside the system directly to IR for biopsy, to make sure all biopsy results are reported to the referring physician and aid the provider should they require assistance in making further referrals for their patient.
- Work two half days a week in the Women's Specialty Clinic to consult with women who have symptomatic fibroids and are interested in the uterine fibroid embolization (UFE) procedure. Assist patients in completing their workup, undergoing the UFE procedure and the recovery period, providing for and/or arranging additional follow-up.

## 2.5.2 Consultation

This core competency is both a skill and an art, and requires knowledge, experience, and an integration of the essential aspects of the CNS role that are brought into clinical practice. The word consultation has also been interchanged with the words clinical consultation, comanagement, referral, supervision, and collaboration.

Examples of consultation could include APRN to APRN, APRN to physician, APRN to staff nurse, or APRN to committee [17].

A few years ago, the hospitalists brought to IR a change they wanted to see happen. At that time all of the outpatients who had gastrostomy tubes placed in IR were staying overnight following their procedure. The hospitalists wanted to see changes for many reasons: (1) patients seemed low risk and the hospitalists assessment was that they could be done as outpatients, (2) patients were not using intravenous pain medication overnight, (3) some were getting their tubes at the start of radiation therapy and so did not need to start tube feeding, and (4) beds were not easy to obtain and this population needed to be evaluated as a possibly to be done on an outpatient basis.

The author reviewed the literature and found that there was scant IR literature about performing this procedure on outpatients. The author went on the Society of Interventional Radiology (SIR) listserv and asked the IR physicians who were performing the gastrostomy tube placement on an outpatient basis about their protocols. A small number of IRs responded and sent the author their protocols. The same amount responded who were not performing this procedure. The author's IR group then developed a protocol and guidelines for the outpatient clinics to follow to get the patients ready for this procedure. Pre- and post-order sets were developed and the procedure moved forward as an outpatient procedure. The amyotrophic lateral sclerosis (ALS) patient population was excluded due to concerns for their airway after the procedure and/or refeeding syndrome. The process has been successful thus far. The author then gave a lecture at a nursing conference in 2017 about the retrospective review and the process we went through to change to the outpatient program. This is just one example of the value of a CNS.

## 2.5.3 System Leadership

The CNS has the ability to manage change and empower others to influence clinical practice and political processes within and across systems [17].

The author developed order sets for the more common procedures, i.e., angiograms, thrombolysis, gastrostomy tube placement, and transjugular intrahepatic portosystemic shunt (TIPS), when she first started in the role in the late 1990s. When a second nurse clinician was hired for IR, one of her responsibilities was to develop order sets for all of the procedures.

Eventually, the order sets became a part of the electronic medical record and now we have over 100 order sets between pre- and post-procedures. This was a time-consuming project and took a couple of years to complete. The author was part of a work group that met with the radiology nurse manager, information technology (IT) manager who is also a nurse, a nurse clinician from a sister hospital in our health care system, and a representative from pharmacy. This work group built upon the existing order sets that had anticoagulation algorithms and antibiotic guidelines. The radiologists then approved the order sets. Because the work group had only developed adult order sets, the author then developed pediatric order sets; these were approved by the pediatric radiologist.

Developing order sets is a task that will never be completed. As processes change, the order sets are updated. The order sets must be reviewed on a regular basis. We fortunately have maintained the same IT manager, a nurse, over the years. This resource has been invaluable to keep the process flowing smoothly.

### 2.5.4 Collaboration

It is working jointly with others to optimize clinical outcomes. The CNS collaborates at an advanced level by committing to authentic engagement and constructive patient, family, system, and population focused problem solving [17].

The hospital system where the author works at has a large cystic fibrosis (CF) population. The CF physicians approached the author because they wanted IR to place gastrostomy tubes as MIC KEY™ buttons at the time of initial placement. This was a change in practice for IR. The author reviewed the literature and found articles for the radiologists to review in support of this change, and in this population they have agreed to perform this procedure. There is also an inpatient CNS for the CF population that the author works with on a regular basis to consult on patients with that are having issues with their buttons. In the outpatient setting there are also resource nurses that the author utilizes regularly.

The author participates in tumor board conferences to discuss patients that are in need of various biopsies. The lung tumor board meets weekly to discuss lung nodules. We review the patient's history—smoking, health issues, previous scans, size of the nodule, how easy is it to biopsy, etc. [27]. If the biopsy is approved, then the author will see the patient in imaging consult clinic to discuss the procedure, prep the patient, and schedule the biopsy. There are two CNSs that work with the pulmonologists and thoracic surgeons, and we manage the patients between tumor board, biopsy, and return of the results.

### 2.5.5 Guidance and Coaching

This core competency is an effective means to engage patients in change leading to healthier lifestyles [17].

One of the populations that frequently need a biopsy are patients that are smokers and they have a lung lesion. The pulmonary CNSs have already coached the patients about quitting. Tools have already been provided to the patients. They are offered pharmacological agents. My role is to inform the patients that a potential complication of lung biopsy is pneumothorax, they may need a chest tube and be admitted to the hospital where they won't be allowed to smoke. The patient needs to be prepared for this scenario and use the tools that the pulmonary CNSs have given them.

### 2.5.6 Research/Evidence-Based Practice

This includes the search for, interpretation of, and use of evidence in clinical practice and quality improvement, as well as active participation in the conduct of research [17].

The author has worked with pharmacy, IT, the radiologists, and a nurse clinician from a sister hospital in our health care system to update and expand algorithms for holding of anticoagulants for various procedures. This was a several month project. We had to review the literature, and found our list of drugs was much more detailed than the list published by SIR. We compared our list to other hospital lists that we found available on-line, brought the lists back to the two different radiology groups, came up with comprises and then agreed on the compromises to develop "the list." This effort will be an ongoing process as new drugs come on the market, new procedures are developed, and new guidelines are published in the literature [28].

The author developed antibiotic guidelines as pre-procedure medications. The guidelines were based upon surgical guidelines and available radiology guidelines. The guidelines are reviewed yearly.

### 2.5.7 Ethical Decision-Making

Identifying, articulating, and taking action on ethical concerns at the patient, family, health care provider, system, community, and public policy levels are concerns for the CNS [17].

In 1996, when the UFE procedure was introduced into the USA, insurance companies in the state of Minnesota did not want to pay for the procedure, stating it was experimental. The lead physician, David Hunter, MD, who the author worked with wrote the state attorney general pleading our case as to why insurance companies should cover this procedure. Patients also wrote the attorney general. After many months, slowly we were able to gain approval. We performed our first case in July 1997. The radiologists and the author have partnered closely with the Women's Health Specialty Clinic to have a formal fibroid program.

## 2.6 The Author's Role

The author has been in her current position for 25 years and over time her responsibilities have changed. The radiologists knew they needed an advanced practice nurse, but they were not sure what to do with one, so the author did not delay in establishing a new role. In the beginning the author strictly had an inpatient presence and made daily rounds.

Nurses have been in the radiology department at the University of Minnesota since 1974 and when the author started in 1994 there were 11 working in radiology, the majority practicing in IR for sedation purposes. There was no formal pre- or post-procedure area. One nurse had developed simple teaching pamphlets for every test. There were no order sets. No patients were called to prepare them for their tests. The author worked in IR for 10 years before the pre/post-sedation unit opened. It was a painful process to get patients ready and recover them until this happened. A pre-call nurse was added about the same time the pre/post-sedation unit opened.

The author developed more in-depth teaching booklets for the more complex procedures, i.e., angiograms, vascular stents, inferior vena cava (IVC) filters, venograms, drainage tubes, gastrostomy tubes, TIPS, port-a-cath, and tunneled central lines. When the hospital opened their own patient learning center, they took over the maintenance of the teaching booklets, eventually putting them all on line.

IR placed internal ureteral stents in women who were undergoing treatment for gynecological cancers. The radiologists dictated in their reports that the patient should be seen every 3 months to follow up on these stents and that the stents should be changed every 9 months. As long as the patients care remained at the University of Minnesota the patients maintained their appointments. However, what the author discovered was that many patients were not getting appropriate follow-up. One of the author's first quality assurance projects was to find the "lost to follow-up" patients and get follow-up care organized. The concern was that the longer the stents are left in place, they could become occluded and/or infected. The author also developed a patient teaching booklet that the patients received at the time of placement to help with education and the author personally followed up with the patients. The author eventually educated the gynecologic oncology inpatient unit and outpatient clinic staff to have support in the follow-up with the patients [29].

The author was the first clinical nurse specialist hired and the first to bill for patients in her organization. The person who was in the billing department was very meticulous with the author about what elements I needed to include in my notes for reimbursement. The author knows billing still scrutinizes the notes that are written for thoroughness.

For many years the author also supported the radiologists in the startup of their consult clinics. We saw patients with vascular malformations, venous and arterial disease, oncology, and lymphedema. Now there are two nurse clinicians who support the radiologists in their practices.

## 2.7 CNS in Other IR Settings

The author has had personal communications with CNSs in the state of Minnesota who have been trained in other facilities to perform venous sclerotherapy procedures by their attending radiologists; they also assist with the laser procedures. Still other CNSs have been trained to perform thoracentesis and paracentesis.

CNSs can be trained to do sinograms and abscess drainage catheter injections and follow-up; chest tube checks and removal; placement of central venous lines, arterial lines, and peripherally inserted central catheters (PICC); arterial catheter removal and achievement of hemostasis; and image-guided procedures including spinal injections, joint infections, aspirations, arthrography, fluid collection/aspiration/drainage procedures, bone/soft tissue biopsy, and chest tube insertion. To obtain privileges, the CNS would need a letter or certification from a training course specific to the procedure or letter from collaborating/sponsoring physician indicating training specific to the procedure has successfully been completed and documentation of 25 cases within the past 24 months for each privilege requested.

## 2.8 CNS in the International Setting

The CNS role was introduced in Canada and the United Kingdom at the same time as in the USA in response to rising complexity and specialization of health care and the need for clinical expertise, education, and leadership to improve care delivery and patient outcomes, develop nursing practice, and support nurses at the point of care. In the 1990s and 2000s the CNS role has been introduced in China, Japan, Hong Kong, New Zealand, Australia, the Republic of Korea, Taiwan, and Thailand. CNS education varies among the countries; titling is inconsistent making it difficult to tell if the nurse is specialized or truly an advanced practice nurse. Like in the US, CNSs provide care in a variety of settings [30].

## 2.9 Conclusion

The author feels that the CNS role in radiology has been enriched by her involvement in the Association for Radiologic and Imaging Nursing (ARIN) [31]. The yearly conferences that the author has attended have allowed her to network with other advanced practice nurses, keep up to date on practice, give lectures, and present posters. The physicians that the author has worked with over the years have been encouraging and supportive when the author was on the ARIN Board of Directors. The CNSs role is very unique in radiology and one has to actively seek out a support system and mentors.

## References

1. Hamric AB. Chapter 1: History and overview of the CNS role. In: Hamric AB, Spross JA, editors. The clinical nurse specialist in theory and practice. 3rd ed. Philadelphia, PA: WB Saunders; 1989. p. 4–5.
2. Reiter F. The nurse clinician. Am J Nurs. 1966;66(2):274–80.
3. Davis AR. Chapter 7: Clinical nurse specialist. In: Davis AR, editor. Advanced practice nurses: education, roles, trends. Boston: Jones and Bartlett Publishers; 1997. p. 81–92.

4. Lusk B, Cockerham AZ, Keeling AW. Chapter 1: Highlights from the history of advanced practice nursing in the United States. In: Tracy MF, O'Grady ET, editors. Hamric & Hanson's advanced practice nursing. 6th ed. St. Louis: Elsevier; 2019. p. 10–15.
5. Critchley DL. Chapter 1: Evolution of the role. In: Critchley DL, Maurin JT, editors. The clinical nurse specialist in psychiatric mental health nursing. New York: Wiley and Sons; 1985. p. 5–22.
6. Peplau HE, editor. Interpersonal relations in nursing: a conceptual frame of reference for psychodynamic nursing. New York: Putnam; 1952.
7. Silk GM. The role and function of the clinical nurse specialist. In: Chaska NL, editor. The nursing profession: a time to speak. New York: McGraw-Hill; 1983. p. 563–79.
8. Peplau HE. Specialization in professional nursing. Nurs Sci. 1965;3:268–87.
9. Hoeffer B, Murphy SA. Specialization in nursing practice. American Nurses Association: Kansas City, MO; 1984.
10. American Nurses Association (ANA), Congress of Nursing Practice 1974. https://www.nursingworld.org/
11. National League for Nursing (NLN). www.nln.org
12. National Association of Clinical Nurse Specialists (NACNS). www.nacns.org
13. Safriet BJ. Still spending dollars, still searching for sense: advanced practice nursing in an era of regulatory and economic turmoil. Adv Pract Nurs Q. 1998;4:24–33.
14. National Association of Clinical Nurse Specialists. Clinical nurse specialist core competencies. National CNS competence task force. 2010. www.nacns.org
15. American Association of Colleges of Nursing (AACN). https://www.aacnnursing.org/
16. National Association of Clinical Nurse Specialists. DNP position statement. July 2015. www.nacns.org
17. Tracy NF, Sendelbach S. Chapter 14: The clinical nurse specialist. In: Tracy MF, O'Grady ET, editors. Hamric & Hanson's advanced practice nursing. 6th ed. St. Louis: Elsevier; 2019. p. 343–73.
18. National Association of Clinical Nurse Specialists. Statement on clinical nurse specialist practice and education. 3rd ed. Harrisburg, PA: National Association of Clinical Nurse Specialists; 2004.
19. American Nurses Credential Center (ANCC). https://www.nursingworld.org/ANCC/Certification
20. National Council of State Boards of Nursing (NCSBN). https://www.ncsbn.org
21. Hamric AB, Tracy MF. Chapter 3: Definition of advanced practice nursing. In: Tracy MF, O'Grady ET, editors. Hamric & Hanson's advanced practice nursing. 6th ed. St. Louis: Elsevier; 2019. p. 61–79.
22. The Accreditation Board for Specialty Nursing Certification (ABSNC). www.nursingcertification.org
23. Sabo JA, Chesney M, Tracy MF, Sendelbach S. APRN consensus model implementation: the Minnesota experience. J Nurs Regul. 2017;8(2):10–16.
24. National Association of Clinical Nurse Specialists. Key findings from the 2016 Clinical Nurse Specialist Census. 2017. www.nacns.org
25. Safriet BJ. Appendix H: Federal options for maximizing the value of advanced practice nurses in providing quality, cost effective health care. In: Institute of Medicine, editors. The future of nursing: leading change, advancing health. Washington, DC: The National Academies Press. 2011, pp. 443–476. https://doi.org/10.17226/12956.
26. Stokowski LA. APRN prescribing law: a state-by-state summary. 2018. http://www.medscape.com.
27. Lehmann S, Frank N. An overview of percutaneous CT guided lung biopsies. J Radiol Nurs. 2018;37(2):2–8.
28. Patel IJ, Davidson JC, Nikolic B, Salazar GM, Schwartzberg MS, Walker G, Saad WE. Addendum of newer anticoagulants to the SIR consensus guideline. J Vasc Interv Radiol. 2013;24:641–45.
29. Lehmann S, Dietz C. The trouble with double J stents. RN. 2014;65(1):54–59.
30. Bryant-Lukosius D, Wong FKY. Chapter 6: International development of advanced practice nursing. In: Tracy MF, O'Grady ET, editors. Hamric & Hanson's advanced practice nursing. 6th ed. St. Louis: Elsevier; 2019. p. 129–41.
31. Association for Radiologic and Imaging Nursing (ARIN). www.arinursing.org

# Radiology Nurse Manager

**3**

Valerie Aarne Grossman and Alexandra Penzias

## 3.1 Introduction

Leading a successful nursing team is a careful balance of evidence-based methods with a high degree of compassion and understanding of a multi-generational group of professionals. Selecting quality candidates, creating appropriate orientation plans for each individual, and working tirelessly to retain team members are essential for every nurse manager. Nurse managers may also be responsible for budgets, incident investigation and resolution, project management, mentoring others, and continual self-reflection and learning. This chapter will assist the reader in learning strategies to be successful in this important role.

## 3.2 Staff Recruitment and Candidate Selection

Radiology nurse managers are presented with the challenge of how to recruit, orient, and retain nursing talent while managing the costs associated with attracting and retaining. Having a clear understanding of the operations scale, complexity, logistical needs, and patient population served, the specific role of the nurse in procedural care as well as the regulations impacting nurse practice in the local jurisdiction all have implications in candidate recruitment, selection, and training.

High-quality orientation is associated with lower attrition [1, 2] and improved patient outcomes [2]. The costs associated with delivering a high-quality orientation are considerable; subsequent analysis of type of radiology practice, complexity, proximity to or association with a medical center, and target patient population should be considered. Nurses working in a large volume, tertiary care interventional radiology department require a different skill set than those working in an exclusively outpatient diagnostic setting. The goal of orientation is to provide nurses with the knowledge, skills, and attitudes to provide safe, high-quality patient care as well as to assimilate into the team and develop as a successful team member.

Radiology nursing requires a vast knowledge base, and a unique skill set [3], inclusive of strong critical thinking and patient advocacy skills. It is a relatively new and emerging specialty and few pre-licensure nursing programs include radiology nursing considerations in their curriculum [4]; subsequently nurse managers in a radiology practice must anticipate providing a comprehensive, competency-based orientation for newly hired nurses.

V. A. Grossman, MALS, BSN, RN (✉)
Department of Radiology,
Highland Hospital (An affiliate of the University of Rochester), Rochester, NY, USA

A. Penzias, DNP, MEd, APRN, ACNS-BC
Cooley Dickinson Hospital, Northampton, MA, USA

Nurses recruited for a diagnostic radiology setting require comprehensive physical assessment, vascular access, and emergency management skills. In contrast, nurses working in a tertiary care interventional setting inclusive of vascular, nonvascular, neuro-interventional, and cardiovascular interventions require additional comprehensive assessment, hemodynamic monitoring, familiarity with care of the ventilated patient, and emergency management skills, as well as an understanding of the major nursing considerations associated with the care of the specific patient populations seen in that setting.

### 3.2.1 Candidate Skills and Characteristics

Recruiting nurses from nursing specialties with similar core competencies ensures a candidate pool with a skill set that is applicable in the radiology setting. This may reduce the duration of orientation and improve the likelihood of success. Candidates with prior knowledge of procedural settings may have the largest transferrable skill set. The comprehensive, high acuity care provided in critical care settings require a skill set like that required by a registered nurse (RN) caring for a high acuity patient undergoing an emergent interventional procedure. RNs with emergency department experience may bring excellent vascular access, critical care skills, and an operational understanding of patient throughput.

Alternatively, some leaders may elect to recruit newly licensed or novice nurses who are inquisitive and show an essential skill set of being a team player. In a competitive employment market, hiring newly licensed or novice nurses may seem financially advantageous; however, this population may require additional time investment during orientation to cultivate both clinical and nonclinical skills necessary for success.

## 3.3 Interviewing

Interviewing presents an opportunity to meet and educate prospective candidates to radiology nursing. Unlike other established specialties, radiology nursing practice is evolving and differs across practice settings; subsequently, the process to recruit and interview nurses should be driven by nursing. All members of the radiology nursing leadership team should be included in the interviewing process as well as representation of the staff nurses, where possible. Each member of the team has unique insights into a candidate that may prove valuable to the process.

### 3.3.1 Pre-interview Process

Following a review of the application and curriculum vitae, the interviewing team should convene to establish the format for the interview, and key questions they would like to ask the candidate. This ensures the greatest yield of candidate information within the context of the interview. The opening phase of the interview consists of introduction of the team, and inquiry regarding candidate interest, posed as an open-ended question. The tone of the interview should be conversational, interactive, and paced to provide multiple opportunities for the candidate to ask questions. Planning and structuring the interview experience allows both the leadership team and the candidate an opportunity to determine if the candidate's attributes are a good fit for the role, the organization, and the radiology team. The goal of any recruitment process is to ensure that the candidate has the knowledge, skills, and attitudes to match the needs of the department, has the aptitude for success, and exhibits the potential to support the mission, vision, and values of the organization.

### 3.3.2 Interview Content

Radiology nursing is unique, and the configuration, size, scale, and specialty practices can be heterogeneous; subsequently even for candidates with prior procedural or radiology nursing experience, or those pursuing an interdepartmental transfer, a description of the department, its leadership structure, services offered, case mix, volume, and patient populations served is beneficial.

Following an overview of the department and description of the role, the use of questions that link the candidate's previous experience with situations that may arise in the radiology setting is both informational for the candidate, while providing an opportunity to evaluate critical thinking, knowledge, and attitudes. In institutions with a strong focus on nursing practice excellence, or process improvement, questions specific to a candidate's desire to pursue certification, advanced degrees, participate in quality and safety initiatives, or a shared governance council can be beneficial in identifying candidates that represent the mission, vision, and values of the organization.

The nurse manager responsible for orientation should be present during the interview to provide the candidate with an orientation overview and transition to practice process. This aspect of the interview provides an opportunity to ask about learning styles, and attributes that might be beneficial to selection of an appropriate preceptor. Additionally, it provides the candidate an idea of the learner expectations, and learning curve required to transition. If possible, including preceptors in the interview process can provide the candidate with the consumer perspective of the orientation experience and insight into the nurse role.

### 3.3.3 Post-interview: Tour and Observation Experience

Following the formal interview, providing a guided tour of the department allows the candidate to synthesize the information received during the interview, and ask additional questions, while meeting other members of the team. If permitted by an institution's human resource department, it is advantageous to provide the candidate with direct contact information for follow-up questions. If permitted by an institution's human resources, security and occupational health policies, offering an observation experience in which the candidate may follow a clinician for a period (4–8 h) after the interview allows the candidate an opportunity to ask clinical staff questions that they may not have had the chance or the courage to ask during an interview. This also provides a chance for departmental staff to be a part of the candidate/team selection process.

## 3.4 Orientation

Careful consideration and development of the structure and process of providing orientation are essential to achieving the goal of cultivating a clinician with the knowledge, skills, and attitudes to support an organization's mission, vision, and values in delivering safe, high-quality care and a positive patient experience. The content of the orientation is influenced by national scope and standards of practice, state boards of nursing, regulatory requirements, such as The Joint Commission, specialty, and additional accreditation standards. Orientation is a learner focused experience. Departmental characteristics, culture, resources, and learner characteristics are driving forces in determining the content and process of delivering orientation education and training. Orientation represents a partnership between the newly hired clinician (orientee), the leadership team, preceptor, and other staff involved in education to prepare an individual for safe entry to practice into a new practice environment.

## 3.5 The Regulatory Landscape

Scope of practice for nurses and advanced practitioners is determined by state boards of nursing in the USA (or international equivalent) and varies across jurisdiction. State scope and practice regulations may have implications for many aspects of a radiology practice operation, from nursing staffing levels, mandates for provider presence in areas where medication are administered, prescribing privileges (absolute and specific) and the level of sedation/analgesia that can be delivered by an RN or certified registered nurse anesthetist (CRNA).

Advanced practitioners (nurse practitioner [NP], clinical nurse specialist [CNS], physician assistant (PA), and CRNA) require further credentialing on an institutional level, with physician oversight. In many jurisdictions across the USA, nurse practitioners and physicians' assistants are recruited and hired interchangeably, while in others, nurse practitioners may practice autonomously [5]. Hiring registered nurses or advanced practitioners across state and federal lines may influence scope of practice, have implications for the depth and breadth of orientation needed, and may be associated with delays in licensure and credentialing.

State funded health agencies determine and monitor the regulations with which institutions must comply in the provision of patient care. These agencies assert both direct and indirect influence on clinician licensure, credentialing, and orientation needs. They also assert direct influence over clinician education through educational mandates to boards of registration. Clinician compliance is critical to an institution's ability to demonstrate compliance with state mandates, subsequently asserting an indirect influence on the orientation needs of newly hired clinicians. In some jurisdictions, independent organizations also credential radiology organizations, such as The Joint Commission [TJC], Det Norske Veritas Healthcare, Inc. (DNV), Healthcare Facilities Accreditation Program (HFAP), or specific programs (American College of Radiologists [ACR]). Participation in these credentialing programs can influence reimbursement for services and market share. In a competitive health care market, maintaining the highest level of credentialing is critical to financial viability, patient safety, and has significant implications for the education needs of clinicians.

## 3.6 Department Characteristics

Radiology practices vary in size, scale, specialty, service affiliation, services provided, and populations served. Departments of larger size and scale may employ advanced practitioners, specifically nurse practitioners (NPs), physicians' assistants (PAs), radiology practitioner assistants (RPAs), and CRNAs, in addition to registered nurses (RNs). As the complexity of a practice increases, so do the regulatory requirements specific to practice, and the education, training, and credentialing need of its clinicians. Through a comprehensive survey of an individual radiology practice, nurse managers can determine what the essential elements of orientation should be for a specific department.

## 3.7 Learner Characteristics

Learning, or the acquisition of knowledge or skill by instruction or study, is essential to the orientation process. Psychologist David Kolb (1984) described learning as the constructive, cumulative, and goal-oriented process that involves creating knowledge through transformation of experience. Malcolm Knowles, referred to as the father of androgogy (adult learning), identified some basic assumptions of adult learning which distinguish it from pedagogy. Adults bring the richness of life experience to the learning environment. According to Knowles, adults are self-directed. An individuals readiness to learn and pursue knowledge is based on what is believed to be relevant, and new knowledge must be immediately applicable to experiences.

While the learning objectives in any given situation will be specific, learning ability, style, and preference are unique to an individual. Fleming [6] identified sensory-based learning. While one learner may respond to reading volumes of material on a topic, another may prefer watching videos, listening to podcasts, or participating in simulation [7]. Adult learners may be able to articulate their learning style directly, or through inventory analysis. For advanced practice leaders responsible for providing education, understanding a clinician learning style is essential to designing an education (orientation and ongoing competency) program that is effective to the dissemination of information and adoption of the skills for practice.

## 3.8 Radiology Societies and Associations

Professional and specialty organizations, such as the Association for Radiologic and Imaging Nursing (ARIN), the American College of Radiology (ACR), the Society of Interventional Radiology (SIR), the Royal College of Radiology (RCR), and the European Society of Radiology (ESR), provide representation for its members, provide standards of practice and education, and promote and disseminate research and publications specific to the specialty. Radiology clinicians are encouraged to use the resources made available by these and other specialty organizations to guide their clinical practice.

## 3.9 Orientation Content

Clinician education and training are critical to providing safe, high-quality patient care and an exemplary patient experience. Specifically, clinicians require didactic education, skills training, and specifically mandated credentialing for each patient population, radiologic procedure, nursing intervention, and phase of care for which they will be responsible. Orientation content specific to institutional, certification, and regulatory requirements must be included. The Association of Radiology Nurses (ARIN) defines the scope and standards for radiology nursing practice and education [8]. Additionally, education and practice standards, and useful curriculums, are available through specialty organizations such as the American Association of Critical Care Nurses (AACN), the Oncology Nurses Society (ONS), the Infusion Nurses Society (INS), the American Society of Perianesthesia Nurses (ASPAN), and the Association of periOperative Registered Nurses (AORN).

Orientation content should be reviewed at established intervals and as necessary to remain current, relevant, and achieving the necessary learner and departmental outcomes. Content should be structured around core objectives that are relevant, achievable, and measurable. Competency statements must be clearly stated. Use terms such as "demonstrates, articulates, states, calibrates," which are observable and measurable. Competency statements should be linked to an approved, established, evidence-based procedure, policy, or protocol. For example, "Demonstrates the care of a patient undergoing moderate sedation in accordance with the Moderate Sedation policy #3.01." In this situation, the statement is linked to a specific policy which delineates the role of the RN.

### 3.9.1 Content Delivery

Successful delivery of orientation content, credentialing, and clinician education begin during the pre-hire phase, at the time of interview, and continues throughout the process of employment. Members of the radiology nursing leadership responsible for education should be present at the time of interview to inquire about the prospective candidate's previous experience with orientation, continuing education, and learning style.

An evidence-based, structured orientation that specifically addresses the education, training credentialing, regulatory requirements of clinicians in a specific context should engage the learner, matching content delivery style with learning style. Pace, content sequencing, and delivery must be done to allow the learner to ask questions and link prior knowledge to new information and experiences. By incorporating multiple learning modalities, allowing the newly hired clinician to directly apply new knowledge and skills in the practice setting, and providing structured feedback, learning is enhanced, and challenges can be identified early.

Orientation is a learner-focused experience, but one that requires the learner to actively engage and prepare for each session, where the classroom experience serves to validate and clarify independent learning. Sequencing of learning opportunities (clinical, didactic, and simulation) in increasing complexity allows the learner to cultivate their knowledge, skills, and critical thinking. Utilization of multiple learning modalities provides a varied and interesting experience that continues to engage the learner and provides educators an opportunity to determine which modality is most effective for each learner.

The emergence and adoption of learning management systems is one method institutions employ to meet regulatory/mandated education requirements. Learning management systems present an efficient means of disseminating information. This method engages the visual/reading learner, can be self-paced, and provides an auditable trail for assignment completion. Interactive learning modules are becoming increasingly sophisticated, engaging learners in learning complex algorithms and processes (e.g., advanced cardiac life support); they are, however, limited in their ability to evaluate highly technical skills and procedures.

Utilization of the lecture-discussion method provides a forum for dissemination of essential information about patient characteristics, pathophysiology, imaging, and intervention and case study analysis provides an opportunity to engage learners to reflect on clinical experiences and demonstrate critical thinking through discussion. Creating case studies based on clinical scenarios that are relevant to a clinical setting can integrate learning about patient, procedure, policy, and protocol related information. Case study analysis can be utilized as a preparatory or an evaluation exercise for clinicians.

Skills sessions utilizing task trainers and simulation manikins are essential in teaching, and evaluating the learning of specific, highly technical skills. This teaching method is well suited to essential skills that require practice, dexterity, and mastery, such as vascular access, suctioning, urinary catheterization, or cardiopulmonary resuscitation. Institutions without simulation facilities may use models for teaching skills such as port access and collaborate with other departments such as endoscopy area to assist orientees in learning vascular access skills or the intensive care unit to learn critical care skills. Learners arrive at the skills session having completed preparatory reading to understand the procedure, protocols and process underlying the skill to be learned. The session serves to synthesize knowledge with the new skill. Processes or situations that are complex, high stakes, and/or team based benefit from the use of high-fidelity simulation. Though cost-intensive, high-fidelity simulation offers learners the best alternative to learning in an actual clinical situation.

### 3.9.2 Clinical Training

Supervised clinical training provides an experiential learning opportunity. To facilitate learning, experiences should increase in complexity as the learner demonstrates mastery, with didactic education and skill sessions preceding clinical experience. The clinical supervisor/preceptor acts as a teacher and serves to facilitate new clinician assimilation into departmental/institutional culture. The clinical supervisor/preceptor is an expert clinician who acts as a departmental role model with an interest in teaching and play a critical role in the new clinician's success.

In conjunction with the department educator, the clinical supervisor/preceptor supports the education experience of the new clinician, providing information, structured feedback, role modeling best practice, patient advocacy, and team behaviors. As skill mastery is achieved, the clinical supervisor/preceptor gradually allows the learner to assume greater responsibility for care of a patient, or patients.

### 3.9.3 Preceptor Development

The preparation of clinicians to supervise or precept capitalizes on clinical expertise to build coaching/mentoring and teaching skills needed to impart both clinical and nonclinical skills on junior clinicians. Clinicians involved in training staff should be proficient or expert clinicians, with a commitment to quality, strong communication and advocacy skills, and have a genuine interest in developing their team. According to Benner [9] proficient clinicians perceive situations, and their decisions are guided by experiences. Proficient nurses can modify a plan of care as needed. By comparison, the expert nurse, with their extensive knowledge base, may have a more intuitive and instinctual grasp on a situation and respond instinctively without the ability to articulate a clinical action in concrete terms. In this respect, a proficient nurse may be a better choice as a preceptor for a novice, whose understanding of a clinical situation is bound by rules, facts, data, and details.

For many established clinicians, supervising new staff presents an opportunity to develop the nonclinical skills needed to pursue leadership roles. Training of staff interested in supervising junior clinicians is essential to assisting the newly hired to develop competency, ensuring positive outcomes and ensuring retention of newly hired staff [2, 10, 11]. Training of supervising clinicians can be achieved through a blended learning model [2]. This model satisfies the needs of different learners and optimizes the use of various modalities for different types of content. Online learning [12] is an efficient means of offering foundational and theoretical content, such as principals of adult learning, learning methods, and principals of teaching. Critical communication and feedback skills are supported through 1:1 coaching with an educator, the use of simulation [13], and a classroom environment for group discussion about clinical situations and nonclinical skills.

The goal of orientation is to provide the orientee with the knowledge, skills, and attitudes need for safe entry to practice into a new specialty. Benner's [9] landmark work, *From Novice to Expert,* based on the Dreyfus Model of Skill Acquisition, provides preceptors with foundational knowledge on how to identify skill/knowledge acquisition. Discussion of Benner's work with potential supervising clinicians provides a foundation for discussing the progression through the orientation process. Additional material about adult learning and learning styles is beneficial to supervising clinicians to support novice clinicians with varying learning styles.

Supervising clinicians must have a clear understanding of the orientation process and expectations, and access to all the resources needed during the orientation period. Challenges common to supervising clinicians include identifying and confronting gaps in practice, how and when to allow the orientee to assume more responsibility for increasingly complex care, and how to provide constructive feedback.

### 3.9.4 Feedback

Feedback, both positive and critical, is essential in high performance organizations [14] and should be an integral element of team communication. Providing feedback, positive and critical, is a skill that can be cultivated. Nurses, particularly those in leadership and supervisory roles, must understand the structure and process of providing both real-time and formal feedback to orientees and staff. Supervising clinicians can cultivate critical communication skills through training inclusive of strategies described in the TEAM STEPPS® [15], or Crucial Conversations/ Crucial Confrontations (VitalSmarts®) programs. These skills assist the clinician in speaking up in high stakes situations, as well as providing feedback in a manner that engages collaboration and minimizes alienation [14].

During the orientation period, written feedback should be submitted weekly to the leadership team by the supervising clinician, with follow-up for any identified learning gaps. Additionally, regular meetings between the orientee, supervising clinician, and the nursing leadership team provide an opportunity to review progress, challenges, practice gaps, and goals. Despite having established criteria for hiring, evidence-based orientation content and processes, not all newly hired clinicians will progress at the same rate [11], some may exhibit unsafe practices, and others may fail to complete orientation. Either by election or due to failure to progress along established milestones, identifying at-risk staff early can reduce institutional risk and costs.

### 3.9.5 End of Orientation

Orientation is complete when all essential milestones have been met, and the orientee demonstrates the integration of knowledge, skills, and attributes for safe entry to practice. Clinicians who have prior experience in a specialty where they had a higher level of mastery will exhibit greater proficiency when familiar situations present themselves. For example, a critical care nurse transfers into the interventional radiology specialty in a tertiary care hospital. At the completion of orientation, they are comfortable with the care process and protocols and can manage the care of elective patients with minimal assistance; when a critically ill patient comes to the department for embolization of gastrointestinal bleed, the new nurse volunteers to assist the team and is able to assist the team with management of the patient utilizing a combination of established critical care skills and their newly acquired radiology nursing knowledge.

A formal meeting between the orientee, supervising clinician, and the nursing leadership team concludes orientation. The structure of the meeting summarizes the goals of orientation and reviews the junior clinicians experience, soliciting both a self-evaluation of their progress, and a summary of feedback. The meeting provides an opportunity to discuss the expectations specific to entry to practice and any additional learning needs the junior clinician may have as they begin practicing autonomously. Soliciting feedback about the orientation process from the junior clinician provides valuable input for continued quality improvement.

### 3.10 Recurrence/Competency Training

The content of ongoing education is driven by department/institutional characteristics, regulatory and accreditation requirements, and ensuring staff competency with "low-frequency/high-risk" procedures/processes. Production pressures of the interventional environment and cost constraints limit resource availability for nonclinical activity; subsequently, ongoing or recurrence education must be provided effectively with flexibility, creativity, and efficiency to reach all staff, regardless of shift assignment, in a manner that reviews all required clinical content and provides an opportunity for essential skills to be validated and documented regularly.

Utilization of learning management systems, peer-to-peer skill review, leveraging staff conference time, and simulation are four modalities for meeting annual education requirements. Learning management systems provide an efficient means to disseminating review of required knowledge. Engaging competent, proficient, and expert staff to support peer-to-peer skills training, such as review of emergency equipment, or point-of-care testing or documentation reviews, empowers senior staff to participate in the quality review and mentorship of staff, while assisting leaders to meet departmental goals. High-fidelity simulation or simulation utilizing standardized patients can evaluate multiple skills, including communication skills or team-based clinical care. Simulation has been determined to help staff learn and utilize both clinical and nonclinical skills [16], identify early signs of clinical deterioration in a safe environment [17], and may be equally valuable as a means of developing competence in nurses [18]. In situ simulation provides a learning experience in a naturalistic setting, minimizing clinician's time away from the department.

### 3.11 Staff Satisfaction

Staff satisfaction and employee engagement are the foundation of everything that happens on your team. A team that is committed to their department and enjoys being part of their "work family" will more naturally participate in projects, clinical ladders, committees, promotional opportunities, national organizations, and support of each other, and as a result customer service will come easily to them. Success with employee engagement begins with hiring the right mix of people to be on your team. Avoid hiring mediocre staff who are critical of others, self-centered, or arrogant just because you need to fill a staffing vacancy;

hire high-energy, positive staff who believe in the concept of "team." Staff satisfaction is a complicated goal for any leader. Employees have their own personal lives and difficulties to deal with, before they even walk into the door of your department. While they know that personal issues should not carry over into their work performance, these are human beings and it is impossible to turn off emotions. Each employee will have their own ability to balance their personal issues and focus on the work in front of them. If someone is unhappy in their personal lives, it may be very difficult to help them be happy in their professional life. The radiology nurse manager must give unending attention to employee engagement if the team is going to ultimately be successful in all that they do for the department. Support may be available through human resource departments, employee assistance programs, as well as private counseling services.

The nurse manager has a duty to be an excellent role model for the staff. Like all staff, the nurse manager is always on stage, every minute of their shift. Staff may watch the manager's every move and evaluate their spoken words. The manager must hold themselves to highest standard, if they want their staff to be held to a high standard as well [19]. Engaged employees will follow the lead of the manager, while disgruntled employees will criticize the manager's actions and words. A calm, positive, "can do" attitude must be set and maintained by the manager, who readily and without complaint spends time in the department and at the bedside. Be on time for work, dress professionally, speak in a professional manner, and round in the department instead of going right to the desk work in your office. Rub elbows with the staff on a regular basis (all shifts), walk in their shoes, and understand the trials and tribulation they endure every minute they are at work. Maintain virtues in yourself that you want to see in your team. An ego that is too large will alienate and break down a team, so instead exhibit and promote humility, integrity, and morality [20]. When problems occur, solve them instead of blaming others or making excuses as this is an opportunity to learn and improve [21].

A manager should plan well to provide their team with the tools to do their job. These include updated policies, working equipment, adequate staffing, work schedules conducive with a healthy personal life (avoid schedules that rotate staff to all three shifts in 1 week!), and ensured meal breaks. Be meticulous with proper staffing levels to meet the departmental needs: when staff repeatedly leave at the end of their shift knowing there are unfinished tasks or that they could not meet the needs of patients and/or team members, it leads to lower team morale and eventually burnout and lower staff retention rates [22]. Through tracking data on patient volume, procedural complexity, and patient acuity, the nurse manager can ensure that staffing levels match departmental characteristics. Adequate staffing levels are associated with higher levels of patient satisfaction, better patient outcomes, and staff satisfaction [23].

A manager must be an advocate for their team members and profoundly loyal to their staff members. Invest in your top performers as they will become role models for other staff members who need to polish their professional and social skills [24]. Have the team develop a list of acceptable and not-acceptable behaviors and hold staff to these behavioral guidelines. Promote team building by holding daily huddles, developing a unit council, allowing staff to eat together when possible, partake in idle "chit chat" during quieter times, promote projects that staff are interested in, and provide for a staff bulletin board where they can post professional pictures, patient comment cards, and other positive items that reflect the overall personality of the team [25]. When staff do present with problems, the nursing leader must listen carefully and attempt to resolve the issue quickly. A leader can't solve problems 100% of the time, but they can certainly *try* 100% of the time. By listening to the team's concerns, and trying to solve the issue, the team will see that the nursing manager validates their professional contribution to the improvement of their team and their environment. Team members are more likely to be loyal to an organization, if they are first loyal to their manager [26]. Promote a "no guilt" department where staff know they can take vacations, ask for days off, change their shifts with others, or say "no" to the manager's request (i.e., picking up an extra shift). Speak naturally of the staff "taking care of the caretaker" with healthy lifestyles, time off, enjoying their free time, and limit overtime, especially in staff that are beginning to appear tired [27].

It is very important for staff to believe their manager appreciates them. Most employees spend more at work than with their own families. To feel fulfilled, staff must believe their investment in their job and the team are meaningful. To be truly engaged in their place of work, employees need to feel as though their managers are genuinely interested in their well-being [28]. There are endless ways a manager can show appreciation to their staff, and they should find what works best with their team. Managers must be willing to change how they show appreciation, as when the team members change and/or mature, so too will the way they receive appreciation [29]. Suggested ways to show appreciation to staff are listed in Table 3.1.

**Table 3.1** Showing appreciation to team members

- Provide a *work schedule* that allows staff to enjoy their own personal lives, while the business needs of the department are met. The reason can't matter to the manager, it is not for the manager to judge (i.e., if someone wants Tuesday evenings off so they can bowl, figure out how they can be off even if you hate bowling!)
- Assure *accurate payroll*. If an employee is counting on their check to pay their bills, and their check is inaccurate, it can be detrimental to employee morale. Maintaining accurate payroll MUST be a priority for the manager
- *Greet your staff* when you see them come in, and say "good bye" when they are leaving
- *Engage conversation* topics of importance to them (the new puppy, the vacation, etc.)
- *Treat staff equally*. (If you bring in snacks for the day shift, be sure to also have something available for those who are working later shifts.)
- *Avoid holding a grudge* towards challenging employees
- Find ways to *lighten the mood* at random times
- Keep a *supply of snacks* in your office. Staff appreciate having a quick snack on those chaotic days or when they are in on call and get hungry
- *Allow the staff to be the individual* professional they strive to be. Everyone is different, they have different goals and perspectives. Find out what they want, what's important to them, and mentor them as they need. When they feel whole, they will more easily support the mission of the organization
- Review attendance records quarterly, and send out letters to those with *perfect attendance*. It is difficult to balance home and work, and for those employees who are able to develop that balance, they appreciate when their manager notices. Discuss the importance of coming to work during the interview (i.e., "some people call in sick when they have a flat tire, others call and say they'll be 2 h late … we hope that you would be the person who comes in 2 h late")
- Take the opportunity after challenging days to send a text or email message to your team *thanking staff* for a job well done
- *Promote loyalty* when you speak to your team. Be loyal to your employer, be loyal to colleagues, and be loyal to your team members. Redirect others who may speak negatively about your team or your employer. *Develop a longevity program*. Suggestions may include an extra weekend off after a year of service, or no call shifts after 5 years of service. Work with the team to create the suggestions, and decide what incentives the department can support and sustain
- Whatever your team needs, be sure they recognize that you appreciate them. They have to believe in their hearts, that they "matter" to the manager. *Leaders must genuinely be interested* in the well-being of their team members
- *Promote their participation* on committees, both departmental and organizational. Plan the schedule for them to have the release time needed to attend their meetings
- *Meet with individual team members* regularly (i.e., quarterly). Find out what is important to them, their goals, and their satisfaction with their current role/schedule/assignment/etc. Because much can change in a short period of time, it is essential for the manager to stay connected with each employee
- When talking with staff, give them *your undivided attention*. Use active listening: pay attention to their nonverbal communication, maintain eye contact, ask clarifying questions when appropriate, validate their feelings, and ask their permission to take notes. Avoid interrupting them, looking at your text messages, answering your phone or door

**Table 3.1** (continued)

- Maintain your office as a "*safe place.*" Whether conversations are regarding positive topics, disciplinary purposes, or any type of conversation: treat your employees as adults and professionals
- *Respond within a timely manner* if your employee leaves you a voicemail, sends a text message or email as this reinforces the importance they play in your daily responsibilities
- If your employee is receiving a company award or a community award, *attend the ceremony*
- Support their *educational advancement* (college, inservices, conferences, etc.)

Adapted from Refs. [28, 30, 31]

Through all of this, the manager must develop certain skills in order to remain satisfied and effective in the leadership role. Honesty is a must; staff must be able to develop trust in their manager in order for the team to truly grow to its fullest potential [32]. Don't sugar coat the difficult conversations, but at the same time don't spread doomsday messages either. Freely give pep talks, be positive. Remind staff that if 90% of their day is challenging and 10% is great, focus on that 10% (and chances are, they'll discover additional things that are positive in their day!). If staff have complaints or concerns regarding a certain action or decision the manager made, lead a professional conversation instead of mounting a defense. Feedback needs to freely flow in both directions between a team member and a manager.

Managers must be good listeners, with a thick skin. Employees should feel safe to come into the manager's office where they can vent (and not all employees know how to vent in a professional manner). Help employees work through their issues and teach them how to communicate their frustrations when necessary. When a manager must counsel an employee, allow them to maintain their dignity and to learn from their mistake (whenever possible). Give employees control whenever and wherever possible; they are adults and professionals. Support their ideas for projects, help them access information and tools they may need, and mentor them as is appropriate. Give them control of their environment where possible such as picking paint colors, adjusting schedules, setting up work areas, or being involved with renovation plans [33]. Managers must also keep an eye out for incivility among the team and intervene quickly and directly. Bullying has been around since the late seventeenth century and it cannot be tolerated in today's work place [34]. Damage to a team can occur quickly if poor behavior is not addressed immediately and adequately.

**Table 3.2** Nurse manager self-reflection and continued growth

- What *worked well today*? What could have worked better and how?
- What *problems* did you see? Solve? Ignore? Delegate to someone else?
- What *patient issues* did you see? How did you/we solve them?
- What equipment issues did you encounter? Are they resolved? What *needs to be addressed tomorrow*?
- If today's world was perfect in your department, what would it have looked like? How can we get there? What do you *need from others or yourself*?
- When you think of your team members, what skills would you like to *mentor* them in developing?
- If your feelings were hurt, assess the circumstances and work to heal those emotions before going back to work. *Avoid holding a grudge*
- *Manage your own mood*, stay positive
- Show your *presence on all shifts* (e.g., go in on off shifts to conduct a performance review, assist with volume surge, computer downtime, etc.)
- *Gather facts* before passing judgment

## 3.12 Manager Self-Reflection

Self-reflection is essential for any manager to be successful. The commute home at the end of a day is a great time to ask yourself the questions in Table 3.2.

The role of the radiology nurse manager is a very difficult one. Maintaining a healthy and professional team who recognizes the honor bestowed upon them each time a patient allows them to provide care is a challenging and rewarding opportunity for the department nursing leadership. Stay fresh, allow yourself to learn every day, and take nothing for granted. Your team and your patients depend on you, to be your very best every day.

## 3.13 Budget Consideration

In many settings, a radiology nurse manager may have a rather small budget in comparison to the budget maintained by the program director and/or chief radiologist [35]. Equipment (scanners, cameras, high tech X-ray machines, etc.) in this setting is costly and outdates quickly [36]. A nurse manager may have a salary budget and perhaps an operational budget which could include office supplies, educational purposes, small equipment (lead aprons, cardiac monitors, procedure carts, critical care equipment, point-of-care equipment, blanket warmer, etc.) and supplies used in the course of a nursing delivery of care (intravenous catheters, oxygen supplies, blood pressure cuffs, etc.).

Creating an accurate and well-planned budget is essential in the financial stability of the department as well as the organization. Creating a budget too small will create difficulties with organizational planning and spending for the next year, while creating a budget that is too large for what your spending actually is may take necessary money away from other departments within the organization [37].

Salary budgets should include accurate full-time equivalent predictions based on historical use, as well as proposed departmental growth. Sick days, personal time, holiday pay, and vacation expenses should be included for accurate salary spending. Also, plan to cover the expense of paid educational days, committee participation, community service, and orientation hours. For example, if the nursing team collectively plans to use 40 weeks of paid vacation for the next year, then the salary budget should plan to include salary dollars for the replacement nurses (per diem, travelers, agency, overtime, etc.). Planning for orientation in the salary budget is essential for fiscal responsibility: for example, if the department averages four new nurses each year, then the salary budget should calculate the anticipated weeks of orientation plan accordingly.

## References

1. Halter M, Pelone F, Boiko O, Beighton C, Harris R, Gale J, Gourlay S, Drennan V. Interventions to reduce adult nursing turnover: a systematic review of systematic reviews. Open Nurs J. 2017;11:108–23. https://doi.org/10.2174/1874434601711010108. Accessed 26 Feb 2019
2. Cotter K, Dieneman J. Professional development of preceptors improves outcomes. J Nurses Prof Dev. 2016;32(4):192–4. https://journals.lww.com/jnsdonline/Fulltext/2016/07000/Professional_Development_of_Preceptors_Improves.4.aspx. Accessed 26 Feb 2019
3. Penzias A. The next generation: introducing prelicensure students to radiology nursing. J Radiol Nurs. 2016;34(2):115.
4. Penzias A, Cadman S, Sullivan A, McIntosh K. Mentoring the nurse of the future: clinical nurse specialist students in the radiology setting. J Radiol Nurs. 2015;34(3):150–6.
5. American Association of Nurse Practitioners. State Practice Environment: Autonomy Map. 2018. https://www.aanp.org/advocacy/state/state-practice-environment. Accessed 24 Feb 2019.
6. Fleming N, Mills C. Not another inventory rather a catalyst for a revolution. J Educ Dev. 1992;11:137–55. https://doi.org/10.1002/j2334-4822.1992.tb00213.x. Accessed 21 Feb 2019
7. Caputi L, Englemann L. Teaching nursing: the art and science (learning styles). In: Evidence based practice for nurses. Glen Ellyn, IL: College of DuPage Press; 2005.
8. ARIN. ARIN Tool Kit—Core Curriculum. 3rd ed. Scope and Standards, & Orientation Manual. 2015. http://www.arinursing.org.
9. Benner P. From novice to expert. Am J Nurs. 1982;82:402–7.
10. Listopad D. Teaching preceptors using the affective domain: part two. J Nurses Prof Dev. 2019;35(1):46–7. https://doi.org/10.1097/NND.0000000000000501.
11. Luhanga F, Myrick F, Young O. Hallmarks of unsafe practice: what preceptors know. J Nurses Prof Dev. 2008;24(6):257–64.
12. Philips J. Preparing preceptors through online education. J Nurses Prof Dev. 2006;22(3):150–6. https://journals.lww.com/jnsdonline/Fulltext/2006/05000/Preparing_Preceptors_Through_Online_Education.10.aspx. Accessed 26 Feb 2019

13. Aveni-Murray L, Buckley K. Using simulation to improve communication skills in nurse practitioner preceptors. J Nurses Prof Dev. 2017;33:33.
14. Penzias A. Management and leadership: management and leadership: speaking up in real time: skills to improve education and safety. J Radiol Nurs. 2016;35(2):159–60.
15. US Department of Health and Human Services. Association of Health Research and Quality (TEAM STEPPS). 2012. https://www.ahrq.gov/teamstepps/index.html. Accessed 26 Feb 2019.
16. Niell B, Kattapuram T, Halperin E, Salazar G, Penzias A, Bonk S, Forde J, Hayden E, Sande M, Minehart R, Gordon J. Prospective analysis of an interprofessional team training program using high-fidelity simulation of contrast reactions. Am J Roentgenol. 2015;204(6):W670–6. https://doi.org/10.2214/AJR.14.13778.
17. Lee C, Mowry JL, Maycock SE, Colaianne-Wolfer ME, Knight SW, Wyse DM. The impact of hospital-based in situ simulation on nurses' recognition and intervention of patient deterioration. J Nurses Prof Dev. 2019;35(1):18–24. https://doi.org/10.1097/NND.0000000000000507.
18. Sofer D. The value of simulation in nursing education. Am J Nurs. 2018;118(4):17–8. https://doi.org/10.1097/01.NAJ.0000532063.79102.19. Accessed 26 Feb 2019
19. Quinn R, Thakor A. Creating a purpose-driven organization. The Harvard Business Review. 2018. https://hbr.org/2018/07/creating-a-purpose-driven-organization. Accessed 24 Feb 2019.
20. Lencioni P. The ideal team player. San Francisco: Jossey-Bass Publishers; 2016.
21. Murli J. Standard work for lean leaders: one of the keys to sustaining performance gains. Lean Enterprise Institute. 2016. www.lean.org/common/display/?o=2493. Accessed 24 Feb 2019.
22. Phillips J, Hebish L, Mann S, Ching J, Blackmore C. Engaging frontline leaders and staff in real-time improvement. Jt Comm J Qual Patient Saf. 2016;42(4):170–8.
23. Buhlman N. Nurse staffing and patient-experience outcomes: a close connection. Am Nurs Today. 2016;11(1):49–52.
24. Wakeman C. The reality-based rules of the workplace. Jossey-Bass Publishers San Francisco 2013.
25. Brass S, Olney G, Glimp R, Lemaire A, Kingston M. Using the patient safety huddle as a tool for high reliability. Jt Comm J Qual Patient Saf. 2018;44:219–26.
26. Maxwell J. The 21 irrefutable laws of leadership. New Delhi: Maanu Graphic Publishers; 1998.
27. Cardillo D. The ultimate career guide for nurses. Falls Church, VA: Gannett Healthcare Group; 2008.
28. Chapman G, White P. The 5 languages of appreciation in the workplace. Chicago, IL: Northfield Publishing; 2012.
29. eConsultancy. 25 Ways to boost employee satisfaction. 2013. https://econsultancy.com/25-ways-to-boost-employee-satisfaction-levels-and-staff-retention/. Accessed 8 Mar 2019.
30. Deschene L. 50 ways to show gratitude for the people in your life. 2012. https://tinybuddha.com/blog/50-ways-to-show-gratitude-for-the-people-in-your-life/. Accessed 13 Apr 2019.
31. Schwartz T. Why appreciation matters so much. Harvard Business Review. 2012. https://hbr.org/2012/01/why-appreciation-matters-so-mu.html. Accessed 13 Apr 2019.
32. Jones DL. Advice from the top. Washington, DC: Casey Strikes Out Publishing; 2018.
33. Shetone A. 7 ways to improve employee satisfaction. 2011. https://www.inc.com/guides/201105/7-ways-to-improve-employee-satisfaction.html. Accessed 26 Feb 2019.
34. Frankenfield R. Recognize and respond to incivility in nursing. 2019. ONS Voice. March, 2019. p. 27
35. Kaufield J. Imaging innovation on a budget. Diagnostic imaging. 2016. www.diagnosticimaging.com/di-executive/imaging-innovation-budget. Accessed 29 Mar 2019.
36. Myrice D. Budgeting for radiology practices—combining science and intuition gives practices more control over their future. Radiol Today. 2011;12(8):10. www.radiologytoday.net/archive/rt0811p10.shtml. Accessed 29 Mar 2019
37. Rundio A. Budget development for nurse managers. Sigma: reflections on nursing leadership. 2016. http://www.reflectionsonnursingleadership.org/features/more-features/budget-development-for-the-nurse-manager. Accessed 29 Mar 2019.

# Section II

# Clinical Patient Care Topics

# X-Ray Interpretation

## 4

Michael Bowen and Tina Sankhla

## 4.1 Introduction

This section will address the history and safety of chest X-rays. A chest radiograph, commonly referred to as a chest X-ray, is a noninvasive test that uses a very low dose of ionizing radiation to produce an image of the heart, lungs, airways, large vessels, and bones in the chest. Chest X-rays are quick, cost effective and readily available at the bedside or in the department of radiology. Chest X-rays are one of the oldest forms of diagnostic imaging. In 1895, the use of X-rays was validated as a diagnostic study [1] and this imaging modality has continued to improve since that time. Chest X-rays remain one of the most commonly ordered imaging tests.

There will be many instances in which the advanced practice providers (APPs) may be called upon to view a chest X-ray in the course of patient care. Common circumstances for chest X-rays to be ordered in the procedural setting include: to evaluate line or tube placement, to assess for pneumothorax, and to assess fluid accumulation. Registered nurses (RNs) and APPs would not be expected to render an official read as this is the responsibility of the radiologist, but as members of the care team they should have a clear functional knowledge of when it is appropriate to order a chest X-ray and how chest X-rays are obtained. RNs and APPs are often the first to see the images and may be required to act upon them. Familiarity with basic interpretation and the ability to recognize some of the most common findings will help to identify urgent findings and will be invaluable in efficient patient care.

In this chapter, we will discuss how chest X-rays are obtained, safety of X-ray imaging, how to approach interpretation, common disease patterns, and emergent findings to always look out for. This chapter will give a basic introduction and is not intended to be a comprehensive guide to interpretation. We will also have a short discussion on next imaging steps if the radiograph has not offered a definitive diagnosis. For further information regarding chest X-ray interpretation, please see the table of references at the end of this chapter.

Chest X-rays are obtained using a small amount of ionizing radiation emitted from an X-ray generator and passing through the area being imaged, in this case the chest. The amount of "safe" radiation is influenced by the patient's age, body habitus, the type of exam, and the technique of acquisition.

According to the Nuclear Regulatory Commission (NRC), the average American receives about 620 millirem (mrem) a year, with approximately 310 mrem being from natural background radiation and the remainder from man-man sources including medical imaging

---

M. Bowen, ANP, RN (✉) · T. Sankhla, MD
Department of Radiology, Emory Healthcare, Atlanta, GA, USA

© Springer Nature Switzerland AG 2020
K. A. Gross (ed.), *Advanced Practice and Leadership in Radiology Nursing*,
https://doi.org/10.1007/978-3-030-32679-1_4

and industrial sources. A single chest X-ray is 10 mrem [2]. Accordingly, the radiation a patient receives from 1 chest X-ray is approximately equal to the amount of background radiation a person receives in 11 days of everyday life from natural background sources. The relative amount of radiation exposure from a single chest X-ray is quite small, and therefore a relatively "safe" radiology exam. You will often see the dose of radiation expressed using the unit of millisieverts (mSv) with a conversion of 100 mrem to 1 mSv.

The impact of ionizing radiation is considered on a scale where cumulative risk is greatest on fetuses and decreases with advancing age [3]. As discussed above, the radiation dose of a diagnostic chest X-ray is small, but is not zero. When working with children especially, the risk versus benefit of ionizing radiation exams should be carefully considered. While one image would not have a significant effect, in children with chronic illness who may be frequently hospitalized and undergo multiple repeated imaging tests, the cumulative dose can quickly become concerning. When working with women of childbearing age, a recent pregnancy test should be reviewed in all nonemergency cases, and if imaging is deemed necessary in a pregnant patient, careful positioning and lead shielding can be used to reduce the risk of unintended harm to a fetus.

While X-ray and computed tomography (CT) use ionizing radiation, other forms of imaging including ultrasound (US) and magnetic resonance imaging (MRI) do not use radiation and may be favored in pregnant women and children when appropriate. Always double check that the correct order has been placed on the correct patient. If there is any question about what type of imaging to order, it is always best to discuss with a colleague or even call the radiology department to verify the best type of imaging for the suspected pathology. A provider should exercise caution when ordering any imaging test, taking care to avoid unnecessary testing and making sure to order the appropriate testing when indicated. By doing so, we can minimize unnecessary radiation exposure to patients and avoid unnecessary cost burden on both our patients and healthcare system.

The American College of Radiology (ACR) has established appropriateness criteria for each type of radiology exam; this has been updated for 2020 [4]. The appropriateness criteria assess the relative risk of ionizing radiation to the relative diagnostic benefit of the individual exam. The ACR has summarized these recommendations in their program for adults entitled "Image Wisely" [5].

Beginning in 2020 the Centers for Medicare and Medicaid Services (CMS) which is part of the United States Department of Health and Human Services will require the use of clinical decision-making software to assist in imaging choices in order for reimbursement of the imaging [3].

## 4.2 Chest X-Ray Image and Acquisition and Positioning

Chest X-rays are obtained by emitting radiation through the body into a cassette. The distance from the emitter to the cassette should be approximately 72 in., but can be as close as 40 in. Increasing distance from the X-ray source to the cassette will cause the image to lose sharpness and will decrease magnification. The loss of sharpness and change in magnification will affect the clarity of the image and make diagnostic interpretation more difficult. The whole area of the chest should be included on the cassette. In order to achieve this, the cassette may have to be turned into a landscape mode or more than one cassette may need to be used to complete the imaging. The distance from the emitter to the cassette is to minimize the exposure of radiation to the patient, optimize the image, and standardize the technique in how the images are acquired [6].

The standard chest X-ray is taken as a posterior anterior (PA) radiograph. The designation of PA is describing the direction of travel of the radiation. In a PA radiograph, the direction of travel would be from posterior to anterior, with the emitter sending X-rays towards the patient's back, through the thorax, and out the chest wall to the cassette. Understanding this standard terminology, the anterior posterior (AP) radiograph is taken with the emitter sending X-rays towards the patient's anterior chest, through the thorax, and out the back to the cassette. The PA is the preferred method of imaging as it is obtained with the patient standing, which allows for better inspiratory effort, and deeper inspiration allows for greater viewing of the structures of the chest. The AP chest X-rays are also often referred to as "portable chest radiographs." They are used for critically ill patients who may not be able to travel to the radiology department. Patients that have limited or no ability to stand and who are unable to travel to the radiology department for their imaging due to their critical status would also be considered appropriate candidates for portable X-rays. AP radiographs are taken with the patient in the hospital bed itself—the technologist will have the patient lie in the supine position (belly up), slide the cassette under the patient's back, and position the portable X-ray generator over the patient's chest.

There are two other positions that are commonly used to help with chest X-ray diagnostic imaging, lateral and decubitus positioning. Lateral images are obtained with the emitter to the patient's right and the cassette to the patients left. Lateral images are obtained to give a clearer image of structures that can be obscured by overlapping anatomy in AP or PA images. The lateral chest X-ray can be particularly useful in looking at the areas of lung posterior to the cardiomediastinal silhouette, and the retrocardiac space, where masses and infection can hide. Lateral images are also useful for bony structures, giving a view of the sternum and vertebral bodies in profile, which can be helpful for identifying fractures and other bony lesions.

In decubitus positioning, the patient is lying down and rolled up onto one side. The general layout of the anatomy will be similar to lateral imaging; however, decubitus positioning makes use of gravity to add further information. For example, decubitus positioning can be particularly useful when assessing for fluid that layers or stays in place, which can help differentiation between a simple versus a complex fluid collection in the chest.

Knowing the different possible positions of the body, and understanding the resulting anatomy you will see with each, will help you understand what diagnostic value each can provide.

## 4.3 Interpretation of X-Ray

Radiation penetrates the body and structures in the body at different rates, with denser structures, like bone, absorbing more of the radiation, and less dense structures, like air-filled lungs, letting more of the X-rays pass through. The image is produced from the X-rays that make it through the body and are registered by the cassette. The resulting image will consist of shades of gray. Bones will appear near-white, as they will absorb the greatest amount of radiation and very little will pass through to be registered by the cassette. Lungs will appear near-black, as a much greater proportion of the X-rays will be allowed to pass through to the cassette. Any metallic object, such as an implanted pacemaker or a retained bullet, will appear even brighter than bone as metal is higher density than bone. Fat and muscle will appear on a spectrum of gray based on their relative densities. Because these intermediate density tissues are all on a spectrum of gray, soft tissues are not well differentiated on X-ray and thus X-ray is a poor modality for evaluating soft tissue lesions. Additionally, if there are two adjacent structures that are the same density, there will not be a line separating them and they may appear continuous. You will only see borders when there are different density structure adjacent to one another.

See Fig. 4.1 below and note how the bones are bright. Compare this to the shade you see in the lung fields and in the cardiomediastinal silhouette. Note how you cannot see individual muscles within the soft tissues.

### 4.3.1 Systematic Approach to Interpretation

Now we will switch gears and approach the topic of interpretation. While this may seem daunting,

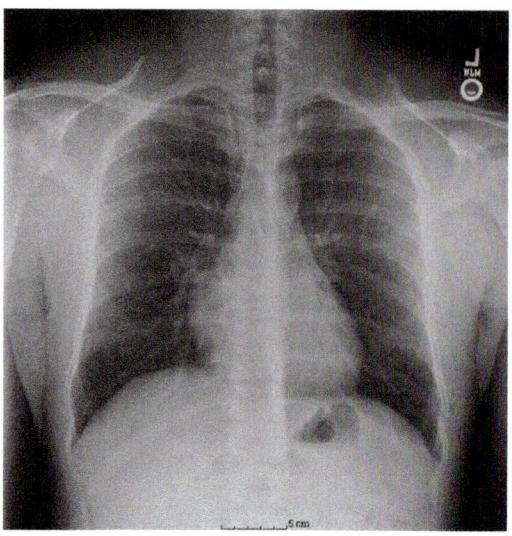

**Fig. 4.1** This is a normal PA chest X-ray. We start by assessing quality of the image. There is adequate penetration as we can see the outline of the vertebral bodies through the heart. The clavicular heads are approximately equidistant from the spinous processes, so we know the patient is not excessively rotated. The entire right and left lung fields are included in the image. There is adequate inspiration as we can count more than six anterior ribs within the lung field. Now that we have confirmed we have adequate quality, we can go through out ABCDEF search pattern. Airways: Our trachea is in the midline and we can follow it down to the carina and see the split into the right and left mainstem bronchi. Bones: There are no apparent fractures or lesions of the clavicles, ribs, vertebrae, or scapulae. Cardiac: Our heart is normal in size and the right and left heart borders are clearly seen. Diaphragms: The bilateral costophrenic angles are crisp and there is no free air under the diaphragm. Extras: There are no lines, tubes, or other support apparatus present. Fields: The lung fields are clear without masses or consolidations and there is no pneumothorax. Go through this pattern with each of the following figure; our captions will report only the irregularities

remember the goal here is not necessarily to pick up the fine details that a seasoned radiologist may comment on in their final report. The goal rather should be to pick up any urgent findings that may have an effect on immediate patient care.

When reviewing a chest radiograph, it is important that you approach your evaluation in a systematic manner and use the same approach or *"search pattern"* every time. Having a consistent *search pattern* will allow you to be sure that you never overlook an important structure. Many patients will have multiple findings, and you must be careful not to think you are done after you make one finding—for example, you may successfully identify an appropriately placed central line, feel satisfied, and neglect to recognize the adjacent pneumothorax. This type of error, referred to as *"satisfaction of search error,"* can have grave consequences. Having a consistent search pattern will allow you to avoid such error.

Below we set forth a simple search pattern that you can follow when looking at any chest radiograph. As you become more experienced, you may choose to adapt this basic structure and develop your own search pattern. *Always remember to compare the current image to any prior imaging that is available* in order to assess whether any abnormal findings are new or already known. And if there is a known abnormality, make sure to assess for stability, for example, if the patient has a known pneumothorax, is larger, smaller, or the same as on the prior?

Remember that due to the way the image is acquired, the radiograph you see is essentially a mirror image with left and right reversed.

### 4.3.2 Assess Quality of Imaging

#### 4.3.2.1 Is There Appropriate Penetration?

Penetration refers to the amount of radiation that travels to your cassette. Too much and the image will be too dark. Too little and the image will be too white. Both extremes will obscure detail, and you may have to ask the technologist to repeat the imaging. In an appropriately penetrated film, you will just barely see the outline of the vertebral bodies through the heart.

#### 4.3.2.2 Is the Patient Rotated?

If a patient is rotated during a scan, this may cause structures to be overlaid obscuring detail or may distort the relative sizes of structures. To assess if a patient is rotated, look at the medial clavicular heads—if the patient is correctly positioned, the bilateral clavicular heads should be equidistant from the spinous processes of the thoracic vertebral bodies.

### 4.3.2.3 Is the Entire Chest Included in the Image?

The film should include the entire lung field. Confirm that you can see from the lung apex, down to the costovertebral angles on both the right and the left sides.

### 4.3.2.4 How Was the Patient's Inspiration?

Poor inspiratory effort will result in low lung volumes, causing crowding of structures within the chest and obscuring detail. Inspiration is assessed by counting the number of ribs in the lung field—there is adequate inspiration when you can count 6 or more anterior ribs in the lung field. As discussed above, PA (posterior to anterior) radiographs will be taken with the patient standing up, allowing for better inspiration compared to an AP (anterior to posterior) where the patient is lying down. A PA radiograph is preferred whenever possible.

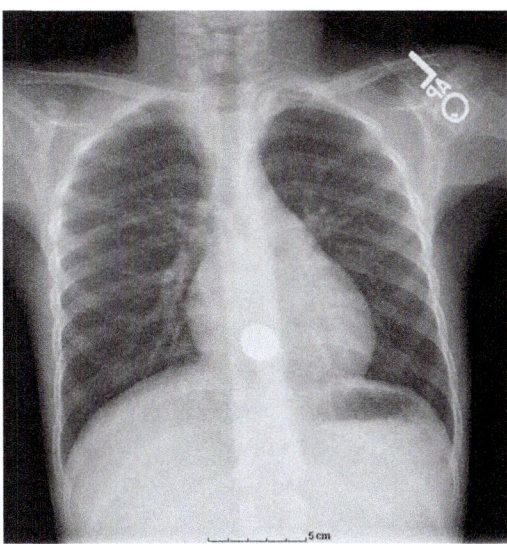

**Fig. 4.2** When assessing your cardiomediastinal silhouette, you will notice there is a round radiopaque object projecting over the heart. We know it is not in the airway this time as we can see the object is below the carina. We can predict that this object is in the esophagus, and our history confirms our suspicion that this child swallowed a coin

### 4.3.3 Assess Structures with Your ABCDEF

- A—Airway—Assess the large airways following the course of the trachea down to the carina and into the left and right mainstem bronchi.

  Check for foreign bodies in the airway, especially in children (Fig. 4.2). If there is an endotracheal tube or tracheostomy tube, confirm that the tube terminates in the mainstem trachea above the level of the carina.

  The trachea normally sits in the midline or slightly offset to the right of midline. If the trachea is abnormally deviated in either direction, think about what could be pulling it (is there a collapsed lung) or pushing it (is there space occupying pathology such as a mass or a large pneumothorax).

- B—Bones—Assess for fractures or bony lesions.

  Make sure to check all bones are included on the chest X-ray, which will include the clavicles, ribs (posterior portion of the rib is the part that appears horizontal on the radiograph), sternum, and vertebra. You should be able to pick up on a displaced rib or clavicle fracture, while a nondisplaced fracture may be hard to see on X-ray. On lateral films, you can check for vertebral fractures or lesions. The chest radiograph field will sometimes include the shoulders—assess the glenohumeral joints to avoid missing a shoulder dislocation. If there is high clinical suspicion for a fracture, but no apparent fracture on the chest X-ray, it is reasonable to consider ordering additional imaging with CT to look for a radiographically occult fracture.

  On lateral films, the spine should get more lucent as you move lower, referred to as the "spine sign" or "more black sign." If it does not get darker and stays the same brightness as you move down, suspect a lesion such as an infection, fluid, or a mass.

- C—Cardiomediastinal silhouette.

  Take a look at the borders of the heart—can you see the right heart border and the left heart border clearly? If a border is obscured, there may be a consolidation from a pneumonia

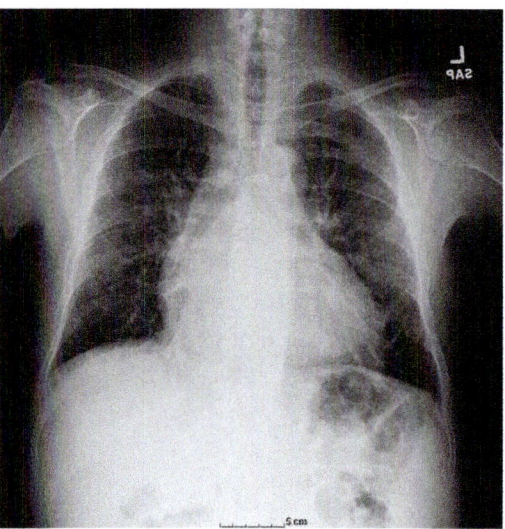

**Fig. 4.3** This patient has cardiomegaly as this is a PA radiograph and the cardiomediastinal silhouette is greater than 1/2 of the width of the lung fields

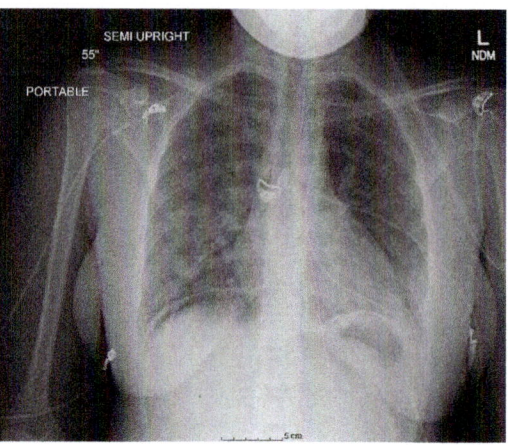

**Fig. 4.4** This patient has air under the left diaphragm, which would be concerning for free air in the abdomen. Note that free air in the abdomen is an emergency if acute, though this may be an expected finding if the patient has recently had abdominal surgery. When assessing the lung fields, we see that there are patchy opacities in the right lung field which could represent pneumonia. When assessing for "extras," we see the patient has an enteric tube that appropriately courses in the expected location of the esophagus, below the diaphragm through the expected location of the GE junction, and terminates beyond the imaged field. The patient also has a left-sided chest tube in place with no apparent residual pneumothorax

(Fig. 4.3). You should also assess the size of the heart. Normal is considered less than 1/2 of the diameter of the lung field on a PA radiograph or less than 2/3 of the diameter of the lung field on an AP radiograph. If the heart is larger than these limits, the patient has cardiomegaly, which may be acute or chronic and should be correlated with the patient's clinical history.

- D—Diaphragm—Follow the course of the left and right hemidiaphragms out to the costovertebral angle.

  Look at the diaphragms. It is normal for the right diaphragm to be mildly elevated relative to the left, as the liver sits under the right diaphragm. The stomach sits under the left diaphragm and you may see the gastric bubble, normal air in the stomach. However, if there is any dark area under the diaphragm, especially on the left between the liver and the diaphragm, this would be concerning for free air in the abdomen from perforated intra-abdominal organ, which would be a critical finding (Fig. 4.4).

  Now follow your diaphragms out laterally to where they meet the lateral chest wall—the cardiophrenic angles are where the lung, diaphragm, and chest wall come together. In a normal setting these angles will be sharp and clearly defined. Fluid in the setting of pleural effusion, most commonly from congestive heart failure and pulmonary edema, will cause a blunting of the cardiophrenic angles. The blunting of the angle begins to occur with around 200–300 $cm^3$ of fluid (Fig. 4.5).

- E—Extras—look for lines, tubes, and other devices.

  Look for any line, tube, or surgical device inserted in the patient.

  - Endotracheal tube (ET tube): An endotracheal tube is inserted in the mouth and terminates in the trachea. If an endotracheal tube is present, make sure the distal tip is in the trachea above the carina, with ideal positioning being 3–6 cm above the carina (Fig. 4.6). If the ET tube terminates in one of the mainstem bronchi, it must be retracted or only one lung will be ventilated.

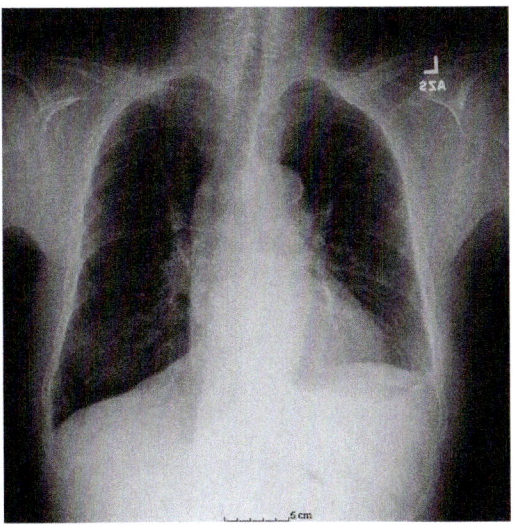

**Fig. 4.5** When you examine the costophrenic angles, the right costophrenic angle appears sharp. In contrast, the left appears blunted with a small pleural effusion

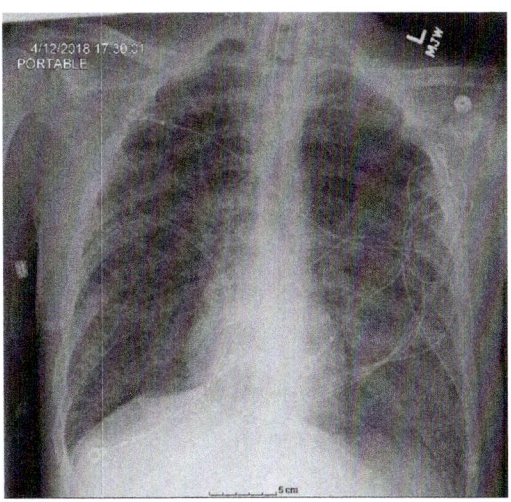

**Fig. 4.7** This is the same patient from Fig. 4.6 a day later, now with a right chest tube in place. You can see how the lung is now re-expanded after placement of the chest tube. Look closely at the right apex and you will see there is still a trace residual pneumothorax

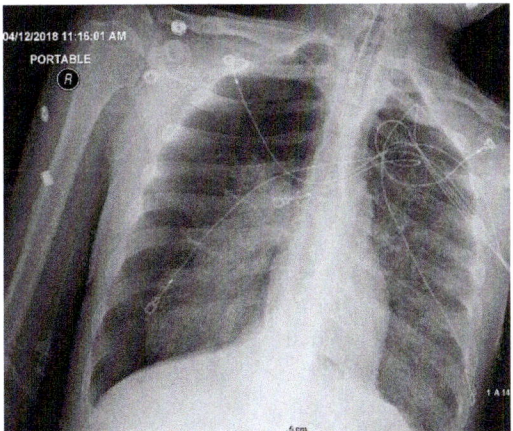

**Fig. 4.6** There is a large region of the right lung field that is dark and without lung markings, representing a large right pneumothorax. There is also an endotracheal tube in place, appropriately terminating in the mid thoracic trachea above the level of the carina. Note also that there are coarsening lung markings in the left lung, which was consistent with this patient's known history of pulmonary fibrosis

- Tracheostomy: A tracheostomy tube is a surgically inserted tube that directly enters the trachea in the low neck and allows ventilation to bypass the oropharynx. Like the ET tube, the tracheostomy tube should terminate beyond the thoracic inlet and above the carina.

- Chest tube: A chest tube is a tube inserted from outside the patient, directly through the chest wall, into the lung field, to treat a pneumothorax or pleural effusion. If there is a chest tube present, make sure the distal tip terminates within the lung field and is not stuck within the soft tissues of the chest wall (Figs. 4.4 and 4.7).
- Central Line: A central line is a large bore catheter that is inserted in a large central vein on the right or left, commonly the internal jugular vein or subclavian vein, and terminates near the cavoatrial junction. Always confirm the course of the central line is as expected. Make sure the central line terminates in the most distal portion of the superior vena cava, or in the proximal portion of right atrium (Fig. 4.8). If it is not in this location, it will likely need to be repositioned.

A possible complication during central line insertion is pneumothorax. A postprocedural pneumothorax will occur on the same side as the access site. This is most common in subclavian central lines, where the initial access may be close to the lung apex. If a patient is asymptomatic, a small pneumothorax may

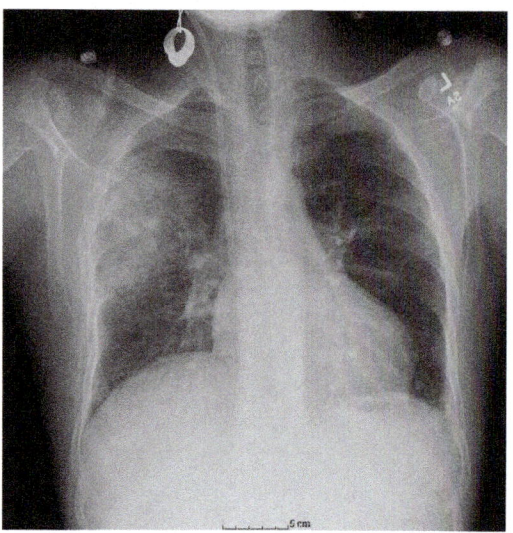 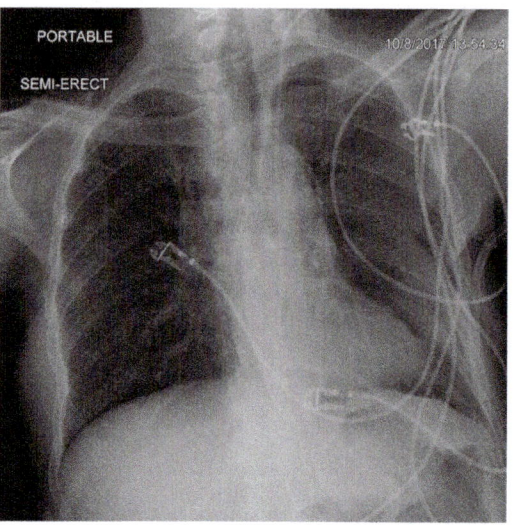

**Fig. 4.8** This patient has a right upper lobe pneumonia. Additionally, note the right internal jugular catheter that terminates appropriately near the expected location of the cavoatrial junction

**Fig. 4.9** This is an example of an accidental arterial insertion. The catheter does not cross the midline and enter the superior vena cava as expected, but rather travels in the expected course of the aorta and has probably inadvertently been inserted in the left internal carotid artery instead of the adjacent left internal jugular vein

resolve on its own and should be monitored with follow-up radiographs. If a pneumothorax appears to be enlarging on follow-up imaging and/or the patient becomes short of breath, a chest tube may need to be placed.

One emergent complication to always look out for is accidental arterial insertion, which is potentially life threatening. If the central line does not follow the expected course of the venous system in the chest and appears to terminate in the aorta, have a high suspicion for arterial insertion (Fig. 4.9). This is an emergency as the arterial system has much high pressures and a patient could massively hemorrhage if a large bore catheter is in their carotid artery. In this scenario, the line should not be moved and vascular surgery should be consulted emergently.

- Peripherally inserted central catheter (PICC Line): A PICC line is a smaller bore catheter that is inserted into a peripheral vein in either arm, and then courses centrally through the subclavian vein to the superior vena cava. Much like the central line discussed above, the PICC line should terminate in the most distal portion of the superior vena cava, or in the proximal portion of right atrium. If it is not in this location, it will likely need to be repositioned.
- Enteric tube: There may be an orogastric tube or a nasogastric tube to provide the patient with enteral feeding. This tube is inserted in the mouth or the nose, which will be above the image field. You will see the tube coursing in the expected location of the esophagus in the mediastinum. The enteric tube should terminate beyond the gastroesophageal junction, either in the stomach or in the small bowel based on indication (Fig. 4.4). It is essential to confirm that the enteric tube passes beyond the gastroesophageal junction into the stomach before initiating feeling. In the worst case scenario, a malpositioned tube can end up in the trachea and feeding can be life threatening due to aspiration of the tube feeds into the lungs.
- Pacemaker: Many patients will have a pacemaker and/or implanted defibrillator. This device will appear as a metal object, brighter than bone, usually projecting over

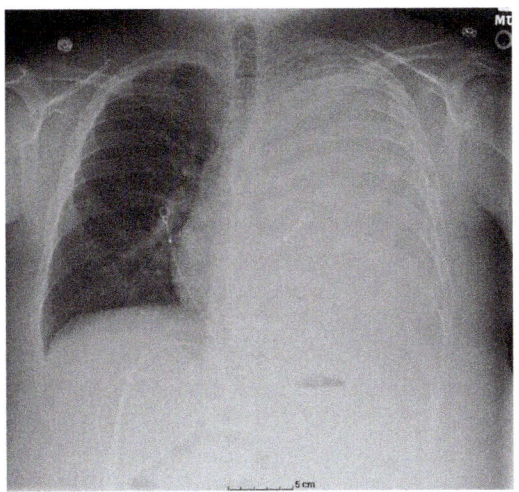

**Fig. 4.10** Here there is a large pleural effusion resulting in complete white out of the entire left lung field, compared to the normal appearing right lung field

the left upper chest. There are many different models of pacemakers and implanted defibrillators that will all appear slightly different, but the most important thing to assess is if any of the leads coming from the pacemaker are discontinuous. Make sure they do not have any breaks.
- F—(Lung) Fields—Look at the upper, middle, and lower lung fields on each side.

Remember the right lung is divided into three lobes, the right upper lobe, the right middle lobe, and the right lower lobe. The left lung is divided into the left upper lobe and the left middle lobe. This leads to two interlobar fissures on the right and one on the left, though these are not usually visible on X-ray.

When looking at the lung fields, start with the upper lung fields, comparing right to left, and then repeat for the middle and lower lung fields. Look for any asymmetries. An asymmetric area of increased density may represent a pneumonia (Figs. 4.4 and 4.5) or pleural effusion (Fig. 4.10). A soft tissue density lesion could represent a mass and would likely need further workup with a CT. Particularly in the peri-procedural setting, it is important to always assess for pneumothorax, air in the lung space. Check the bilateral lung apices—if there is a pneumothorax, there will be a dark area with absent lung markings at the apex, and likely a lucent line delineating the displaced lung border (Figs. 4.6 and 4.7).

During assessment of the chest X-ray, you may notice a finding that is unrelated to the reason for ordering the exam. These are commonly referred to "*incidentalomas.*" When these are noted they are required to be followed up and investigated, most commonly done by cross-sectional imaging to further delineate the findings.

## 4.4 Application

Please review the previous images to apply your new found knowledge. The findings are described under the imaging for your reference after you feel confident in your findings.

## 4.5 Other Modalities

As useful and accessible as chest X-rays are, they do not answer all diagnostic dilemmas. Other modalities to consider include ultrasound (US), computed tomography (CT), and magnetic resonance imaging (MRI). These modalities each have their own strengths, limitations, and considerations for selection.

We have discussed previously the issue of radiation, which can have an impact on the choice of imaging modality. CT has a significantly higher radiation dosing than chest X-ray. The radiation dose of a chest CT is approximately 70 times the dose of a chest X-ray, at 7 mSv for a chest CT compared to 0.1 mSv for a chest X-ray. The use of non-radiating modalities such as ultrasound and MRI can be especially important options for use in children and pregnant women as discussed previously. The way in which the images are acquired and processed in ultrasound, CT, and MRI can provide different and additional information when compared to simple chest X-ray.

As an example of how CT can provide additional information compared to chest X-ray, chest CT has been demonstrated to be a more effective tool for lung cancer screening. It is now the recommendation for people ages 55–80 with a 30 pack year history to be screened with low dose CT scanning. The resolution of small nodules is significantly better in CT. The ability to identify and track small lesions has been demonstrated to improve outcomes, and is cost effective [7]. The use of screening CT is just one example of the information that CT can offer.

Ultrasound, for instance, can be used to identify septations in pleural fluid to establish the fact the fluid may be more complex. The septations are not generally seen in CT, but can be seen in MRI. Ultrasound is also a useful tool for procedures as it can be used for real-time image guidance. This makes for generally safer procedures, but ultrasound has some limitations in regard to depth of imaging and ability to penetrate air-filled structures. Ultrasound can also be used to assess lymph nodes, and other soft tissue structures in the chest. Ultrasound is also a powerful tool for assessing cardiac structure and function. Ultrasound is a readily portable modality and can easily be taken to the bedside for evaluations and procedures.

MRI uses radio waves and magnets to alter atomic alignments, and is best used for detailed evaluation of soft tissue structures. MRI can be used to assess primary disease and extent of spread and invasion to surrounding soft tissues. MRI can also be used to assess structures of the heart, such as valves and vessels. MRI, because it can be used for dynamic imaging, can assess ejection fraction and wall motion of the heart and flow rate within vessels. The exquisite soft tissue detail that can be seen with MRI can also allow for identification of lymph nodes and masses that may not be evident on chest radiographs and CT images.

The disadvantages of MRI include the high cost and the long length of time needed to acquire MRI imaging. MRI makes use of magnetic fields, so unfortunately patients with metal hardware (i.e., some pacemakers, valve replacements, retained shrapnel), cannot get MRI scans. The metal can heat up and can move, causing damage to surrounding structures. The majority of newer devices and surgical hardware however are made from non-ferromagnetic materials and therefore MRI compatible. Every patient must undergo a pre-screening to verify that they will be safe in the scanner. Additionally, MRI scans require the patient to be within the scanner for a longer length of time compared to CT, which can be difficult for patients who are claustrophobic. Patients that have claustrophobia may require anxiolytics in order to manage those symptoms. Additionally, because MRIs can take a long time, it can be dangerous to send a patient who is in unstable or critical condition into the MRI scanner.

This brief summary of additional imaging modalities should not be considered complete, but is offered as an example to demonstrate the varying values and limitations of other imaging modalities. Choosing the correct imaging modality will be dependent on the pathology in question and should be considered carefully with input from the radiology department if there is any uncertainty.

## 4.6 Conclusion

Chest X-rays are an easily accessible, inexpensive, and generally safe diagnostic tool that are highly useful in a wide variety of medical settings. Having a clear understanding of how images are acquired, how to address radiation risk, and how to systematically approach the interpretation of chest X-rays will prove to be very useful in your career. These skills will facilitate high-quality patient care and improve the outcomes for patients.

This chapter has provided an introduction to the basic concepts of chest X-ray acquisition and interpretation. We encourage you to look at as many chest X-rays as possible and practice using our ABCDEF method to become more confident in your interpretation skills. These skills will continue to improve with practice. Make sure to personally review any radiographs available for your patients and take a few extra moments to compare your own interpretation to the final radiologist's report to continue honing your skills. See Table 4.1 for additional resources.

**Table 4.1** Further resources for interpretation

Additional readings to improve diagnostic chest X-ray skills
1. Corne J, Kumaran M. Chest X-ray made easy. 4th ed. London: Elsevier Health Sciences; 2015
2. Felson B. Chest roentgenology. India: Atbs Publisher; 2011
3. Goodman L. Felson's principles of chest roentgenology, a programmed text. 4th Edition Revised. London: Elsevier Health Sciences; 2015
4. Forrest JV, Feigin DJ. Essentials of chest radiology, Philadelphia: W.B. Saunders Co.; 1982
5. Lillington GA, Jamplis RW. A diagnostic approach to chest diseases: differential diagnoses based on roentgenographic patterns. 3rd ed. Baltimore: Williams and Wilkins Co.; 1987
6. Mettler F. Essentials of radiology. London: Elsevier Health Sciences; 2018, 1996
7. Novelline R. Squire's fundamentals of roentgenology 2018. 7th ed. Cambridge: Harvard University Press; 1982
8. Squire LF, Colaice WM, Strutynsky N. Exercises in diagnostic radiology. Vol. 1: The chest; 1972
9. Mettler F. Essentials of radiology. 3rd ed. Philadelphia: W.B. Saunders Co.; 2013
10. www.auntminnie.com (Registration is free)

# References

1. Howell J. Early clinical use of the X-ray. Trans Am Clin Climatol Assoc. 2016;127:341–9.
2. "NRC: Doses in Our Daily Lives" U.S.NRC United States Nuclear Regulatory Commission: Protecting People and the Environment. United States Government 10/2/2017. www.nrc.gov/about-nrc/radiation/around-us/doses-daily-lives.html
3. Appropriate Use Criteria Program. https://www.cms.gov/Medicare/Quality-Initiatives-Patient-Assessment-Instruments/Appropriate-Use-Criteria-Program/index.html.
4. American College of Radiology. ACR Appropriateness Criteria®. https://acsearch.acr.org/list.
5. Image Wisely is a joint initiative of the American College of Radiology, Radiological Society of North America, American Society of Radiological Technologists and American Association of Physicists in Medicine. https://www.imagewisely.org/.
6. Ravin CE, Chotas HG. Chest radiography. Radiology. 1997;204:593–600.
7. U.S. Preventive Services Task Force. Final recommendation statement. Lung cancer: screening. U.S. Preventive Services Task Force. 2014. http://www.uspreventiveservicestaskforce.org/Page/Document/RecommendationStatementFinal/lung-cancer-screening. Accessed 15 Mar 2019.

# Point-of-Care Laboratory Testing in Radiology

## 5

Kent B. Lewandrowski

## 5.1 Introduction

Point-of-care testing (POCT) (a.k.a. near-patient testing, bedside testing, point-of-service testing) has been defined by Nichols as "laboratory diagnostic testing performed at or near the site where clinical care is delivered" [1]. Typically, the testing is performed by non-laboratory personnel including physicians, nurses, and practice assistants. POCT is widespread in both the hospital and outpatient settings where a rapid test result is needed to expedite clinical care. For a general review of POCT the reader is referred to ref. [2]. In radiology, there are four common applications of POCT:

1. Activated clotting time (ACT) to monitor high-dose heparin anticoagulation in interventional radiology, prothrombin time international normalized ratio (PT-INR) and activated partial thromboplastin time (aPTT) for monitoring coumadin and heparin anticoagulation, respectively.
2. Whole blood creatinine testing to screen patients for renal insufficiency prior to administering intravascular contrast agents or gadolinium contrast agents in magnetic resonance imaging.
3. Blood or urine pregnancy testing to screen patients prior to exposure to X-rays.
4. Capillary blood glucose testing that may be required pre, intra, or post procedure or when patient emergencies occur in the department.

This chapter will describe the role of POCT in radiology including regulatory compliance (in the United States), program management, and clinical applications.

## 5.2 Regulatory Compliance in the United States

Laboratory testing is one of the most highly regulated segments in the American health care system. The aim of most of these regulations is to ensure the quality and timeliness of laboratory test results regardless of where the test(s) are performed. At a minimum, sites performing laboratory testing must meet the requirements stipulated under federal law in the Clinical Laboratory Improvement Amendment of 1988 (CLIA-88) (see https://www.cms.gov/Regulations-and-Guidance/Legislation/CLIA/index.html?redirect=/CLIA/05_CLIA_Brochures.asp) and its subsequent revisions (Table 5.1). CLIA-88 is overseen by the Centers for Medicare and Medicaid Services (CMS). In addition, health care accrediting organizations such

K. B. Lewandrowski, MD
Division of Clinical Laboratories and Molecular Medicine, Department of Pathology, Massachusetts General Hospital, Boston, MA, USA

Harvard Medical School, Boston, MA, USA

**Table 5.1** Categories of requirements for laboratory testing mandated by CLIA-88

- Personnel requirements and qualifications
- Quality control requirements
- Quality systems and quality assurance
- Patient test management
- Proficiency testing requirements

**Table 5.2** Types of CLIA certificates

| Certificate | Test complexity and method of certification |
|---|---|
| Waiver | Issued only to laboratories that perform waived testing |
| PPM | Issued to sites where a physician, midlevel practitioner, or dentist performs only selected microscopic tests. The PPM certificate is a special category of moderate complexity testing. PPM sites can also perform waived testing |
| Registration | Issued to sites performing moderate or high complexity testing prior to the site being inspected and found to be in compliance with CLIA regulations |
| Compliance | Issued to a laboratory that has been inspected by CMS or state health agency and is determined to be in compliance with CLIA regulations |
| Accreditation | Issued to a laboratory that has been inspected by an accreditation organization approved by CMS (deemed status organization) and is determined to be in compliance with CLIA regulations |

*PPM* provider performed microscopy, *CMS* Centers for Medicare and Medicaid Services

as The Joint Commission (TJC), the College of American Pathologists (CAP), and the Commission on Office Laboratory Accreditation (COLA) have additional requirements for POCT as do some individual states.

Before a testing site "laboratory" can perform laboratory testing it must first obtain a CLIA certificate from CMS (Table 5.2). The type of CLIA certificate that is required depends on the complexity of the test menu (CLIA waived testing, provider performed microscopy, moderate and high complexity testing) and the method of certification. According to the Centers for Disease Control and Prevention (CDC), waived tests are "simple tests with a low risk for error or patient harm from an incorrect result. They include:

- Certain tests listed in the CLIA regulations
- Tests cleared by the FDA for home use
- Tests where the manufacturer has applied to the FDA for waived status by providing scientific data that verifies that the CLIA waiver criteria have been met.

Sites that perform only waived testing must have a CLIA certificate of waiver and follow the manufacturer's instructions; other CLIA requirements do not apply [3]. Typical examples of waived tests include urine pregnancy tests, dipstick urinalysis, and fecal occult blood. Of note, both TJC and the CAP do have requirements for waived testing beyond those mandated by CLIA-88 as do some states. For a list of CLIA waived tests as of 4/1/2019 see ref. [4]. Of note, this list is periodically updated. In practice, manufacturers typically state if their test is CLIA waived in the package insert as this confers a commercially competitive advantage over non-waived tests. For testing sites that are not subject to TJC or CAP accreditation, the waived status of a test is of great importance as it frees the site from routine inspections every 2 years to document compliance with the CLIA regulations. These sites may, however, receive ad hoc inspections for a variety of reasons. For sites performing only waived tests there must be a designated site director but there are no other personnel, quality control, or other requirements except that the site must follow manufacturer's guidelines [5]. A typical example of a waived POCT test in radiology would be a visually read urine pregnancy test strip. However, if the site is part of an organization that will be accredited by either TJC or the CAP, there are additional requirements for waived testing in the accreditation standards. In the case of TJC the following are required.

1. There must be a CLIA site director.
2. There must be written policies and procedures to address all aspects of specimen collection, reagents and quality control, instrument maintenance, test performance and reporting and other requirements. These policies must be approved by the CLIA site director (or designee) at inception and at periodic intervals thereafter.

3. Staff performing testing must demonstrate competency by at least two methods on initial hire, at 6 months and annually thereafter.
4. Appropriate quality control must be performed for both instrumented and non-instrumented tests.

For further details the reader is referred to the Comprehensive Accreditation Manual for Laboratory and Point-of-Care Testing available from The Joint Commission (Oakbrook Terrace, IL 60181).

For sites performing non-waived testing the facility must obtain the appropriate CLIA certificate for moderate and/or high complexity testing and be inspected every 2 years to ensure compliance with CLIA and with any other requirements stipulated by the accreditation agency (e.g., TJC, CAP). There are essentially no high complexity POCT tests in radiology, so this discussion will be limited to the requirements for moderate complexity testing such as the activated clotting time. The main categories of CLIA requirements for moderately complex testing are as follows. For a more complete description of the regulatory requirements see the Comprehensive Accreditation Manual for Laboratory and Point-of-Care Testing available from TJC.

1. Personnel: CLIA stipulates specific qualifications and training requirements for laboratory directors, technical consultants, clinical consultants, and testing personnel.
2. Competency assessment of testing personnel: At initial hire and then at 6 months and at 1 year followed by annual assessment after the first year. Competence must be assessed by at least six methods.
3. Method performance verification to ensure the method is accurate and precise and to establish the reference range and reportable range for the test
4. A complete policy and standard operating procedure as described above
5. Quality control
6. Quality systems: procedures must be in place to ensure the quality of testing throughout the preanalytical (specimen collection), analytical, and postanalytical (results reporting) phases of testing
7. Patient Test Management
8. Proficiency Testing (PT); Also known as external quality control, CLIA requires PT for all tests where a PT program exists or the use of an alternate means of establishing accurate performance when PT specimens are not available. PT consists of enrolling in a PT program (usually through the CAP) where unknown samples are sent to the lab at specified intervals. The lab performs the tests in the exact same manner as patient samples and reports their results to the PT program. The PT program evaluates the results and determines through statistical analysis of peer reporting data whether the results from the laboratory are satisfactory or unsatisfactory. PT failures must be evaluated to determine the cause of the error. Repeated failures may result in the site being suspended from performing testing.

Based on the description outlined above it is clear that the regulations for moderate complexity testing are considerably more complex and cumbersome than those for waived testing. This alone tends to discourage many sites from performing moderately complex testing unless it is absolutely necessary. Most hospitals have a POCT management team based in the clinical laboratory to provide regulatory oversight for POCT. Sites considering POCT should contact their respective POCT coordinator to arrange for assistance and consultation.

## 5.3 POCT Tests in Radiology

This section will briefly describe the major applications of POCT tests in radiology.

### 5.3.1 Pregnancy Testing

Pregnancy testing is performed in radiology to avoid exposing a fetus to ionizing radiation. Testing can be performed on urine specimens, plasma, serum, or whole blood. Most pregnancy tests are based on sandwich (noncompetitive) immunoassays employing a capture antibody against human chorionic gonadotropin (hCG) followed by a labelled antibody to permit either a visual read (positive or negative) or an instrument read (either qualitative or quantitative). Testing may be performed in the central laboratory if the results for STAT testing are sufficiently rapid or at the point of care. Most POCT pregnancy test strips are sandwich assays based on lateral flow technology. Recently whole blood POCT pregnancy tests have become available eliminating the need to centrifuge blood samples to obtain plasma or serum. The main disadvantage of these whole blood assays is the need to perform phlebotomy, a skill that might not be readily available. In contrast, urine pregnancy tests require that a bathroom be available for the patient to collect a sample. Soon pregnancy tests that use a finger-stick capillary blood sample will become available. Urine pregnancy tests can usually detect hCG levels down to 20–25 mIU/mL whereas serum POCT hCG tests can detect down to approximately 10 mIU/mL. Most sources recommend waiting until the first day of a missed period before performing the urine pregnancy test although some tests are more sensitive than others. As such false negative results may be observed in early pregnancy (false positive results may also occur for a variety of reasons). Blood-based tests are more sensitive and may detect pregnancy as early as 6–8 days after ovulation.

### 5.3.2 Creatinine Testing and Calculation of the Estimated Glomerular Filtration Rate (eGFR)

Measurement of creatinine and eGFR are widely used in radiology to identify patients with chronic kidney disease who are at risk for contrast-induced acute kidney injury and nephrogenic systemic fibrosis [6]. Frequently patients present for their scans but do not have recent creatinine/eGFR values necessitating either cancelling the scan or performing the study without contrast. In most cases the creatinine/eGFR is normal on these patients and the scan can be performed as ordered [6]. Several POCT creatinine-measuring devices are available using either whole blood or capillary finger-stick blood. These devices permit a rapid measurement of the patient's creatinine and calculation of the eGFR directly in the radiology unit. Unlike most central laboratory creatinine assays that employ a colorimetric measurement of creatinine (Jaffe method) the most common POCT devices are configured to utilize electrochemical methods.

### 5.3.3 Anticoagulation Monitoring and Activated Clotting Time (ACT) in Interventional Radiology

Assessment of a patient's anticoagulation status is important both before and in some cases during the performance of invasive procedures. The prothrombin time/international normalized ratio (PT-INR) is used to assess patients receiving coumadin whereas the activated partial thromboplastin time (aPTT) is used to monitor patients on heparin. Several POCT devices are available to measure PT-INR from a finger-stick blood sample. Devices for measuring the aPTT at the POC are also available. POCT devices may be employed to assess a patient's baseline anticoagulation status before the start of an invasive procedure. In some patients, rapid reversal of anticoagulation is required [7] and in this setting POCT devices may be advantages in that they reduce the turnaround time of the test result when compared to the central laboratory. The aPTT is not suitable for measuring anticoagulation status in patients on high-dose heparin during invasive procedures. In this setting the ACT test is used. The ACT is a rapid POCT that measures the clotting time of whole blood when exposed to a strong activator (either celite or kaolin) of the intrinsic coagulation pathway. Usually a target ACT value is established that is specific to the type of invasive procedure. ACT values from different devices are not equivalent and each hospital must carefully establish its own target values for both the device and the procedure.

### 5.3.4 Capillary Blood Glucose Tests

Diabetic patients may need to have their blood glucose checked before, during, or after procedures in the radiology department particularly when emergencies occur suggesting hypoglycemia. Radiology departments typically use the same "professional use" glucose meter that is used throughout the hospital for routine monitoring of diabetic patients. Unlike home-use meters, these professional use meters have a number of built-in safety checks to ensure accurate test results. These include lockout of untrained operators, lockout if daily quality control has not been successfully performed, lockout of expired test strips, electronic or wireless download of results into the electronic medical record and other features.

## 5.4 Outcomes for POCT in Radiology

There are only a few studies reporting improved outcomes from the use of POCT in radiology [6, 8]. In a study of the use of POCT creatinine/eGFR, the authors reported a significant improvement in the timeliness and efficiency of outpatient radiology procedures following implementation of POCT creatinine/eGFR testing [6]. In another study by Nichols et al., the authors reported significant improvements in the availability of test results before certain procedures again resulting in improved timeliness and efficiency before interventional procedures [8].

## 5.5 Conclusion

Point-of-care laboratory testing is firmly established in radiology for selected applications including anticoagulation monitoring, assessment of renal function, tests rule out pregnancy, and glucose monitoring in diabetic patients. These tests are important to ensure patient safety and to improve the efficiency of the radiology operation.

## References

1. Nichols J. Point-of-care testing. Clin Lab Med. 2007;27:893–908.
2. Lewandrowski K, editor. Point -of-care testing. Clin Lab Med. 2009;29:421–622.
3. https://wwwn.cdc.gov/clia/resources/testcomplexities.aspx. Accessed 28 Feb 2019
4. https://www.cms.gov/Regulations-and-Guidance/Guidance/Transmittals/2017Downloads/R3902CP.pdf
5. Ehrmeyer S, Laessig R. Regulatory compliance for point-of-care testing: 2009 United States perspective. Clin Lab Med. 2009;29:463–78.
6. Lee-Lewandrowski E, Chang C, Gregory K, Lewandrowski K. Evaluation of rapid point-of-care creatinine testing in the radiology service of a large academic medical center: impact on clinical operations and patient disposition. Clin Chem Acta. 2012;413:88–92.
7. Blaze C. Anticoagulation management. Seminars Intervent Radiol. 2010;27:360–7.
8. Nichols J, Kicker T, Dyer K, Humbertson S, Cooper P, Maughan W, Oechsle D. Clinical outcome of point-of-care testing in the interventional radiology and invasive cardiology setting. Clin Chem. 2000;46:543–50.

# Pre- and Post-Procedure Nursing Care

Patricia Tuck and Dina A. Krenzischek

## 6.1 Introduction

The development of new tools and technologies have allowed more complex procedures to be done as minimally invasive procedures in the operating room and interventional radiology [1, 2]. Although these interventions have greatly improved, the psychological preparation (in addition to the physical preparation) for patients remains to be addressed. Patient's coping mechanism and compounding sources of stress contribute to increase anxiety and distress as the patient prepares for surgery or non-invasive procedures. Evidence has shown that the preparation of the patient undergoing a surgery/procedure can significantly be reduced by using an individualized approach in managing patient's coping mechanism and addressing sources of distress [3]. A study has shown that too much or too little information during patient's education in preparation for procedure can increase anxiety. However, comparing pre education and after education has shown decreased anxiety and increased satisfaction. So, needs-based education helps determine the appropriate patient education [4].

Patients are encouraged to implement some basic approaches in overcoming the impact of anxiety on psychological and recovery process such as [1, 5–7]:

1. Read reliable medical sources such as information provided by the provider or by professional societies such as the Association for Radiologic and Imaging Nursing (ARIN), the American College of Radiology (ACR), or the Society of Interventional Radiology (SIR). Some hospitals offer YouTube videos for common procedures.
2. Prepare a list of questions or concerns, such as potential complications or limitations post-procedure.
3. Speak with provider about: medical history, consent and ensure that it is clear and understandable; availability of medical drugs before surgery; type of anesthesia or sedation medications; and share list of all home medications and over the counter medications.
4. Discuss post-procedure pain management after surgery and at home (for outpatient).
5. Submit all required documents requested by the providers' office, hospital, or outpatient facility where procedure will be performed.
6. Practice deep breathing exercises or other relaxation techniques, such as listening to music. Plan for family/friend assistance when going home. Some procedures will necessitate that the patient have someone with them for 12–24 h after discharge.

P. Tuck, MSN, RN, NE-BC (✉)
Interventional Radiology Department, Mercy Medical Center, Baltimore, MD, USA

D. A. Krenzischek, PhD, RN, MAS, CPAN, CFRE, FAAN, FASPAN
Patient Care Service, Mercy Medical Center, Baltimore, MD, USA

### 6.1.1 Definitions

Key definitions to understand in this chapter include:

*Pre-procedure care*—the nursing roles in this phase focus on validating existing information, eliciting additional or new information, reinforcing preoperative/procedure teaching, reviewing discharge instructions and providing nursing care to complete preparation for the experience [1].

*Post-procedure care*—the nursing roles in this phase focus on providing post-anesthesia/procedure nursing in the immediate post-procedure and transitioning the patient's transfer to the inpatient unit or to home. If patient goes home, the necessary preparation for discharge to home needs to be implemented. Constant vigilance is required during this phase [1].

*Provider*—includes the radiologist, nurse practitioner (NP), clinical nurse specialist (CNS), or radiology physician assistant (RPA).

## 6.2 Pre-procedure Care (But Not Limited To) [1, 7–9]

Follow all individual institutional policies and procedures in the pre-procedure care of the patient.

### 6.2.1 Assessment

1. Confirm patient identification with wrist band using two identifiers and allergy and fall precaution bracelets, if applicable.
2. Verify consent is done in advance. If done on the day of the procedure, the nurse may sign the consent as a witness to the patient's signature. Ask the patient to verify the procedure site (right or left) as needed. Encourage patient to ask questions.
3. Review medical notes and history (hypertension, cardiac, respiratory, diabetes, endocrine, renal diseases, blood problems e.g., sickle cell disease, anemia), difficulty of voiding, lung problems (e.g., COPD, asthma, obstructive sleep apnea, or airway problems), neuro assessment, current problems, and any previous procedures and surgery responses to anesthesia or sedation and relevant social history (including substance use). Note height and weight per facility policy. The date of the history and physical is important to note. Regulatory agencies may require a date of less than 30 days with a note on the day of the procedure stating no changes.
4. Review all other required documents such as advance directives, X-ray film/disk with patient and labeled as indicated, electrocardiogram, and laboratory test results (hematology, chemistry, coagulation, pregnancy testing, and others) and note any abnormalities.
5. Note medication reconciliation form and include medication ordered before procedure, home medication list including herbals and over the counter medications (OTCs). Assess last dose of *all* medications including anticoagulant, insulin/oral medication, and pain medication as indicated.
6. Inquire about allergies to medications and any history of reaction to contrast media (and treatment, if known), latex, tape, or other bandage products.
7. Review relevant presurgical/procedure status including:
   (a) Anesthesia/sedation plan with airway assessment, including American Society of Anesthesiologists (ASA) Physical Status
   (b) Vital signs, oxygen saturation, airway problems
   (c) Baseline pain and discomfort
   (d) Psychological, emotional, and spiritual needs
   (e) Nothing by mouth (NPO) status per guidelines; some medicines maybe permitted with sips of water
   (f) Language barriers and need for an interpreter
   (g) Mobility and need for walker, cane, wheelchair, or any device
8. Review readiness of presurgical /procedure patient's teaching, sedation plan, and discharge planning based on patient's needs.

9. Confirm availability of safe transport if patient will be going home or arrangements for an inpatient hospital bed. If appropriate, inquire about attendance overnight.

### 6.2.2 Intervention

1. Introduce nurse, providers, and other health care team members interacting with patient and family members.
2. Verify and confirm patient's identification using two identifiers.
3. Assist physician in obtaining consent if not taken before surgery/procedure. Confirm site marking by provider, if appropriate.
4. Facilitate the availability of interpreter or other means to assist patient in communicating and understanding the consent and care.
5. Obtain vital signs and implement any intervention as ordered based on clinical assessment and provide emotional, psychological, and spiritual support. Inform providers if additional information is obtained. Implement clinical monitoring.
   Assess peripheral pulses prior to angiogram procedure/mark site and document clearly as this will be used for post-procedure comparisons. Note if pulses are palpable or by Doppler, quality, extremity temperature, and sensation. If a radial access site/other is anticipated, perform the appropriate tests for meeting criteria.
6. Insert intravenous access (IV) line, if ordered for procedure. (20 or 18 gauge maybe preferred.) Some interventional procedures, e.g., thrombolysis case or embolization for gastrointestinal bleeding, may require more than one IV access.
7. Administer premedication, e.g., antibiotic, and document last dose of anticoagulant as indicated.
8. Insert urinary drainage catheter as ordered.
9. Implement additional laboratory testing as ordered, e.g., international normalized ratio (INR), partial thromboplastin time (PTT)/prothrombin time (PT), platelets, creatinine, type, and screen.
10. Validate patient's understanding of preoperative/procedure teaching including sedation and discharge planning. Include family members in the patient teaching if available.
11. Implement sedation as ordered or assist anesthesia provider as needed.
12. Implement radiation safety procedures.
13. Prepare special equipment appropriate for the procedure.
14. Take patient belonging inventory and store patient's belongings and valuables in a secure area. Jewelry, eyeglasses (contact lenses), hair pins, dentures, hearing aids, etc. should be removed per facility policy.
15. Instruct and educate family members where to wait, any patient tracking system or communication update system.
16. Complete checklist for procedure room readiness and document on record. Inform the patient about the "Time-Out" procedure that will be done in the procedure room.

### 6.2.3 Outcome

1. Patient meets all the requirements to undergo procedure with anesthesia, sedation, or local anesthesia as indicated.
2. Patient validates understanding of consent procedure, expectations, and patient's teaching including discharge planning.

## 6.3 Post-procedure Care (But Not Limited To) [1, 7–9]

Follow all individual institutional policies and procedures in the post-procedure care of the patient.

### 6.3.1 Assessment

1. Determine patient destination post-procedure (radiology recovery area, post-anesthesia care unit (PACU), home after recovery, or transfer to an inpatient area).

2. Confirm patient identification using two identifiers.
3. Review data received from transfer of care.
4. Review presurgical/procedure assessment and interventions.
   (a) Obtain vital signs, oxygen saturation, breathing, airway, circulation, consciousness/sedation level, peripheral pulses where appropriate, and pain level. Assess distal pulses every 15 min × 4, every 30 min × 4, then every 60 min until discharge/transfer or per physician's orders.
   (b) Notify physician for the following conditions:
      - Decrease or change in strength of pulses in affected extremities
      - Extremity is cold or cool to touch or color change
      - Pain or nausea
      - Inability to move extremity/sensory, temperature, or color change
      - Change in vital signs, including level of consciousness (LOC)
      - Bleeding or hematoma at the puncture site or dressing site
      - Procedure-specific change in condition (e.g., increased hematuria after tube placement, short of breath after lung biopsy).
5. Assist with hemostasis if surgical suture or plug is not used for hemostasis.
   (a) Maintain bed rest for a period of time as prescribed by the physician.
   (b) May logroll patient 10–15° from side to side. Head of bed may be elevated no greater than 30° during bed rest if manual hemostasis for femoral access (see Chap. 9).
6. Assess pain and discomfort, nausea and vomiting, dressing, bleeding, or any complications.
7. Note presence of drainage tubes, patency, characteristics of drainage as indicated and drainage output.
8. Note estimated fluid deficit or blood lost where appropriate.
9. Assess patient's emotional and psychological status.

## 6.3.2 Intervention

1. Verify patient's identification using two identifiers.
2. Connect patient to monitoring device(s).
3. Obtain hand off report from providers/procedure staff.
4. Obtain vital signs and oxygen saturation.
5. Provide emotional and psychological support.
6. Educate patient including care plan, expectations, and discharge planning. Include family member or significant other if available.
7. Provide written discharge instructions and obtain signature of patient after teaching, verification of understanding, and respond to patient's questions. Instructions should include what to do in the case of questions, concerns, or in an emergency, whom and how to contact provider. Also included will be information about any follow-up appointments needed status post-procedure (e.g., routine tube exchange appointment).
8. Implement post-procedure orders.
9. Provide safe transport of patient to receiving unit or to the car if ambulatory.
10. Arrange safe transportation to home.

## 6.3.3 Outcome

1. Patient meets discharge criteria for transfer to the receiving unit or home.
2. Patient is safely transported to the receiving unit or home.

## 6.4 Discharge Criteria

The post-procedure nurse follows standardized minimum criteria in collaboration with the proceduralist and/or anesthesia provider. The expected outcomes before patient is transferred or discharged are:

1. The established criteria must be met or assessment is comparable to pre-procedure status to safely transfer care to an inpatient unit or discharge the patient to home.

2. The anesthesia provider or proceduralist (for non-anesthesia patients) need to order patient's discharge per criteria.

Nursing responsibilities include cultural, developmental, and age-specific assessment, diagnosis, intervention, and evaluation of individuals who have received sedation/analgesia and/or anesthesia for surgical, diagnostic, or therapeutic procedures. In the absence of the physician responsible for discharge, post-anesthesia care unit (PACU) nurses shall determine that the patient meets discharge criteria based on established criteria.

The provider (physician) is responsible for general medical supervision and coordination of patient care in the recovery area (PACU or radiology recovery area), management of complications and resuscitation, and discharge of patients from these areas. In collaboration with PACU RNs, the providers develop discharge criteria that are approved by the department of anesthesiology and medical staff to safely discharge patients from the post-anesthesia/procedure area.

### 6.4.1 Criteria (But Not Limited To)

1. Activity: Able to ambulate and move all extremities at preoperative level or as expected.
2. Oxygen saturation: Oxygen saturation by pulse oximeter upon discharge to home or nasal cannula for transfer to inpatient unit is at patient's preoperative/procedure baseline.
3. Respirations: Able to cough and deep breathe freely or within 20% of preoperative/procedure rate.
4. Pulse: Within 20% of preoperative /procedure rate.
5. Blood pressure: Within 20% of preoperative/procedure baseline with two consecutive blood pressures 15 min apart.
6. Temperature: Equal to or greater than 36.0 °C/96.8 F.
7. Consciousness/mental status: Level of consciousness and orientation has returned to preoperative/procedure baseline.
8. Pain: Tolerable with basic function or at a reasonable level for the patient, and it has been at least 30 min since the last dose of intravenous narcotics/sedatives were administered.
9. Nausea: Nausea/vomiting is absent or minimized with no active vomiting.
10. Surgical bleeding: Consistent with procedure, bleeding, drainage, swelling, or inflammation is minimal.
11. Reversal agents: Reversal agents have not been administered within 120 min of discharge.

### 6.4.2 Considerations

All criteria must be met with "Yes" or comparable to pre-procedure condition. If any assessment of the above criteria has "No" answer, the nurse may not discharge the patient from the post-procedure area without consultation from the anesthesia provider or designee. Discharge criteria should be developed in consultation with the anesthesia department using the above assessment parameters but not limited to. Discharge criteria must be approved by the department of anesthesiology and the medical staff.

## 6.5 Common Procedures/Special Care/Complications

### 6.5.1 Arteriogram [10]

An **arteriogram** (angiogram or arteriography) is performed to evaluate various vascular conditions, such as an aneurysm, stenosis, or blockages.

Arteriograms can be used in many areas of the body. Some of the more common types are: aortic angiography, cerebral angiography, coronary angiography, extremity arteriography, fluorescein angiography, pulmonary angiography, and renal arteriography.

## Special Care

Assess the arterial puncture site frequently or per physician's orders. At each interval assess the patient for:

1. Bleeding—Check dressing for any oozing or bleeding from the puncture site and mark the size/diameter of any hematoma with a surgical marking pen. Always check for bleeding after the patient coughs or vomits. In the case of a femoral approach a hematoma around the puncture site can also be indicative of internal bleeding into the thigh, pelvis, or retroperitoneal space. If bleeding does occur, place pressure directly over the site manually until hemostasis occurs and report to practitioner.
2. Circulation—Monitor pulses in the extremity used for access for presence and quality. Compare to baseline.
3. Position—On average the patient will remain on bed rest for 2 h following radial catheterization until hemostasis wristband is deflated and removed. If procedure is done through the femoral artery bed rest is usually 4 h post-diagnostic catheterization and at least 6 h post-interventional catheterization with head of bed at 30°. If a surgical closure device or plug is used, follow the manufacturer's instructions for care.
4. Cardiovascular status—Monitor closely for any arrhythmias, chest pain, or signs of stroke.
5. Medications—After the arteriogram patients may resume most medications. The providers should note when to resume anticoagulants or medications with those properties.
6. Other—Drink plenty of fluids; resume a regular diet; not perform any strenuous activity or lifting for 2 days; and not take a hot bath for 12 h. Additional care for the procedure site, for 1 or 2 days, includes keeping a bandage/dressing over the spot where the catheter was inserted; put ice or a cold pack on the area for 10–20 min at a time to help with soreness or swelling; and may shower 24–48 h after the procedure, or as ordered by the physician. Patients should have a responsible adult drive them home and stay with them for the first 24 h.

## Complications

General risks of an arteriogram include pain, bleeding, infection at the place where the catheter was inserted, blood clots, hematoma, and damage to blood vessels. Other risks include distal embolization, loss of peripheral pulse, retroperitoneal hemorrhage, pseudo aneurysm, allergic reaction, or renal injury due to the contrast media used. Specific types of arteriograms may carry additional risks.

### 6.5.2 Cardiac Catheterization
[8, 9, 11]

A diagnostic cardiac catheterization (often referred to as a cath) uses either a radial or femoral artery approach to study coronary vessels and left ventricle of the heart. Contrast is injected under fluoroscopy to examine the vessels for blockage and evaluate the contractility of the left ventricle. Additionally, the femoral or brachial vein can be accessed using a Swan-Ganz catheter to evaluate the right side of the heart. Samples of blood can be taken to evaluate the oxygen content of the heart. An interventional cardiac cath encompasses aspects of the diagnostic cath with the addition of an intervention such as angioplasty and stenting to open blocked arteries and restore blood flow to the area of the heart that the vessel feeds.

## Special Care

Assess the arterial puncture site frequently or per post-cath physician orders.

1. Monitor closely for any cardiac arrhythmias, chest pain, or signs of stroke.
2. Monitor as for any arterial angiography as described in general angiography.

## Complications

Although rare, a coronary arteriography might lead to low blood pressure, a stroke, or a heart attack. However, serious complication rates are very low.

### 6.5.3 Percutaneous Drainage Procedures [11–17]

Percutaneous drainage is sometimes recommended to treat fluid or air collections which produce symptoms. Recurrent fluid collections (e.g., seroma) maybe treated by medication installation. Drainage catheters are a minimally invasive method of draining abscesses. Drains are commonly made of latex, polyvinyl chloride, or silicone and placed within either wounds or body cavities. Drains may also be used postoperatively to form hollow connections from internal organs to the outside to drain a body fluid, such as the T-tube for bile drainage, nephrostomy, gastrostomy, jejunostomy, and cecostomy tubes. Drains within wounds are removed when the amount of drainage decreases over a period of days or, rarely, weeks. Body fluid drains are often left in for longer periods of time.

Drains and catheters are procedure specific but all require maintenance and due diligence. Proper catheter/drain management post-procedure is an extremely important part of the patient's plan of care (POC). The nurse will be responsible to teach the patient and caregivers home care and assess their ability to properly manage the catheter/drain, and possibly record drainage amounts while at home.

All complications are procedure specific however in general; drainage interventions may include pain, bleeding or hematoma formation, local arterial thrombus, sepsis, perforation and failure of procedure to provide relief of symptoms or improve outcomes. Accidental early removal may result in caustic drainage leaking within the tissues. The risk is reduced within 7–10 days when a wall of fibrous tissue has been formed. If a drainage catheter is accidentally dislodged, the patient should know that if the catheter is still needed, it should be replaced as soon as possible so the track does not close and to ensure the easiest replacement.

#### 6.5.3.1 Nephrostomy Tube Placement [14, 18–20]

Percutaneous nephrostomy (PCN) is an image-guided placement of a catheter into the renal collecting system to provide permanent or temporary urinary drainage or to relieve ureteric obstruction. Indications for nephrostomy tubes are to remove renal calculi, to decompress an obstructed system, and to maintain or improve renal function following ureteric obstruction caused by malignant tumor. PCN is used to access the renal pelvis for radiological procedures such as an insertion of an antegrade stent.

**Special Care**

All percutaneous interventions are considered clean-contaminated procedures but are most often contaminated when an obstruction is present. Follow the antibiotic prophylaxis guidelines recommended by the Society of Interventional Radiology (SIR). The nurse should pay special attention during the "allergy" review in anticipation of pre-procedure administration of antibiotics. Pertinent lab results would be anticoagulation studies, complete blood count with platelets, urine culture, electrolyte assessment, and creatinine per protocols. Ask the patient if they are taking any anticoagulants and the last dose; check the medication administration record for all inpatients. Contraindications to the procedure are bleeding diathesis such as hemophilia or thrombocytopenia, uncontrolled hypertension, and/or anticoagulant use such as warfarin. A urine specimen may be taken during the procedure for culture and sensitivity. Post-procedure, most patients have bloody urine for several hours. Normally this bleeding will resolve spontaneously. The nurse should report any clots noted. As stated above the most important role of the nurse pre- and post-procedure is that of an educator, instructing the patient and the family on the management, care, and flushing of the nephrostomy tube. Patient (and caregiver) education should emphasize the following points:

1. The patient (or caregiver) can demonstrate how to connect and disconnect tube from drainage bag.
2. The drainage bag should be kept lower than the insertion site and drainage catheter to enable gravity drainage.
3. The nephrostomy tube can be held in place with a special catheter-holding device, and then secured to clothing using a safety pin. The catheter can be secured to the leg using a leg bag with straps. There should be a little slack in the tubing to allow for different positioning.
4. Nephrostomy tubes may require flushing to maintain patency. Usually 10 mL of sterile saline is *forward flushed* gently. Specific flushing instructions will be provided per the provider. Aspiration *should not* be attempted without explicit instruction from the provider. The patient will need a prescription for the necessary supplies for flushing.
5. Dressing care and skin care at the insertion site should be given per the provider's preference and instructions. Wet or soiled dressings should be replaced.
6. Instructions will need to include information on activities of daily living and taking care not to dislodge the catheter. If the catheter is accidently dislodged it should be immediately reported. The longer the catheter is out, the more difficult it can become to reinsert as the established tract will close.
7. Drainage bags should not be overfilled; therefore they may need frequent emptying. The nephrostomy tube leg bags can be connected to larger bags for overnight drainage.
8. Patient should know the signs of a blocked drainage catheter and to report any signs of infection such as fever, purulent discharge, skin breakdown, or leaking around the catheter at the insertion site.
9. Patients should also be aware that there will be routine scheduled tube changes every 4–6 weeks or as needed if the nephrostomy has to remain in place for a long period of time. Patients should be encouraged to schedule appointments in advance and adjust if needed.

**Complications**

Bleeding and sepsis are the two most serious complications of percutaneous nephrostomy which will be the same for any intervention that requires a drain/catheter placement. All general complications listed for any drains/catheter also pertain.

### 6.5.3.2 Biliary Tube Placement [13, 16, 17, 21, 22]

Bile is produced by the liver and aids in the breakdown of food and flows from the liver, through the bile ducts, and into the intestines. When the bile ducts become blocked due to inflammation, tumors, or infection, bile backs up into the liver. This build-up can cause sepsis, nausea and vomiting, anorexia, and fever. It causes jaundice, pruritus, and dark urine. Biliary drainage requires the insertion of a catheter into the bile duct and t drainage tube into one of the bile ducts in the liver to allow bile out. A biliary drain allows bile to flow from the liver into either a bag or the intestines depending on the procedure. Percutaneous transhepatic biliary drainage (PTBD) is often related to ongoing care of the oncology patient but plays an essential part in the treatment of biliary obstruction whatever the cause.

**Special Care**

Prior to the procedure the patient's international normalized ratio (INR) and platelet count should be reviewed. At many institutions 1.5 is the maximum INR and the minimum platelet count is 50 per microliter for the initial placement. Institutions may vary on these parameters. Any percutaneous procedure involving infected drainage and the passage of a tube through highly vascularized organs has an increased risk of sepsis. Prevention is the best treatment for sepsis. The standard of care is the administration of pre-procedure broad spectrum antibiotics to all patients unless contraindications prohibit it.

Proper catheter/drain management is an extremely important part of the patient's plan of care (POC). The nurse will be responsible to teach the patient and any caregivers present pertinent after care and assess their ability to properly manage the drain at home. Education should include the following:

1. Check dressing and catheter daily. Change dressing if it is loose, soiled, or saturated. Inspect the insertion site while dressing is off. There should not be redness, swelling, or leaking fluids.
2. Flush catheter daily with 10 mL sterile saline using sterile technique. *Flush forward only.* Stop if there is resistance, pain, or leaking around the insertion site and notify the provider. Provide a prescription for all necessary supplies for flushing.
3. Manage drainage. Empty and measure the drainage as necessary. Record the amount of drainage. If more than 500 mL in a 24 h period notify provider.
4. Report fever/chills or sudden lack of drainage.
5. Follow-up care includes routine drain changes in IR, usually 8–12 weeks or as needed. Patients should be encouraged to schedule appointment in advance and adjust if needed.

**Complications**
Minor:

1. Fever, chills, and rigors can be treated with antibiotics, antipyretics, and possibly meperidine to control rigors
2. Bile leakage into the surrounding tissue which can be alleviated with proper flushing technique.
3. Surgical pain at the insertion site which can be anticipated and usually resolves within a 48–72 h period.

Major:

1. Sepsis can be a life-threatening complication if not treated. Administration of prophylactic antibiotics pre procedure is one of the best ways to prevent infection from turning into a sepsis situation.
2. Bleeding excessively, either venous or arterial, must be promptly recognized and treated. Signs of bleeding are rapid accumulation of blood into the drainage bag, excessive bleeding around the dressing, or spurting blood. The patient may require an embolization (see embolization) in IR to treat the blood flow or have surgery for correction of the cause. Recognition and proper management of these rare but potential complications are an essential part of the IR nurse's skill set.

### 6.5.3.3 Abscess Drainage [15–17, 20]

Historically, intra-abdominal abscesses were treated with surgical drainage. This intraoperative method of drainage was associated with substantial morbidity and mortality. Over the last 20 years advances in image-guided percutaneous drainage have provided a more effective and safer choice than surgical debridement, while in fact being classified now as the treatment of choice. Image-guided percutaneous abscess drainage (IGPAD) is minimally invasive and the relatively simple choice to avert development of sepsis, thereby reducing the hospital length of stay (LOS), reducing the cost of treatment, and often able to be done on an outpatient basis. Ultrasound (US) and CT are the most commonly used imaging modalities to guide IGPAD and fluoroscopy is also used to guide serial dilatation and drain placement following successful needle access.

**Special Care**
Prophylactic antibiotics may be considered prior to drain insertion. Positioning is variable depending on the location of the abscess. Depending on the location and size of the abscess local anesthesia may be sufficient but moderate sedation is often used as the patient is already experiencing pain caused by the abscess. As described above (see nephrostomy tube) catheter/drain management post-procedure is an extremely important part of the patient's plan of care (POC). The nurse will be responsible to teach the patient and caregivers home care and assess their ability to properly manage the catheter/drain at home. Drainage from the catheter should be measured and emptied every 8–12 h. Amount of flush and frequency is decided per provider. Follow up abscessogram, which is an injection of a small amount of contrast media through the drainage catheter followed by digital fluoroscopy or CT. Examination is done at routine intervals (weekly, bi weekly, monthly) to assess the decrease in the abscess

size and characteristics. Often when there are less than 20 mL returned in a 24 h period, the drain can be removed by the provider.

**Complications**

Patient and caregivers are instructed to notify the provider immediately if:

1. Temperature is greater than 101.5 F, chills, nausea, and or vomiting (sepsis/peritonitis).
2. Swelling, redness, increased warmth, or drainage/leakage at the procedure site (local infection, sepsis, peritonitis).
3. Excessive pain or bleeding at the site or drainage in catheter becomes bloody (hemorrhage).
4. Sudden increase in drainage (>50 mL daily) could indicate the development of a fistula.
5. If sutures break or become loose, drain falls out, drainage stops, or resistance is met when flushing.

## 6.5.4 Percutaneous Biopsy [12, 14, 17, 23, 24]

Percutaneous biopsy is one of the most common procedures done in interventional radiology. A tissue sample can differentiate a benign or malignant tumor. Common biopsy sites include the thyroid, muscles, lungs, abdominal structures (liver, kidney), pelvic organs, lymph nodes, and bone. The type and location of the target lesion determines what image modality will be used. Ultrasound (US), fluoroscopy, computed tomography (CT), and magnetic resonance imaging (MRI) are all utilized for biopsy procedures. For the most part there are very few contraindications to performing a biopsy under local anesthetic; however, sedation may be necessary for the patient to remain still during the procedure. Patients must understand that test results may not be available on the day of the procedure. If the test results are not available, the patient will be instructed to make an appointment with the referring physician to discuss the results. The patient should be told not to assume everything is normal if they have not been contacted by the physician or the medical facility as test result time varies.

Emphasis should be on the importance of following up on all test results.

### 6.5.4.1 Liver Biopsy [17, 20, 23, 25]

US- and CT-guided liver biopsies are commonly used for diagnosing and staging many chronic liver diseases. Due to coagulopathies that commonly occur in patients with hepatic disease, bleeding is the most common and potentially critical complication. In some instances the interventionalist will use a transjugular approach. Transjugular liver biopsy (TJLB) is the alternative to a percutaneous approach in hepatic patients with diffuse liver disease, coagulopathy, and ascites. With this approach there is a decrease in the potential for bleeding afterward and pressure measurements may be done during the biopsy that can determine the degree of portal hypertension.

**Special Care**

1. Perform usual procedural workup with special attention to blood work (complete blood count/platelets, chemistries, and coagulation studies).
2. Anticipate moderate sedation for anxiety and pain relief. It is important to go over everything that will happen in a calm and assuring manner. Many patients actually feel the biopsy being retrieved and it can be frightful. Informing them ahead of time without great detail allows them to be prepared and know that this is normal for the procedure.
3. After the procedure patients will lay on their right side with an ice pack over the biopsy site. Patient remains NPO until cleared by physician in case of any complication.
4. Studies indicate that most complications occur within 2 h post-procedure but can occur up to 24 h later. The recovery time varies from institution to institution. Anywhere from 1 to 5 h could be considered normal.
5. Patients should have a responsible adult drive them home and stay with them for the first 24 h.
6. Instruct the patient not to lift more than five pounds or play contact sports for 2 weeks.
7. Instruct patient not to drive for 24 h.

8. Instruct the patient to resume medications per provider's order.
9. Ensure understanding of dressing changes as directed.

**Complications**

Minor:

1. Localized and temporary discomfort at the site of the biopsy.
2. Pain that requires an analgesic (referred pain to shoulder may occur).
3. Low blood pressure due to a vasovagal response.

Major:

1. Intraperitoneal hemorrhage.
2. Intrahepatic or subcapsular hematoma.
3. Biliary peritonitis.

### 6.5.4.2 Lung Biopsy [12–14, 24]

CT-guided percutaneous lung biopsy is the minimally invasive method to obtain tissue for histopathology and microbiologic analysis from pulmonary lesions suspected to be malignant or infectious in nature. The technique uses a needle passed through an intercostal space to obtain tissue from peripheral pulmonary lesions. There is a great degree of accuracy, sensitivity, and specificity in detecting malignancy, explicitly a primary lung or metastatic disease. An on-site cytology technologist may be desired to assure an adequate tissue sample. A lung biopsy can diagnose bacterial, mycobacterial, viral, or fungal infections that have been intractable to a standard treatment regimen. Lung specimens can be valuable in clarifying the diagnosis and response to treatment in the case of chronic lung disease such as sarcoidosis, pulmonary fibrosis, or rheumatoid lung disease.

**Special Care**

Pre-procedure planning will include having a recent CT or positron emission tomography (PET) scan of the chest and any available relevant images that the radiologist can use to determine appropriateness of the proposed biopsy and gauge rate of growth, size, and location of the lesion. These will help determine whether the percutaneous approach is feasible and will be the most effective. At the time of scheduling the patient will be instructed to hold any anticoagulant for 3–5 days prior to the procedure. Relevant labs will be ordered. The provider will determine safe lab levels for proceeding with the procedure. It is imperative that the patient is able to remain still for this procedure, therefore nurse administered sedation or anesthesia is needed. Contraindications for this procedure include an uncooperative patient, patient with altered mental status, intractable cough, patients using positive pressure ventilation, severe respiratory compromise such as patients with prior pneumonectomy, severe interstitial disease, or pulmonary hypertension.

In the pre-procedure area the patient is prepped in the usual fashion. Lab results, history, and physical are checked by the pre-op nurse, provider, and sedation provider/anesthesia. As in all interventional procedures the nurse's ability to educate the patient about what to expect intra-op and post-op is paramount to having a successful outcome. Post-procedure the patient will remain 2–4 h for recovery. The patient will be in a "biopsy" side down position. A chest X-ray is done immediately post-procedure and then 2 h later. If the patient experiences chest pain and or shortness of breath, a comparison between the two will show any pneumothorax progression and whether a chest tube is warranted for re-inflation of the lung.

**Complications**

Most complications occur immediately or within the first 2 hours but can occur after discharge.

Minor:

1. Pneumothorax: Average of 20% patients develop a pneumothorax of some degree. Most resolve without intervention; however, 5% require chest tube placement and admission for subsequent days. A Heimlich valve with chest tube is used [24].
2. Hemoptysis: Lung tissue becomes irritated with the biopsy and small amounts of blood

are released into the airways. This may cause the patient to cough up small bits of blood; this resolves without intervention in most cases.
3. Localized hemorrhage: Biopsy gun fires and a shock wave is formed distal to the needle. The mild hemorrhage or hematoma resolves on its own.

Major (Rare):

1. Chest wall hematoma: Rare but significant chest wall hematoma and hemothorax may develop if the intercostal or internal mammary arteries are injured during the biopsy. This will most likely require surgical intervention and evacuation.
2. Massive hemorrhage: Very rare but will require immediate resuscitative interventions. Patient will be hypoxic and is at risk for asphyxiation and death.
3. Tumor seeding: Seeding is a risk that tumor will spread along the track of the needle biopsy when a core biopsy is taken. Risk is very rare.
4. Air embolism: This can be fatal. Reported incidences are less than 0.003% [26].

## 6.6 Embolization [17, 25–28]

Embolization is a minimally invasive treatment that blocks one or more blood vessels or abnormal vascular channels. In a catheter embolization procedure, medications (liquid embolic or sclerosing agents) or synthetic materials called embolic agents (coils, particles, microspheres/beads, plug or absorbable gelatin compressed sponge such as Gelfoam®) are placed through a catheter into a blood vessel to prevent blood flow to the area. Catheter embolization can be applied to almost any part of the body to control or prevent abnormal bleeding. Embolization is commonly the first line of treatment in gastrointestinal bleeding of any cause. Hemorrhage from trauma maybe treated using embolization versus open surgery. Uterine fibroids which can cause heavy menstrual bleeding and bulk symptoms can be treated by uterine artery embolization (UAE) in some cases. UAE is also utilized for post-partum hemorrhage (see Sect. 6.3.3). Embolization is performed for arteriovenous malformations (in brain, lungs, other). Embolization may be used alone or combined with other treatments such as surgery or radiation.

Embolizations require arterial access either trans-femoral or radial. As such much of the care pre-procedure and post-procedure are the same as routine arteriography care, no matter what type of embolization is being done (see Chap. 9).

**Pre-procedure**

1. Refer to Sect. 6.6.2. Additional pre-procedure assessment and intervention comments are below.
2. All outpatients will be made aware that they may be admitted post-procedure or, if discharged to home, made aware that a responsible adult should be available to take the patient home and stay overnight with the patient.
3. Radial artery approach:

Assess left radial artery only. Perform a Barbeau test and document the waveform. For a radial approach, the intravenous access site should be on right side if no patient contraindications.

**Post-procedure**

1. Refer to Sect. 6.6.3 for a femoral approach.
2. For a radial approach and hemostasis refer to Chap. 9

### 6.6.1 Chemoembolization [29, 30]

Trans-arterial chemoembolization (TACE) is the combination of local delivery of chemotherapy and embolization to treat cancer, most often of the liver. In chemoembolization, anticancer drugs are injected directly into the blood vessel feeding a cancerous tumor. In addition, synthetic material called an embolic agent is placed inside the blood vessels that supply blood to the tumor, in effect trapping the chemotherapy in the tumor. This method is often used to treat inoperable tumors in the liver. Approach can be trans-femoral or radial artery. Chemo handling and disposal policies and procedures should be followed by the IR team.

**Special Care**

Often patients have disease-related pain which is difficult to control, chemotherapy-induced nausea, vomiting, fatigue, and anxiety. Systemic chemotherapy agents can affect the immune system increasing chances of bleeding and/or infection. As the IR nurse preparing a patient for TACE (or any interventional oncology procedure), it is important that there is awareness of the implications the patient's systemic disease may have pre- and post-procedure. Laboratory values can be affected by a patient's disease process or systemic treatment which can exacerbate the symptoms of the procedure. Understanding the clinical presentation and communicating it to the interventional radiology team allow for optimal management.

All elements of pre-procedure and post-procedure care for embolization with arterial access are outlined in Sect. 6.6. Attention to the most recent blood work (platelet counts, absolute neutrophil count, liver/renal function and anticoagulation values) is needed. Administration of antiemetics and pain medications is important. Chemotherapy precautions are followed intra-procedure. There is no special precautions post-procedure related to chemotherapy as the drug is not systemic.

Liver-directed therapies such as TACE can levy or exacerbate already present symptoms in many patients such as fatigue, pain, and nausea and vomiting. There are also effects from TACE on liver function or the contrast medium effects on the kidneys. These values can become elevated post-TACE and need close monitoring. Understanding the potential symptoms and risks patients can have allows the IR nurse to adequately assess and manage the patient before, during, and after the procedure with guidance from the interventional radiologist.

**Complications**

Minor:

1. Most TACE patients experience post-embolization syndrome (PES). It most probably occurs due to the anti-inflammatory responses to tumor ischemia/necrosis and chemotherapy agents. Symptoms of low-grade fever, abdominal pain, and nausea and vomiting can occur within the first 24–72 h after the procedure and last up to a week. Symptom management with antiemetics, narcotics, and fluids are the treatment of choice until the sequelae passes. Acetaminophen is contraindicated for pain due to its hepatic toxicity.

Major:

1. Liver failure.
2. Biloma (an encapsulated bile collection outside the biliary tree due to a bile leak) is a rare but potentially life-threatening complication if it is symptomatic. Timely and appropriate management, including percutaneous drainage, partial hepatectomy, and antibiotic administration, should be performed in the case of any signs of infection [29].
3. Liver Abscess.
4. Nontargeted extra-hepatic embolization can occur when chemotherapeutic or embolic agents are delivered to the gastrointestinal mucosa, gall bladder, diaphragm, or skin.

### 6.6.2 Radio Embolization
[17, 20, 26, 31]

Yttrium-90 ($^{90}Y$) microspheres are tiny spheres loaded with $^{90}Y$, a radioisotope that emits pure beta radiation. $^{90}Y$ has a half-life of about 64 h. The radiation from $^{90}Y$ is largely confined to a tissue depth of 2–3 mm. After injection into the artery supplying blood to the tumors, the spheres are trapped in the tumor's vascular bed, where they destroy the tumor cells by delivering the beta radiation. Normal tissue is not affected.

Most of the radiation emitted from the tumor is contained within the patient's body, and external radiation is so low that it does not present a significant risk to others. Because the spheres may have trace amounts of free $^{90}Y$ on their surface, only very small amounts of $^{90}Y$ can be excreted in the urine. This is a palliative and not curative procedure [29].

### Special Care
The patient is NPO for the procedure but may take maintenance meds in the morning with a sip of water. IV hydration may be included in the pre-procedure orders; all elements of pre-procedure and post-procedure care for embolization with arterial access are outlined in Sect. 6.6.

Post-procedure, the patient may experience fever, lethargy, fatigue, nausea, and abdominal pain (PES). Despite these potential side effects, typically patients who receive $^{90}Y$ therapy are discharged the same day. On discharge, prescriptions are given for a proton pump inhibitor, steroids, antiemetic, and pain medications. $^{90}Y$ microspheres are a source of radioactivity. There is a small amount of radioactivity around the liver. Therefore, if a patient goes to the emergency department within 3 days of $^{90}Y$ treatment, they should be instructed to identify that they have had a recent radioembolization. All bodily fluids must be properly disposed in the first 24 h. Hands should be washed after using the restroom and any spill should be wiped and flushed. Patients do not need to restrict close contact with household members, unless a caregiver/family member is pregnant or under the age of 10. In those specific instances you must remain at arms-length for 72 h.

### Complications
Minor:

1. Post-embolization syndrome (PES) as described in Sect. 6.6.
2. Gastric or duodenal ulceration which can be minor or major depending on the symptomology. Patient can be treated with prophylactic proton pump inhibitors to decrease the likelihood of this.

Major:

1. Radiation pneumonitis (seen 2–3 months after procedure).
2. Radiation hepatitis (seen 2–3 months after procedure).
3. Acute pancreatitis.

### 6.6.3 Uterine Artery Embolization
[27, 28, 32]

Uterine artery embolization (UAE) is often used to treat pelvic hemorrhage secondary to trauma, malignancy; radiation induced bleeding and postpartum hemorrhage. Early vascular intervention can delay or avoid the need for hysterectomy. Done in this manner the procedure is considered emergent. UAE is performed by accessing the right femoral artery and guiding a catheter under fluoroscopy into position in the distal uterine artery. Embolization is performed using a gelatin sponge material (Gelfoam®) mixed with saline and contrast for opacification. Complete embolization is reached once stasis of blood flow in the uterine artery has been achieved.

Secondly, UAE is done to treat uterine fibroids which cause heavy menstrual bleeding, pain, and pressure on the bladder and bowel. When done to treat fibroids the procedure is also known as a uterine fibroid embolization (UFE). UFE is an elective procedure and as such the patient should have a prior consult with the radiologist. One of the major contraindications to the procedure is the desire to maintain childbearing potential. While not impossible to have successful pregnancy after UAE or UFE, studies show increased risks of spontaneous abortion, abnormal placenta position, and postpartum hemorrhage. The patient and the clinician must do a careful risk/reward analysis prior to the procedure.

### Special Care
A pregnancy test should be performed on the day of the procedure; serum pregnancy is more sensitive. The patient is NPO for the procedure but may take maintenance meds in the morn-

ing with a sip of water. Local anesthetic and/or moderate sedation will be used for the procedure. A pain pump may be started during the procedure for pain control. Preparation should be made in advance. All elements of pre-procedure and post-procedure care for embolization with arterial access are outlined in Sect. 6.6. A urinary drainage catheter is usually inserted to keep the bladder deflated during the procedure. It will be removed after the procedure. The patient may stay overnight for symptom control but often is done as an outpatient. In the acute post-procedural period, immediate complications may relate to vascular access, thromboembolic events, infection, and pain management. As with all embolization, post-procedure, the patient may develop post-embolization syndrome (PES), experiencing fever, lethargy, fatigue, nausea, as well as abdominal pain and pelvic cramping. Symptom management with antiemetics, narcotics, and IV fluids are the treatment of choice until the symptoms resolve. There can be a high rate of constipation post-procedure in this group of patients due to fibroids pressing on bowel and opioids for pain management. Over the counter stool softeners and good hydration maybe ordered.

**Complications**
Awareness of the known complications of UFE may allow more rapid diagnosis and effective therapeutic responses to complications when they occur.

Minor

1. Post-embolization syndrome (PES).
2. Expulsion of fibroid tissue.
3. Altered ovarian and sexual function.
4. Subcutaneous tissue necrosis.
5. Treatment failure.

Major

1. Pulmonary embolus.
2. Uterine ischemia, necrosis.
3. Sepsis.
4. Death.

## 6.7 Radiofrequency Ablation [33]

Radiofrequency ablation (RFA) maybe indicated for lung, liver, renal, and bone malignancies. Thermal ablation with RFA, cryoablation or microwave ablation (MWA), a newer technique, may be done. Ablation is often a palliative treatment for patients who are poor surgical candidates due to comorbidities. Computed tomography (CT) is the preferred modality. Ultrasound (US) or magnetic resonance imaging (MRI) guidance (for cryoablation) can be done.

Careful team assessment and planning is needed prior to this procedure. Absolute and relative contraindications should be considered. The patient should be screened for metallic implants and pacemakers. It is preferable to have more than one large bore intravenous access. Nursing care will involve care as per procedures that require sedation and analgesia/anesthesia. Antiplatelet and anticoagulation medications are held per physician order. Additional laboratory tests, e.g., serum tumor markers, may be requested. Pre-procedure antibiotics are given. Patient education is an important part of nursing care for patients undergoing ablations.

**Special Care**
Pain management is an important consideration as the procedure is painful and the patient needs to lie still during the procedure.

Intraprocedural care for thermal ablation involves the use of grounding pads, usually placed horizontally on the patient's thighs. These are used to prevent skin burns. Cool packs may be used on the grounding pads, if needed. Procedures can be lengthy, so careful positioning of the patient for the procedure is needed for comfort and for prevention of skin/nerve injuries.

Patient vital signs should be monitored closely post-procedure for signs of bleeding. Patients often are hospitalized overnight for pain control and observation. Patients should be informed post-ablation syndrome is common after thermal ablation, 1–2 days post-procedure and for 1 week. Symptoms include low-grade temperature, mild myalgia, and fatigue. Treatment is supportive.

Patient discharge instructions should emphasize the importance of follow-up, e.g., by CT or other modality.

**Complications**

Complications include infection, bleeding, injury to tissue adjacent to the target area, nontarget ablation (e.g., ureteral injury, psoas muscle, bowel injury after renal ablation), post-ablation syndrome (expected), skin burns, or others according to area on which the procedure was done. Hematuria may occur after renal interventions. Pyeloperfusion may be done to prevent thermal injury during some renal ablations. Hydrodissection, by infusing normal saline, to separate target and nontarget tissue may be done.

## 6.8 Conclusion [25, 34, 35]

As an extension of perioperative services, IR follows the guidelines and care standards of ASPAN and ARIN. Guidelines by the Association of PeriOperative Registered Nurses (AORN) are also useful for perioperative and intraprocedure care of the patient. The role of the IR nurse, with a background in a critical care or perioperative area involves assessment, planning, care, and education of patients who undergo diagnostic, interventional, and therapeutic procedures. Radiology nurses must have high level of technical and clinical skills garnered by a strong grasp of anatomy, physiology, and radiologic science. Critical thinking and planning, along with the ability to balance, organize high workload demands (clinically and operationally), and care for patients with a variety of procedures is a necessity to manage the rapid turnover of a hospital or ambulatory center intertwined with the needs of the most critical of patients.

## References

1. ASPAN. Perianesthesia nursing standards, practice recommendations and interpretive statements. 2019–2020. https://www.aspan.org/Clinical-Practice/ASPAN-Standards. Accessed 1 Feb 2019.
2. Hybrid ORs and Imaging Techniques: Advances in Minimally Invasive Procedure. 2015. https://www.mdedge.com/.../hybrid-ors-and-imaging-techniques-advances-. Accessed 1 Feb 2019.
3. Augmented Reality for Minimally Invasive Surgery: Overview and Some Recent Advances. 2010. https://www.intechopen.com/.../augmented-reality-for-minimally-invasive-surgery-ov. Accessed 1 Feb 2019.
4. How to Mentally Prepare for Surgery and Recover Faster | Psychology. 2017. https://www.psychologytoday.com/.../how-mentally-prepare-surgery-and-recover-fast. Accessed 1 Feb 2019.
5. Wongkietkachorn A, Wongkietkachorn N, Rhursiri P. Preoperative needs-based education to reduce anxiety, increase satisfaction and decrease time spent in day of surgery: a randomized controlled trial. World J Surg. 2018;42(3):666–874. https://doi.org/10.1007/s00268-017-4207-0.
6. Zener R, Johnson P, Wiseman D, Pandey S, Mujoomdar A. Informed consent for radiation in interventional radiology procedure. Can Assoc Radiol J. 2018;69(1):30–7. https://doi.org/10.1016/j.carj2017.07.002.
7. Powell R, Scott NV, Manyande A, Bruce J, Vogele C, Byrwe-Davis LM, Unsworth M, Osner C, Johsnton M. Psychological preparation and post surgical outcomes for adult undergoing surgery under general anesthesia. Cochrane Database Syst Rev. 2016;26(5):cdoo8646. https://doi.org/10.1002/14651858. cd008646, pub2
8. Inge C, Koetser J, Wwrenburg SM, Boermester MA, Vanlienden KP. Cardiovasc interventional. Radiology. 2013;36:12–319. https://doi.org/10.1007/s00270-012-0395.
9. Rafiei P, Walser EM, Duncan JR, Rana H, Ross JR, Kerlan RK Jr, Gross KA, Balter S, Bartal G, Abi-Jaoudeh N, Stecker MS, Cohen AM, Dixon RG, Thornton RH, Nikolic B, Society of Interventional Radiology Health and Safety Committee. Society of interventional radiology IR pre-procedure patient safety checklist by the safety and health committee. J Vasc Interv Radiol. 2016;27:695–9. https://doi.org/10.1016/j.jvir.2016.03.002.
10. Arteriogram: Types, Procedure, and Results—Healthline. 2017. https://www.healthline.com/health/arteriogram. Accessed 1 Feb 2019.
11. Cardiovascular and Interventional Society of Europe(CISE). Drainage. 2019. https://www.cirse.org/patients/ir-procedures/drainage/. Accessed 20 Apr 2019.
12. Jones S, Taylor E. Imaging for nurses. Hoboken, NJ: Blackwell Publishing; 2006.
13. Clifford T, Daley K. Chapter 17: Medical imaging and interventional radiology. In: A competency based orientation and credentialing program for the registered nurse in the perianesthesia setting. Cherry Hill, NJ: American Society of Perianesthesia Nurses; 2016. https://www.aspan.org/Clinical-Practice/Competency-Based-Orientation-RN. Accessed 20 Feb 2019.

14. Gross K. Interventional radiology procedure. In: Stannard D, Krenzischek D, editors. PeriAnesthesia nursing care: a bedside guide for safe recovery. Sudbury Massachusetts: Jones and Bartlett Learning; 2012. p. 329–35.
15. Hearns WC. Abscess drainage. Semin Intervent Radiol. 2012;29:325–36. https://doi.org/10.1055/s-0032-1330068.
16. Jaffe TA, Nelson RC. Image-guided percutaneous drainage: a review. Abdom Radiol (NY). 2016;41:629. https://doi.org/10.1007/s00261-016-0649-3.
17. Khadir M, Syed L. Abscess drainage, percutaneous biopsies, and nephrostomy tube. In: Grossman VA, editor. Fastfacts for the radiology nurse. New York: Springer Publishing Company LLC; 2014. p. 193–4.
18. HaufmanS. Nephrostomy. 2018. https://emedicine.medscape.com/article/445893/. Accessed 30 Mar 2019.
19. Echenrique A, DeJesus L, Abisch A. Under the beam: nursing considerations on patient undergoing a nephrostomy tube placement. J Radiol Nurs. 2016;35(3):248–51. https://doi.org/10.1016/j.jradnu.2016.06.003. Accessed 3 Mar 2019
20. Nettina S. Lippincott manual of nursing practice. 10th ed. Philadelphia: Wolters Kluwer Health/Lippincott Williams & Wilkins; 2013.
21. Phillipe S, Graham C, Almeda J. Biliary catheter placement in interventional radiology for oncology care. J Radiol Nurs. 2018;37:268–70. https://doi.org/10.1016/j.jradnu.2018.09.002.
22. Biliary Drainage—InsideRadiology. 2017. https://www.insideradiology.com.au/biliary-drainage. Accessed 1 Feb 2019.
23. Nodarse-Perez PO, Perez-Menendez R, Heredia-Andrade E, Noa-Pedroso G, Araluce-Cordovi R, Fernandez-Sotolongo J. Safety of reducing the recovery time after percutaneous and laparoscopic liver biopsy. Cir Cir. 2016;84:196–202.
24. Lehmann S, Frank N. An overview of percutaneous ct-guided lung biopsies. J Radiol Nurs. 2018;37(1):2–8. https://doi.org/10.1016/j.radnu.2017.12.002.
25. Wempe E. Expanding the role of the registered nurse in interventional oncology. Inter Oncol. 2014;2(8):E63–6. https://www.iolearning.com/article/expanding-role-registered-nurse-interventional-oncology. Accessed 9 May 2019
26. RadiologyInfo.org: Radiological Society of North America. 2018. https://www.radiologyinfo.org/en/info.cfm?pg=cathembol. Accessed 2 May 2019.
27. Myers T. Uterine artery embolization for postpartum hemorrhage. J Radiol Nurs. 2016;35:142–5. https://doi.org/10.1016/j.jradnu.2016.01.008. Accessed 4 Apr 2019
28. Binkurian T, Linnane M, Browne F. Nursing care of the patient undergoing uterine fibroid embolization in the radiology department. J Radiol Nurs. 2015;34:143–9. https://doi.org/10.1016/j.jradnu.2015.06.005.
29. Sur BW, Sharma A. Transarterial chemoembolization for hepatocellular carcinoma. J Radiol Nurs. 2017; https://doi.org/10.1016/jradnu.2017.12.004.
30. Zhang B, Guo Y, Wu K, Shan H. Intrahepatic biloma following transcatheter arterial chemoembolization for hepatocellular carcinoma: incidence, imaging features and management. Mol Clin Oncol. 2017;6(6):937–43. https://doi.org/10.3892/mco.2017.1235. Accessed 9 May 2019
31. Tiwari T, Malone C, Foltz G, Akinwande O, Ramaswamy R. Yttrium-90 radioembolization: current clinical practice and review of the recent literature. J Radiol Nurs. 2019;38(2):86–91. https://doi.org/10.1016/j.jradnu.2019.03.004.
32. Schirf BE, Vogelzang RL, Chrisman HB. Complications of uterine fibroid embolization. Semin Intervent Radiol. 2006;23(2):143–9. https://doi.org/10.1055/s-2006-941444.
33. Arellano RS. Ablation of renal cell carcinoma: an assessment of currently available techniques. J Radiol Nurs. 2018;37(1):30–5. https://doi.org/10.1016/j.jradnu.2017.11.003.
34. Lockeretz ML. Visionary treatment: today's interventional radiology (IR). J Legal Nurse Consult. 2017;28(2):8–11. http://www.aalnc.org/page/journal-v2.0. Accessed 1 May 2019
35. Association of periOperative Registered Nurses (AORN). https://www.aorn.org/

# Procedural Sedation and Analgesia in Radiology

Michael J. Long and Lois Elaine Stewart

## 7.1 Introduction

Advances in technology, increasing procedure complexity, and a growing older population have contributed to the explosion of interventional and diagnostic procedures requiring sedation. Procedural sedation and analgesia (PSA) is a continuum of stages that encompasses minimal, moderate, and deep sedation (Fig. 7.1). This continuum has been further defined by the American Society of Anesthesiologists (ASA) that comprises all levels of sedation plus monitored anesthesia care (MAC—is a moniker used for the specific act of administration of sedation/analgesia by anesthesia practitioners and does not describe the stage of sedation) and general anesthesia. Within this continuum, movement between the stages is possible regardless of pharmacological agent and familiarity with rescue techniques associated with the intended level of sedation and the next corresponding stage is essential for the practitioner providing sedation. For this reason, deep sedation is often relegated to patients under the care of anesthesia providers with advanced airway skills. Understandably, some radiology departments choose anesthesia services for procedures requiring more than just moderate PSA. The practice of deep sedation and its administrator is presently a hot debatable issue in current literature; however, the practice of deep sedation is within the radiologist's and registered nurse's scope, and a growing body of literature in other departments like endoscopy, intensive care units, and emergency rooms demonstrate the safety of deep PSA by appropriately trained multidisciplinary teams.

In radiology settings, PSA is provided by either a radiology nurse, a licensed independent practitioner (LIP-nurse practitioner or physician assistant), an anesthesia practitioner (anesthesiologist, nurse anesthetist, or anesthesiologist assistant), or a radiologist. As defined by the ASA's *"Practice Guidelines for Moderate Procedural Sedation and Analgesia 2018,"* minimal sedation is performed using a pharmacological agent and the patient is able to respond to verbal commands and their cardiopulmonary functions are intact [1]. In moderate PSA, the patient responds "purposefully" to verbal instructions or tactile stimulation, independently maintains airway and ventilatory drive but may need cardiovascular support. In deep PSA, the patient is unconscious, responding only to repeated verbal prompts or pain, and may require ventilatory and cardiovascular support. Defining each stage utilizing subjective terminology like "purposively" leads to its wide interpretation and therefore variations in moderate PSA exist. Due to current guidelines, approved by the

M. J. Long, DNP, CRNA (✉)
L. E. Stewart, PhD, CRNA
Community Health Network Anesthesia,
Indianapolis, IN, USA

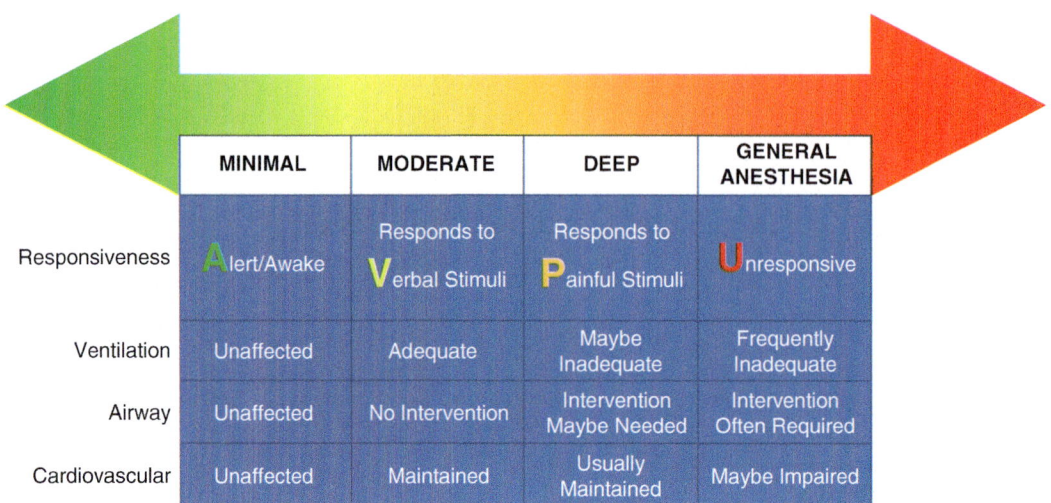

**Fig. 7.1** Sedation continuum (adapted from ASA's Continuum of Depth of Sedation, Definition of General Anesthesia, and Levels of Sedation/Analgesia Table ([1], p. 463)

American College of Radiologists (ACR) and the Society of Interventional Radiologists (SIR), the following sections of this chapter will generally pertain to moderate PSA unless specifically noted otherwise [1].

## 7.2 Indication and Goals

PSA is an important service offered to patients in radiology and imaging settings. Patient comfort and satisfaction remain the primary goals of PSA. The main objectives of PSA target anxiolysis, amnesia, and/or analgesia. However, not one pharmacological agent possesses all these attributes and not all procedures necessitate all three.

Lengthy procedures, inability to hold oneself still, and the need for precision/accuracy are other reasons for utilizing PSA for relatively painless procedures or those that can be feasibly performed under local anesthesia infiltration. Having to remain immobile for lengthy period of time is almost an impossible task, even among the healthiest of patients. Also, many procedures performed by diagnostic or interventional radiologists require precision for accurate diagnoses, and the need for an immobile patient becomes paramount. PSA is an option that can facilitate procedural completion and may improve diagnostic outcomes compared with the awake patient that is unwilling to remain motionless. Nevertheless, only administer the drug necessary for the procedure and the amount that is required for procedure completion and patient comfort. Unwarranted or excessive administration of sedatives or analgesics can delay recovery or push the patient further along the sedation continuum. Polypharmacy, the use of multiple drugs (opioid + benzodiazepine + alpha-2 agonist + H1 receptor blocker) in the delivery of sedation, or different combinations of the same class of drug (opioid 1 + opioid 2 and benzodiazepine) is strongly discouraged. Ultimately, procedural knowledge and good communication with the proceduralist can ensure a successful PSA practice.

Finally, it is important to be mindful of sedation's limitations, particularly in procedures that are extremely painful or complex. Conversion to anesthesia due to the inability to provide adequate PSA or oversedation can be avoided by intimate knowledge of the procedure and sedation pharmacology. Appropriate training and knowledge of the procedures is vital prior to allowing anyone (physician, LIP, or nurse) to administer PSA. A provider's credentials do not translate to competence and every department's leadership should have in place a process that properly vets and trains each PSA practitioner prior to allowing them access to patients. This includes and is not limited to: sedation pharmacology, radiology procedures, infusion pump technology, vital signs monitor technology, capnography interpretation, department workflow, handoff techniques, medication safety practices, airway management to include bag-valve-mask technique, and the Joint Commission's standards for moderate sedation practice.

## 7.3 Preprocedure Evaluation

A preprocedure evaluation, in conjunction with a physical examination, should be performed prior to initiating PSA and includes all of the following: a medical/surgical/social history, current medications (both prescribed and over the counter), airway evaluation, level of consciousness, food and drug allergies, and previous experiences with sedation or anesthesia. It is an additional means for identifying information that may have changed or missed since meeting with the physician in the office. Finally, it provides the sedating practitioner with baseline characteristics such as pain scores, level of consciousness, or unique patient characteristics that would require alterations during PSA. The physical examination and evaluation are performed by either the LIP or the radiologist. Finally, informed consent for the procedure is obtained prior to the administration of PSA and should include the PSA plan, its risks, benefits, and alternatives if any are available.

### 7.3.1 Patient Selection and Setting

Every patient should be evaluated for their appropriateness for PSA by assigning an ASA Physical Status (ASAPS) classification number (Table 7.1). Its purpose is to grade the patient's overall health status prior to surgery or procedure and has been identified as an independent predictor of morbidity and mortality when classified correctly [2]. ASAPS 1 and 2 is at lowest risk for the development of complications and therefore appropriate for PSA. Patients classified as ASAPS 3 or 4 may require consultation with

**Table 7.1** ASA physical status classification

| Class | Definition | Examples |
|---|---|---|
| 1 | Healthy patient | 30-year-old nonsmoking nonpregnant woman with no systemic disease |
| 2 | Mild or moderate systemic disease | Smoker<br>42-year-old with HTN (well controlled)<br>Pregnant woman |
| 3 | Multiple systemic diseases or major systemic disease that affects activity | Morbid obesity (BMI > 40)<br>Chronic renal failure on dialysis |
| 4 | Life-threatening severe systems disorders | Symptomatic CHF<br>Recent MI |
| 5 | Moribund patients with little chance of survival without surgery | Ruptured aneurysm<br>Major trauma |
| 6 | Organ donor | |

*E*—denotes emergency when paired with the class number
*HTN* hypertension, *BMI* body mass index, *CHF* congestive heart failure, *MI* myocardial infarction
ASA Physical Status Classification, adapted from the ASA Physical Status Classification Table published online at https://www.asahq.org/standards-and-guidelines/asa-physical-status-classification-system

the anesthesia department to identify any additional considerations or their appropriateness for PSA. Any patient classified as an ASAPS 5 are not appropriate candidates for PSA without an anesthesia practitioner and therefore should not be performed by a sedation nurse.

Another condition that should not be performed without an anesthesia practitioner is a patient with susceptibility to malignant hyperthermia (MH). MH is an autosomal dominant pharmacogenetic disorder that is triggered by inhalational anesthetics and the muscle relaxant succinylcholine, often used during emergent intubation scenarios. Once exposed, the patient experiences a progressive hyperdynamic metabolic state characterized by muscle rigidity, hyperthermia, and rhabdomyolysis. Without treatment with dantrolene, the only known antidote, mortality is extremely high. Even without exposure to triggering agents, MH-susceptible patients have exhibited symptoms and therefore require ongoing intensive evaluation. Identifying these patients prior to any procedure and referral to anesthesia services is key to their survival. Any patient exhibiting tachycardia, masseter muscle spasm, hypercarbia, and hyperthermia of an unknown etiology during a procedure should alert the sedating practitioner to the potential for this disorder and immediate consultation with anesthesia is warranted.

## 7.3.2 Risk Assessment and Prevention

In addition to assigning an ASAPS score, the immediate preprocedure evaluation is that final moment to identify certain physiological, historical, or social characteristics, previously missed, that would make them a poor candidate for PSA or increase their risk for complications related to the sedation pharmacology. Although these characteristics have the potential for significant morbidity and mortality, not all are contraindications for PSA. Identification of these risk factors and appreciation of their associated complications prior to the procedure allows time for patient optimization and the appropriate alterations to the PSA plan (Table 7.2). Factors that predispose a patient to complications can be related to all of the following: patient, procedure, proceduralist, pharmacological agent, sedating practitioner, and environment.

**Table 7.2** Complications and risk factors

| Complication | Risk factors/characteristics |
|---|---|
| Aspiration of gastric contents | Gastroesophageal reflux<br>Diabetes mellitus<br>Cerebral vascular accident<br>Obesity<br>Pregnancy<br>Oversedation |
| Airway obstruction | Large tongue<br>Edentulous<br>Oral abnormalities; loose tooth/teeth |
| Respiratory complications | COPD<br>Patient position<br>Oversedation<br>Inadequate sedation |
| Cardiovascular complications | History of heart failure<br>History of poorly controlled HTN<br>Patient position<br>Dehydration<br>Extremes of age |
| Oversedation | Extremes of age<br>Inexperienced sedation provider |
| Inadequate sedation | Opioid dependence/tolerance<br>Inexperienced sedation provider |
| Neurological complications | Elderly<br>Polypharmacy |
| Nausea and vomiting (N/V) | History of N/V<br>Infants and children<br>Nonsmoking females |
| Drug interactions/reactions | Known sensitivity<br>Polypharmacy |
| Difficult bag-mask ventilation | MOANS |

*HTN* hypertension, *COPD* chronic obstructive pulmonary disease

## 7.3.3 Airway Assessment

The purpose of the airway assessment is to identify physical characteristics that may contribute to difficult bag-mask ventilation and intubation. For the patient undergoing PSA, without an anesthesia provider, the ability to bag-mask ventilation is arguably more important than identifying whether it would be difficult to emergently intubate; if you can ventilate with a bag-valve-mask (BVM) oxygen can be delivered to the lungs. However, the Modified Mallampati Classification has low specificity in identifying patients that are difficult to mask ventilate [3].

Modified Mallampati classification (Fig. 7.2) stratifies patients based on oropharyngeal characteristics. Patients should be instructed to sit upright and protrude the tongue as far as possible with a wide-open mouth. It is important for the patient to perform this maneuver without phonation (saying AH!) which can provide an inaccurate Mallampati assessment. Mallampati scores 1 and 2 are not associated with difficult intubations; however, this should not preclude the possibility of a difficult airway. Difficult intubations (93%) and difficult mask ventilations (94%) were unanticipated in a Denmark study of over 180,000 patients [4]. A Mallampati 3 or 4 may

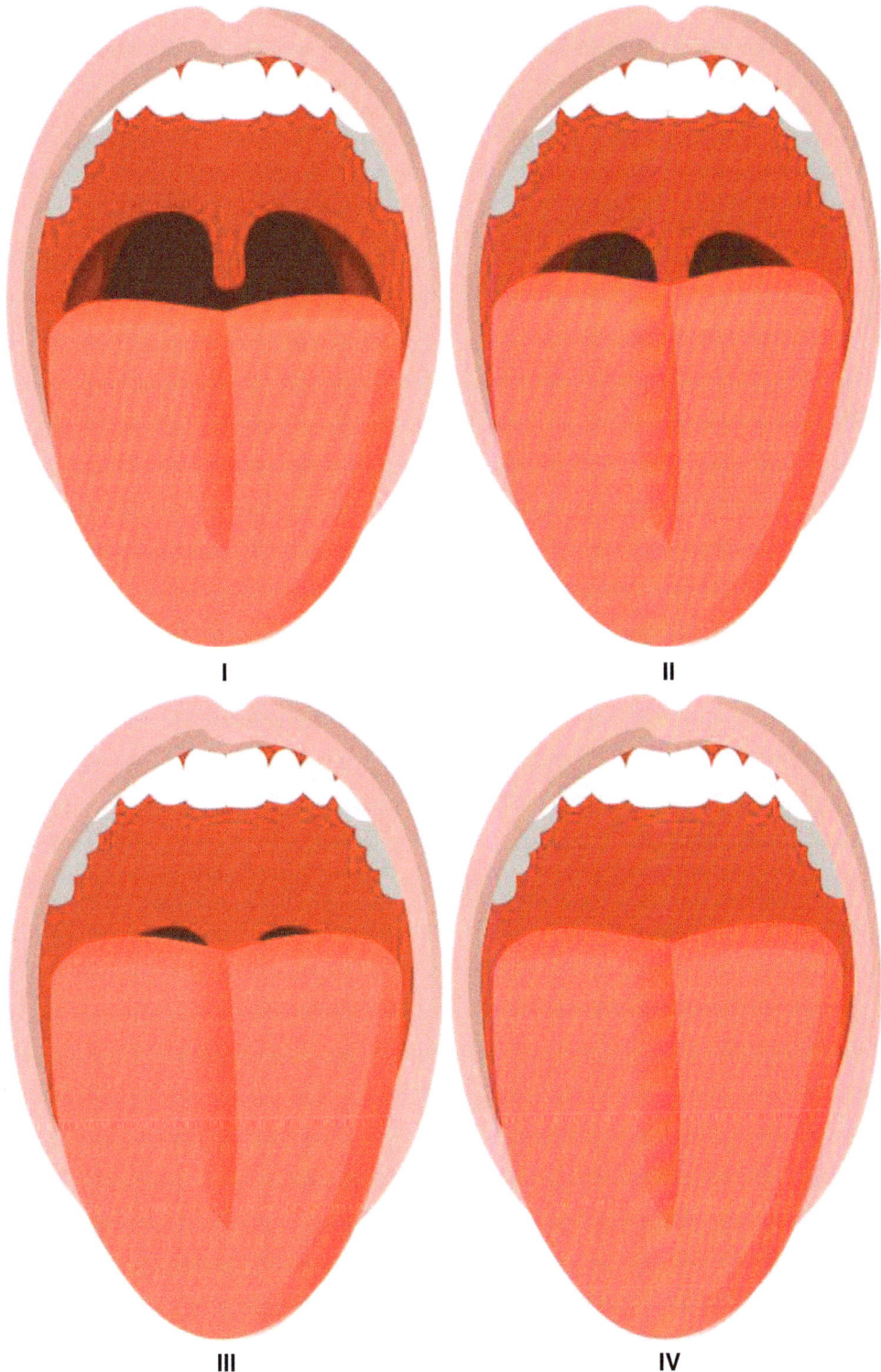

**Fig. 7.2** Modified Mallampati. This image is licensed under the Creative Commons Attribution-ShareAlike3.0Unported (CC BY-SA 3.0)

require an anesthesia consult before proceeding with PSA. In addition to the Mallampati score, look for other physical characteristics that can contribute to difficult mask ventilation utilizing the *MOANS* mnemonic. *M*—Mask seal difficulty (e.g., beard, nasogastric tubes, acromegaly); *O*—Obesity (BMI > 30); *A*—Age extremes; *N*—No teeth; *S*—Snoring or stiff lungs.

### 7.3.4 Preprocedural Fasting

Pulmonary aspiration of gastric contents is a potential complication that has serious and potentially deadly consequences in those patients at risk. This results from the loss of innate protective airway reflexes that are lost during deeper levels of sedation. There is no finite method of predicting when this occurs; therefore, care must be taken through preventative measures. Fasting, in addition to avoiding oversedation, potentially offers a means to ameliorate this condition. Current fasting recommendations include:

- Solid foods: at least 6 h of fasting.
- Clear liquids: at least 2 h of fasting.
- Breast milk: at least 4 h of fasting.
- Nonhuman milk: at least 6 h of fasting.

It is important to note that these times are based on healthy adult patients, and patients with delayed gastric emptying (e.g., history of stroke, diabetes) may require longer fasting times. In addition, during emergent procedures requiring PSA, a risk-benefit analysis in favor of procedure completion may necessitate forgoing these guidelines.

## 7.4 Periprocedure Considerations

### 7.4.1 Equipment and Monitoring

Selection of appropriate equipment and monitoring are essential in preventing and treating complications associated with PSA. It is impossible and unreasonable to prepare for every possible scenario that could possibly occur; however, certain resources are critical in ensuring safety during PSA. The most important resource is a team appropriately trained in the interpretation of certain types of monitoring modalities and the competence to act accordingly should an emergency arise. Of course, total reliance on monitoring should not replace vigilance which can lull the provider into a false sense of security. Therefore, it is imperative that the provider administering the PSA not have any other responsibilities except those that are specific to the administration and monitoring of the patient receiving PSA.

Supplemental oxygen should be utilized during PSA unless a patient's condition contraindicates its usage. Current recommendations, supported by high-level evidence, support its use during PSA; however, method of administration (mask versus nasal cannula) and the rate of oxygen flow should be based on clinical judgment and institutional policy [1].

### 7.4.2 Monitoring

Monitoring a patient periprocedurally is an essential nursing function that should include but not limited to blood pressure, heart rate and rhythm, ventilation, arterial oxygenation, pain level, and level and response to sedation. Ideally, these should be performed and documented every 5–15 min. New practice recommendations suggest every 5 min, however, in radiology settings the need for protective sequestering outside of the procedure room may not permit this time interval and therefore the sedation practitioner should use clinical judgement in these special circumstances. Standard monitoring (electrocardiogram, noninvasive blood pressure, pulse oximetry, and temperature) recommendations now include capnography which provides real-time information about the patient's ventilatory status. Pulse oximetry, a poor surrogate for a patient's ventilation, more accurately assesses arterial oxygenation. The most recent evidence, a meta-analysis from 13 randomized controlled trials, showed that the use of capnography during PSA decreased the incidence of respiratory compromise and arterial desaturation and may avoid the need for assisted ventilation [5]. Like other standard monitors it is important to educate the sedation provider on capnography waveform interpretation and troubleshooting potential issues that arise with gas sampling. Shadowing anesthesia providers performing MAC (monitored anesthesia care) is a potential method in providing this specialized education.

### 7.4.3 Postprocedure

The purpose of PSA postprocedural monitoring is to provide an environment in which the patient can recover from the procedure and the medications utilized and to ensure the patient has returned to preprocedure function prior to discharge. A patient receiving sedation outside the operating room (OR) should receive the same standard of care as surgical patients and therefore postprocedure polices should mirror those used by the perioperative services. Resources for standards or recommendations for postprocedural care can be obtained from the following organizations: Association of periOperative Registered Nurses (AORN), American Society of PeriAnesthesia Nurses (ASPAN), American Association of Nurse Anesthetists (AANA), American Society of Anesthesiologists (ASA), and the American Academy of Anesthesiology Assistants (AAAA).

## 7.5 Pharmacotherapeutics

Pharmacological choices are highly dependent on the procedure, patient history, setting, and the experience of the practitioner providing the sedation. Historically, many different classes of drugs have been used successfully for the provision of PSA including barbiturates and chloral hydrate, but narrow therapeutic indices have driven the pharmaceutical industry to produce pharmacological preparations with better safety profiles. In addition to safety, many practitioners prefer these newer preparations especially with their predictability and desirable pharmacokinetics. Although some nurse practice acts allow administration of sedatives that can produce anesthesia, like propofol and ketamine, current practice recommendations, supported by the ACR and SIR, have deemed these agents outside the scope of moderate PSA practice. Therefore, classes of drugs identified for deep sedation and general anesthesia will not be discussed in this section. For further information about the legality of these drugs when given by nurses under the supervision of qualified health care providers please refer to https://sedationcertification.com/resources/position-statements/position-statements-by-state/ (see Sect. 7.8). Also, due to the infrequency of other methods of administration (e.g., intramuscular, subcutaneous, transnasally) for PSA, discussion of each class of drug will be associated with intravenous route of administration.

Every PSA regimen should include the use of non-opioid adjuvants, patient history, and physical assessment permitting to decrease opioid consumption during the procedure. Examples include acetaminophen, nonsteroidal anti-inflammatory drugs (ketorolac, celecoxib), and local anesthetics (lidocaine, bupivacaine). It is imperative that the sedation provider be intimately familiar with the pharmacokinetics and dynamics of the drugs that they administer especially as it relates to indications, contraindications, duration of action, and side effects (Table 7.3).

Hemodynamics such as blood pressure and heart rate should be maintained within 20% of the patient's baseline to ensure adequate perfusion to vital organs. Many of the agents utilized during PSA have the propensity to alter hemodynamics that can be profound in susceptible patients. Therefore, the availability of vasoactive pharmacotherapeutics should be immediately available within the procedure room to counteract these alterations. The choice of drugs is highly dependent on each institution's formulary.

### 7.5.1 Benzodiazepines

Benzodiazepines are a class of drug most commonly associated with PSA. They exert their effects by binding to the GABA receptor, a major

**Table 7.3** Sedation pharmacology

| Drug | Dose (IV) | Pharmacokinetics | Elimination |
|---|---|---|---|
| Midazolam (Versed) | 0.5–5 mg | Onset: 0.5–1 min<br>Peak: 3–5 min<br>Duration: 15–80 min | Renal |
| Lorazepam (Ativan) | 1–4 mg | Onset: 1–5 min<br>Peak: 15–20 min<br>Duration: 6–10 h | Hepatic and renal |
| Diazepam (Valium) | 2–10 mg | Onset: <2 min<br>Peak: 3–4 min<br>Duration: 15–60 min | Hepatic |
| Fentanyl (Sublimaze) | 25–100 mcg | Onset: <0.5 min<br>Peak: 5–15 min<br>Duration: 30–60 min | Hepatic and pulmonary |
| Morphine | 2.5–15 mg | Onset: <1 min<br>Peak: 5–20 min<br>Duration: 2–7 h | Hepatic |
| Hydromorphone (Dilaudid) | 0.5–2 mg | Onset: <0.5 min<br>Peak: 5–20 min<br>Duration: 2–4 h | Hepatic |
| Meperidine (Demerol) (Analgesia) | 25–100 mg | Onset: <1 min<br>Peak: <60 min<br>Duration: 2–4 h | Hepatic |
| Meperidine (Shivering) | 12.5 mg | | |
| Dexmedetomidine (Precedex) | Loading dose: 1 mcg/kg<br>Infusion: 0.2–1 mcg/kg/h | Onset: <5 min<br>Peak: 15 min<br>Duration: N/A | Hepatic<br>Renal <1% |
| Diphenhydramine (Benadryl) | 10–50 mg | Onset: Within minutes<br>Peak: 60 min to 3 h<br>Duration: 4–6 h | Hepatic |
| Scopolamine | 0.2–0.65 mg | Onset: Immediate<br>Peak: 50–80 min<br>Duration: 120 min | Hepatic, renal |

Doses are given in ranges and therefore amounts are patient specific and titrating dosing should be utilized to avoid overdose

inhibitory compound, within the central nervous system (CNS). This class of drugs has the ability to produce anxiolysis, hypnosis, skeletal muscle relaxation, and anterograde amnesia but is devoid of analgesic effects and many of the negative side effects seen with opioids like nausea, vomiting, and constipation. Also, due to their action on inhibitory neurotransmitters within the CNS and the ability to raise the seizure threshold, this class of drug is often used for the prevention and treatment of seizures. All benzodiazepines are metabolized by the liver and most produce active metabolites except for midazolam, making it the preferential choice for PSA. Dose-dependent respiratory depression can occur with this class of drug and particular attention to dosing is warranted in patients with liver disease, the elderly and when used in combination with opioids due to synergistic effects. This synergy allows for lower dosing of both classes of drugs to produce greater effects. Common prescribed benzodiazepines used for PSA are midazolam, lorazepam, and diazepam.

### 7.5.1.1 Reversal

Flumazenil (Romazicon) provides reversal for the effects of benzodiazepines in a dose-dependent fashion. The duration of action of flumazenil is shorter than that of benzodiazepines and particular attention to the reemergence of respiratory depression or somnolence may be warranted. Flumazenil should also be used sparingly in patients with a history of seizures due to its ability to lower the seizure threshold in susceptible patients. Arguably, its use in patients on antiepileptics is contraindicated. Reversal agents are important to have immediately available but education about the importance of careful titration can avoid the negative precipitating events than are associated with abrupt reversal.

## 7.5.2 Opioids

Opioids are analgesics that act on opioid receptors within and outside the CNS. The beneficial and untoward effects of opioids are highly dependent on its affinity to a particular opioid receptor (mu, kappa, delta). Opioids with a high affinity for mu receptors exhibit the highest analgesic effects. Kappa and delta receptor affinity produces less analgesia compared with mu receptor activation. It is these receptors within the CNS that also produce the negative effects attributable to opioids like respiratory depression. This respiratory depression is dose dependent and is compounded in patients at higher risk for respiratory compromise. It is important that the sedation practitioner understand the effect of pairing opioids with benzodiazepines like midazolam. The effect of this combination is not additive (1 + 1 = 2) as one would surmise. Contrariwise, the pairing exhibits synergism (1 + 1 = 3) and decreased doses may be required to avoid oversedation or adverse reactions resulting from this synergy.

Opioid receptors are found throughout the body which translates to their large side-effect profile which include nausea, vomiting, constipation, chest wall rigidity, urinary retention, and sphincter of Oddi spasm. Opioids that have been used in PSA are morphine, fentanyl, meperidine, and hydromorphone. Fentanyl has become the most common intravenous opioid utilized for PSA. Fentanyl's lipophilic properties exhibit higher predictability in regard to onset and duration of action making it ideal for procedural sedation. Morphine and hydromorphone are hydrophilic and therefore have longer duration of actions and delayed onset of actions. Meperidine, an opioid commonplace in PSA, is now primarily used for postprocedural shivering. Its use is limited by active metabolites and their adverse CNS effects in susceptible populations.

### 7.5.2.1 Reversal

Reversal of respiratory depression caused by opioids is performed by administering naloxone (Narcan) which acts on opioid receptors antagonistically. Care should be taken when administering opioid reversal due to the reemergence of respiratory depression after naloxone's short duration of action when compared with longer acting opioid agonists like morphine. More importantly, due to the reversal of the analgesic effects and the potential for hyperalgesia, care should be given when reversing opioids in patients with chronic pain or with painful procedures. Ultimately, reversal agents should be immediately available, only used sparingly for emergent situations and only when patient stimulation and bag-mask ventilation is unsuccessful.

## 7.5.3 Alpha-2 Agonists

The newest drug appropriate for PSA in radiology and imaging settings is dexmedetomidine (Precedex). Dexmedetomidine is a highly selective alpha-2 agonist that exerts its action in the locus ceruleus at the level of the spinal cord. This unique action produces anxiolysis, sedation, and analgesia without the respiratory depression that occurs with other agents used in PSA. Dexmedetomidine induces sleep that is comparable to natural sleep and patients are often easily arousable during continuous administration. Its use and safety is well documented in all age groups and the critically ill. Dexmedetomidine usually requires a loading dose administered over 10 min followed by a continuous infusion. Cardiovascular side effects, like bradycardia and hypotension, are the main side effects typically seen with dexmedetomidine. The sedative effects of dexmedetomidine vary and dosing should be adjusted accordingly. Less neurocognitive dysfunction seen with other sedatives remains the primary benefit of dexmedetomidine.

Clonidine is another alpha-2 agonist used for its sedating properties; however, the sedation it produces is mild limiting its use for moderate sedation.

#### 7.5.3.1 Reversal

Atipamezole (Antisedan) is an alpha-2 antagonist which provides rapid reversal of the effects of dexmedetomidine should the need arise.

### 7.5.4 Other Adjuncts

*Diphenhydramine.* Used for its sedating effects, diphenhydramine (Benadryl), an $H_1$ receptor antagonist, exerts its effect by crossing the blood brain barrier into the CNS promoting drowsiness. Paradoxical reactions (insomnia, restlessness, euphoria, seizures), especially in children and elderly patients, have been reported.

*Scopolamine.* Scopolamine, an anticholinergic, like diphenhydramine has the ability to cross the blood brain barrier and exert CNS effects promoting sedation and in some instances amnesia. The side effects related to central anticholinergic syndrome limit its routine use during PSA which can be reversed with physostigmine.

## 7.6 PSA Training and Certification

Procedural sedation is not usually part of a nursing program's core clinical curriculum. Therefore, additional training is needed to prepare nurses and LIPs who are not anesthesia practitioners for this specialized practice. For those departments that do not have the resources for PSA training or lack a PSA training program, training and/or certification is available from numerous proprietary and nonprofit organizations that are too many to list. Below are a list of a few organizations offering training and/or certification in moderate and deep PSA.

### 7.6.1 Moderate Sedation Training/Certification

SSTmoderate—offered by the ASA, the professional organization representing anesthesiologists. This course is approved by the Montana Nurses Association for continuing education credit, an approved accreditor by the American Nurses Credentialing Center's (ANCC) Commission on Accreditation (COA). https://www.asahq.org

Adult Moderate Sedation—offered by the National Sedation Center (NSC), an accredited program approved for continuing education credits by the Association of periOperative Registered Nurses (AORN), an approved accreditor by the ANCC, and the American Medical Association (AMA). https://www.nationalsedationcenter.com

Safe Administration of Moderate Sedation—offered by AORN, an approved accreditor by the ANCC. https://www.aorn.org

Sedation Certification—offered by https://sedationcertification.com and is approved for continuing education credit by ANCC. It also offers complimentary membership to the American Association of Moderate Sedation Nurses (AAMSN).

### 7.6.2 Deep Sedation Training/Certification

No deep PSA training or certification programs are available for LIPs or nurses. Training is available on the ASA educational website (asahq.org) for physicians who are not anesthesiologists and is termed

SSTdeep. It requires the successful completion of the SSTmoderate within 2 years and two options are available, a less expensive online didactic and a more comprehensive module which includes a mentored clinical component with simulation. The cost of the programs are currently $199 and $3399, respectively. (See https://www.asahq.org.)

## 7.7 Practice Recommendations/Guidelines

Practice guidelines and/or recommendations are utilized often to guide clinical decisions especially in the age of evidence-based practice. This paradigm has replaced the provider preference model of practice and is the preferred method of practice in the United States. From a legal perspective, practice guidelines/recommendations can be introduced into legal proceedings to establish negligence or breach of duty but do not provide a legal standard for practice. Autonomous clinical judgement should be part of the clinical decision-making process when providing care for any patient based on the provider's experience and the patient's history and physical.

### 7.7.1 Practice Guidelines for Moderate PSA 2018 (ASA)

Current guidelines define moderate PSA, the most common sedation technique provided by nurses in radiology settings, as a "drug-induced depression of consciousness during which patients respond purposefully to verbal commands" and analgesia as the "management of patient pain or discomfort during and after procedures requiring moderate sedation" [1]. These guidelines were developed and published by the ASA with approval from other professional physician organizations including the Society of Interventional Radiologists (SIR) and the American College of Radiology (ACR).

Recommendations include:

- Preprocedure evaluation and preparation.
- Continuous capnography as a standard monitor.
- Presence of an individual in the procedure room properly trained to respond to airway complications and emergencies.
- Identification of drugs used for moderate and deep sedation.
- Recovery care.
- Quality improvement initiatives and reporting.

### 7.7.2 ACR/SIR Practice Parameter for Sedation and Analgesia 2015

The *"Practice Parameter for Sedation and Analgesia"* was a joint venture by ACR and SIR, published in 2015, to provide guidance to assist its members on the safe administration of minimal and moderate PSA in radiology and imaging settings [6]. They describe moderate PSA as a "minimally depressed level of consciousness induced by the administration of pharmacologic agents in which the patient retains a continuous and independent ability to maintain protective reflexes and a patent airway and to be aroused by physical or verbal stimulation." This practice parameter does not provide any recommendations for deep PSA.

Recommendations include:

- Scope of practice.
- Qualifications of responsibilities of personnel.
- Patient selection.
- Risk factors.
- Patient evaluation and management.
- Sedation-related documentation.
- Discharge criteria.
- Equipment.
- Quality control and improvement, infection control, and patient education.

### 7.7.3 SIR Position Statement: Staffing Guidelines for the Interventional Radiology Suite 2016

The "Staffing Guidelines for the Interventional Radiology Suite" was a guideline published in 2016 by SIR to provide its members with a resource about staffing (pre-, intra-, postprocedure) within interventional radiology departments [7].

Recommendations include staffing considerations as they pertain to:

- Preprocedure and recovery.
- Interventional radiology.
- Off hours (on-call).
- Special considerations.

### 7.7.4 ARIN Clinical Practice Guideline: Capnography During PSA

The Association for Radiologic and Imaging Nursing (ARIN) developed a position statement and clinical practice guideline for its members about the use of continuous capnography during PSA in radiology and imaging settings [8].

Recommendation:

- Continuous capnography should be utilized during PSA unless a patient's condition precludes its usage.

## 7.8 Scope of Practice and Regulations

Variations in federal, organizational, state, and institutional policies create differences in PSA practices throughout the United States (US).

### 7.8.1 Federal

The Centers for Medicare & Medicaid Services (CMS) specifically addresses provider certification as it relates to PSA [9]. The Conditions of Participation (CoP) for Anesthesia Services provides guidance that hospitals must comply with in order to receive reimbursement for anesthesia services. CMS utilizes the standards, definitions, and language created by the ASA. Therefore, it is important to cognizant of the aforementioned. Specifically mentioned in the CoP is the differentiation of anesthesia which, in congruence with the ASA recommendations, includes deep sedation and general anesthesia. This is controversial especially with other professionals already engaged in deep sedation practices which may not be in compliance with current CMS CoP requirements.

### 7.8.2 State

State regulation of nurses and advanced practice nurses engaging in PSA is the purview of state nursing boards and practice acts. Due to state rights, each state develops and adopts standards that meet their unique needs. Therefore, practice can vary quite dramatically between neighboring states. The key factor with state boards and practice acts is identifying what pharmacotherapeutics are within a nurse's scope of practice. While one state may allow nurses to administer ketamine, a neighboring state may restrict it to only physicians and LIPs. A great resource for all these variations can be found on the sedationcertification.com website.

### 7.8.3 Organizational

The Joint Commission (TJC) provides standards for hospitals that ultimately influence reimbursement. Therefore, TJC wields considerable power over a hospital's accreditation and the standards they elect to adopt. TJC provides recommendations for moderate sedation that ambiguously address the credentials of the sedation provider while not actually stating what those credentials should be [10].

Practice recommendations, produced by various previously mentioned professional organizations, influence institutional adoption of PSA standards. It remains the institution's responsibility to choose those recommendations that best fit their culture. Crego [10] states that regulation in the U.S. is fragmented which is further compounded by variation in regulatory standards, lack of research about nurses proving sedation, and absent national standards for PSA. This is alarming especially with the increased utilization of PSA outside of operating rooms.

## 7.9 Conclusion

PSA by non-anesthesia trained professionals is increasing and remains an important part of meeting the healthcare needs of our population. It is essential for those providing sedation services to be intimately familiar with the complexities that come with PSA. Ensuring a successful and safe PSA practice requires a multidisciplinary approach with all vested professionals and should include anesthesia practitioners, registered nurses, LIPs, administration, technologists, pharmacists, and proceduralists.

## References

1. Practice Guidelines for Moderate Procedural Sedation andAnalgesia 2018: A Report by the American Society of Anesthesiologists Task Force on Moderate Procedural Sedation and Analgesia, the American Association of Oral and Maxillofacial Surgeons, American College of Radiology, American Dental Association, American Society of Dentist Anesthesiologists, and Society of Interventional Radiology. Anesthesiology. 2018;128(3):437–79.
2. Hackett NJ, De Oliveira GS, Jain UK, Kim JYS. ASA class is a reliable independent predictor of medical complications and mortality following surgery. Int J Surg. 2015;18:184–90.
3. Green SM, Roback MG. Is the Mallampati score useful for emergency department airway management or procedural sedation? Ann Emerg Med. 2019;74(2):251–9. https://doi.org/10.1016/j.annemergmed.2018.12.021.
4. Nørskov AK, Rosenstock CV, Wetterslev J, Astrup G, Afshari A, Lundstrøm LH. Diagnostic accuracy of anaesthesiologists' prediction of difficult airway management in daily clinical practice: a cohort study of 188 064 patients registered in the Danish Anaesthesia Database. Anaesthesia. 2015;70(3):272–81. https://doi.org/10.1111/anae.12955.
5. Saunders R, Struys MMRF, Pollock RF, Mestek M, Lightdale JR. Patient safety during procedural sedation using capnography monitoring: a systematic review and meta-analysis. BMJ Open. 2017;7(6):e013402. https://doi.org/10.1136/bmjopen-2016-013402.
6. ACR/SIR Practice Parameter for Sedation and Analgesia. 2015. https://www.acr.org/-/media/acr/files/practice-parameters/sed-analgesia.pdf. Accessed 3 May 2019.
7. Baerlocher MO, Kennedy SA, Ward TJ, Nikolic B, Bakal CW, Lewis CA, et al. Society of Interventional Radiology position statement: staffing guidelines for the interventional radiology suite. J Vasc Interv Radiol. 2016;27(5):618–22. https://doi.org/10.1016/j.jvir.2016.02.010.
8. Pella L, Lambert C, McArthur B, West C, Hernandez M, Green K, et al. Systematic review to develop the clinical practice guideline for the use of capnography during procedural sedation in radiology and imaging settings: a report of the Association for Radiologic & Imaging Nursing capnography task force. J Radiol Nurs. 2018;37(3):163–72.
9. CMS Provider Certification. 2011. https://www.cms.gov/Regulations-and-Guidance/Guidance/Transmittals/downloads/R74SOMA.pdf. Accessed 3 May 2019.
10. Crego N. Procedural sedation practice: a review of current nursing standards. J Nurs Regul. 2015;6(1):50–6.

# Positioning the Patient for Procedures

## 8

Lois Elaine Stewart and Michael J. Long

## 8.1 Introduction

Many aspects of care across the entire spectrum of procedural sedation require careful assessment, planning, and collaboration [1]. Proper patient positioning is one aspect of this care. Positioning during procedural sedation should facilitate the technical ease of the necessary procedure, while minimizing the physiological impact upon the patient. Specific patient positions impose related and predictable physiological changes upon all patients. Such changes can be exacerbated by sedation and anesthesia, as well as the time needed to complete the procedure requiring sedation. These factors may combine to form a risk of injury due to procedural positioning. The risk of iatrogenic injury may also be influenced by intrinsic patient factors and extrinsic process factors [2].

Safe and effective procedural sedation is best accomplished through proactive vigilance and teamwork. This teamwork is facilitated by clear and consistent communication at each stage of procedural care: pre-sedation assessment, intra-procedural care, and post-sedation assessment [1]. Conscientious hand-off communication must be maintained at each care interval. The prevention of complications that may be imposed related to patient positioning is a significant responsibility shared by the entire procedural team. At times, strong patient advocacy is required to achieve a compromise between procedural efficacy and patient safety, to find the best positioning alternative to balance these concerns.

### 8.1.1 Importance of Positioning Safety

Patient safety should always be an utmost priority of healthcare providers. The normal human has protective reflexes that function unconsciously to minimize physical harm to vital systems. Examples of these reflexes include rapid withdrawal from painful stimuli, the corneal reflex, and the cough reflex [3]. Reflexive protection of bodily integrity can also involve the movement of an extremity that is static for too long to be comfortable. The discomfort can often be due to an overly stretched, flexed, or compressed position. Medications used for sedation, especially in combination with any preexistent disease states, can greatly alter the constellation of protective reflexes a patient may normally possess [4].

The sedation provider must assume primary responsibility for preventing harm during the time the patient's sensorium is altered. In essence, the sedation provider and the procedural

L. E. Stewart, PhD, CRNA (✉) · M. J. Long, DNP, CRNA
Community Health Network Anesthesia, Indianapolis, IN, USA

team must function as protective reflexes for the sedated patient. Bony projections should be protected, and normal curvatures should be maintained in the spine as possible [2]. Extreme or unusual positions may be required, and could be unnatural or need to be maintained past the point of comfort. Time spent in these types of positions should be limited as much as possible. At other times position changes may be required during the procedure. Care must be taken to avoid mechanical injuries to the patient from changes in position, such as a hand becoming caught in a table mechanism when reclining or inclining the head of the table. All pressure points in contact with surfaces should be protected in some manner. This can be accomplished through mattresses, foam padding, pillows, or specifically designed positioning devices. Common strategies have emerged for specific positions that may be encountered during procedures, based on anecdotal and scientific data; these will be covered later in this chapter.

### 8.1.2 Alterations in Physiology due to Procedural Positioning During Moderate Sedation

In addition to the risk of iatrogenic injury, procedural positioning also can impose physiological changes in several bodily systems. The extent of these physiological changes is dependent upon several main factors: the necessary procedure, the length of the procedure, the physical status of the patient, concurrent medication regimen, the necessary position, the positioning devices used, and the type of sedation or anesthesia utilized, among others [4]. The bodily systems most commonly affected by positioning include the respiratory system, the cardiovascular system, the neurological system, and exposed or susceptible areas of skin and tissue.

#### 8.1.2.1 Respiratory System Effects: Procedural Sedation and Positioning

Medications used for procedural sedation are commonly known to depress respiratory function in various ways. During moderate sedation, the goals for the respiratory system encompass the maintenance of a patent airway supporting spontaneous ventilation, with avoidance of hypoxemia and excessive levels of hypercarbia [5]. Supplemental oxygen is very often supplied for improved safety in sedated patients, and ventilation should be monitored in pursuit of these respiratory goals. Position changes naturally affect factors that support adequate airway maintenance, ventilation, and oxygenation. The respiratory alterations from procedural positioning may be reasonably anticipated and attenuated in a majority of moderate sedation cases. This is not as easily accomplished with general anesthesia, which introduces several more variables.

Adequate pulmonary function depends first upon a patent airway. Airway patency is primarily affected by patient neural and anatomic factors, airway muscle tone, bulbar reflexes, and level of consciousness [5]. Moderate sedation can alter the state of most of these patient factors, as can changes in patient positioning via the effects of gravity. Diminished muscular control of the oropharyngeal structures of the airway can lead to varying degrees of airway obstruction, and eventually will cause hypoxemia, hypercarbia, and apnea [2]. Gravity can either exacerbate or diminish the airway obstruction present due to sedation, dependent upon the patient position assumed in the procedure. In general, airway patency is improved during sedation in the sitting, lateral, and prone positions, and is diminished to variable degrees in the supine position [3, 4].

Normal exchange of gases during pulmonary function depends on ventilation of the lungs, perfusion of the lungs, and a reasonable matching or balance between these two processes [3]. Ventilation and perfusion patterns depend upon intrinsic properties of the thorax/abdomen and extrinsic factors the lungs must accommodate. Intrinsic properties include chest wall and lung tissue compliance, lung volumes, intrathoracic pressures, diaphragm function, and abdominal compartment pressure [2, 3]. Extrinsically, gravity affects the distribution of ventilation and perfusion in the lungs, diaphragm function, and the distribution of abdominal contents [2, 3]. Because gravity can be a substantial factor altering pulmonary dynamics, positioning can significantly alter respiratory performance in sedated patients. These effects may be more pronounced in patients with preexisting pulmonary disease [4].

The sitting position generally produces few significant effects upon pulmonary dynamics and so is usually well tolerated. The supine position imposes notable reductions in lung volumes and capacities which can lead to altered gas exchange and decreased oxygen reserve [4]. The lateral position can lead to gravitational ventilation-perfusion mismatching. This potentially diminishes oxygenation in susceptible patients in the lateral position [4]. Compensation of lateral ventilation-perfusion mismatching is readily accomplished in patients without significant pulmonary disease. The pulmonary effects of prone positioning can be varied. If the weight of the body or a positioning device compresses the stomach in the prone position, abdominal compartment contents and pressure can limit diaphragmatic excursion and lung volumes [2]. If the abdomen is allowed to be free of pressure, the prone position can have advantageous effects upon lung compliance, lung volumes, ventilation-perfusion matching, and overall pulmonary function [2].

#### 8.1.2.2 Cardiovascular System Effects: Procedural Sedation and Positioning

The overall function of the cardiovascular system is to produce an adequate supply of oxygenated cardiac output to furnish the various tissue oxygenation needs of the body. The maintenance of cardiac output and tissue perfusion are largely dependent upon the factors of vascular preload, heart rate, myocardial contractility, and systemic vascular resistance (SVR), also termed afterload [2]. Hemodynamic feedback systems and volume/pressure reflexes function to compensate for shortfalls in these critical factors and act to preserve cardiovascular stability [4]. For example, if mean arterial pressure falls, heart rate and SVR are increased to preserve tissue perfusion.

Alterations in some of these critical factors can occur merely from postural changes imposing the effects of gravity on the cardiovascular system [2]. These effects are normally compensated for by the physiological reflexes mentioned above. However, these mechanisms can be blunted or interfered with by disease states, treatment regimens, and the administration of sedation medications, among other factors [4]. Therefore, during procedural sedation, hemodynamic support may be necessary due to the combined effects of positioning and sedation upon the patient [4]. This is especially true of patients who may be intravascularly dehydrated, elderly, on cardiovascular medication, or with preexisting cardiovascular disease.

Anticipating postural changes in perfusion is predictable on a baseline normal model. As a general rule of thumb, mean arterial pressure changes around 2 mmHg for each inch of difference between the level of the heart and a body part [4], in the opposite direction. In other words, as the position of the head rises as compared to the heart, mean arterial pressure in the cranial vascular tree falls by 2 mmHg for each inch of elevation [4]. Therefore, postural hemodynamic changes in the supine and lateral positions are usually of little effect. Any position with legs in a dependent state can lead to hypotension, owing to gravitational pooling of blood in the venous system of the legs [3]. This would include the sitting and flexed lateral positions. Any position with the legs elevated above the level of the heart would increase venous preload and improve arterial pressures at least initially [3]. This would include the lithotomy and Trendelenburg positions. Prone positioning has the potential to diminish cardiac output due to increased intrathoracic pressure but is often well tolerated hemodynamically. Prone positioning devices that are rigid and increase pressures in the abdomen and thorax are more likely to affect the hemodynamic stability of patients [4].

### 8.1.3 Patient Comfort and Anxiety Effects

Many patients who require procedural sedation may have difficulty achieving or maintaining the required position, due to age or comorbidity factors. The patient should be informed of the position that is necessary for conducting the procedure, and information regarding potential concerns should be drawn out from the pre-procedure interview. A plan for positioning can be discussed proactively and should include the patient, procedural provider, the team members, and the sedation provider. Often the patient will have significant anxiety regarding aspects of the procedure, including positioning. Patient comfort can be optimized, complications avoided, and anxiety diminished by the creation of a plan with the procedural team and the patient. Compromises with positioning should be made if at all possible, in deference to any preexisting limitations. Once the plan is agreed upon, an explanation given to the patient will also greatly mitigate the level of anxiety present.

### 8.1.4 Incidence and Medicolegal Implications of Positioning Injuries

As stated previously, the bodily systems most susceptible to untoward effects due to procedural positioning include the respiratory system, the cardiovascular system, the neurological system, and exposed or susceptible areas of skin and tissue. The most common neurological injury suffered due to positioning is perioperative peripheral nerve injury [6]. The overall incidence of perioperative peripheral nerve injury is difficult to quantify, but it is thought to be well below 1% of sedation and anesthesia cases [2, 3, 6]. The incidence of perioperative peripheral nerve injury among cases with known complications, by review of anesthesia literature reveals a large collection of data in the American Society of Anesthesiologists Closed Claim Project, encompassing the data years 1990–2007 [6]. This body of work shows that peripheral nerve injuries account for 22% of the closed claims cases in the database; the only more common closed claim is the complication of death [2].

Among common injuries to susceptible skin and tissue are perioperative pressure injuries, which can include pressure or shear force ischemia, skin tears, and joint stresses [7]. Effective sedation can at times mask patient symptoms that would reveal a risk of skin, tissue, or joint injury. Preventing pressure injuries is a high priority for healthcare providers as these injuries can impart a large burden of morbidity and cost [7]. Literature regarding the well-defined incidence of such injuries related to either procedural sedation or anesthesia is scant and variably defined.

### 8.2 General Principles of Patient Safety for Procedural Sedation

A planned and proactive approach to assessment and intervention in the prevention of positioning injury is the best strategy, including the use of proven preventative adjuncts. The mattress type most often associated with pressure injuries seems to be gel mattresses, while the standard operating room (OR) and procedural table mattresses performed better [7]. Additional padding can be accomplished through the use of appropriately sized pillows, foam rubber pads, or warmed gel pads [7]. A key factor in the application of additional padding is not to produce compression to the structures from the bulk of the protective padding. If specialized positioning devices are to be used, it is imperative to know and follow the manufacturer's recommendations [1]. Proactive assessment and planning for positioning should occur during the following phases of care: pre-procedure, intra-procedure, and post-procedure.

### 8.2.1 Pre-procedure Phase

This phase should include a thorough assessment of intrinsic patient risk factors for complications, extrinsic/procedural risk factors, and documentation of any preexisting deficits or physiological alterations in the patient baseline status [1]. This should especially include peripheral nerve function or dysfunction, skin condition, joint range of motion limitations, and peripheral pulses. Documentation of the pre-procedural assessment and effective hand-off communication between team members is key to the prevention of positioning injury.

Collaboration among all team members and the patient regarding the positioning plan, as mentioned before, is key and should occur at this point in time. Planning for specific positioning devices, protective padding and effective monitoring should also take place, and specifically be led by the sedation provider [4]. An effective measure of imposed positioning stress can occur at this point, by having the patient conduct a trial assumption of the needed position necessary during the pre-assessment [3]. This can reveal the patient's physiological tolerance of the required position. Finally, staff members of sufficient number and specific expertise should be regularly scheduled as needed for the procedure and patient safety needs.

### 8.2.2 Intra-procedure Phase

Prompt and accurate communication among members of the intra-procedural team is very important. The execution of the positioning strategy should include the use of any special positioning equipment within the manufacturer's guidelines. Protective padding or support of all vulnerable areas should occur as needed, including bony prominences, joints, spinal curvatures, eyes, nose, breast, and genitalia [2]. Safety straps should be employed per the facility protocol. If the procedure requires the sedation provider be removed in distance from the patient's bedside, the placement of a visual clue to indicate adequate chest respiratory movement can be an excellent monitoring intervention. A visual clue could be as simple as a fluffed 4 × 4 gauze taped to the portion of the patient's chest wall that has the most respiratory excursion. The sedation provider must exercise consistent vigilance in initial positioning and subsequent monitoring to prevent injury [8]. Immediate re-assessment should occur with planned or accidental repositioning of the patient during the sedation. If extreme positions must be maintained for a prolonged time period, planned positioning breaks in a more anatomically neutral position should occur at agreed-upon intervals [1]. Standard re-assessment of positioning and injury prevention should occur at a regular basis during the sedation interval, including peripheral pulse assessment distal to areas of potential compression.

### 8.2.3 Post-procedure Phase

Vigilant assessment and monitoring should continue during the recovery, or post-procedure phase of care. The hand-off communication should include the length of the procedure, the position maintained during the sedation, and any relevant risk factors for positioning injury [1]. Preexisting alterations in physiologic status uncovered in the pre-procedure assessment should be emphasized as well. Once sedation has worn off, accurate documentation of any alteration in baseline function should take place and will be valuable for monitoring symptom progression and in diagnosis [7]. Any such alteration should be brought to the attention of the procedural provider and the team as soon as possible.

## 8.3 Descriptions of Commonly Required Patient Positions

### 8.3.1 Physiologic Alterations/Iatrogenic Risk

Positioning for radiological procedures may vary due to modality, type of procedure, patient condition, available equipment, and facility-specific requirements. The following descriptions of commonly required positions are the foundation from which some modifications may ensue, given that patient safety is observed.

### 8.3.2 Supine Position (Dorsal Decubitus)

The supine position is very frequently used for procedures requiring sedation and anesthesia. A patient in the supine position is lying recumbent, back flat on the mattress, facing upward. The head should be supported, and the neck maintained in a neutral position, by the use of a pillow or small positioning device such as a gel or foam donut [4]. Arms may be positioned at the patient's sides or may be placed on padded arm boards. If arm boards are used, the patient's arms should be abducted less than 90° at the shoulder, and the forearm should be placed in the supinated position [4]. When a single arm is abducted it is important to avoid rotation of the head, most especially to the side opposite the abducted arm [1]. If the arms are tucked and secured at the patient's sides, the elbows should be supported and not allowed to hang over the edge of the table [3]. In the arms tucked position, the hands should be in a neutral position with the thumbs up and the palms inward [4]. The legs should remain uncrossed, and, if possible, a pillow should be placed under the patient's knees for comfort. Bony prominences of concern include the heels, areas of the thoracic/lumbar/sacral/coccygeal spinal column, scapulae, elbows, and the back of the cranium [1]. In a case projected to last longer than 1 h, heel pads should be strongly considered. Figure 8.1 shows a patient positioned supine for a procedure.

### 8.3.3 Lateral Decubitus Position

The patient in the lateral decubitus position is essentially in a side-lying position, with the side down noted by preceding the term "lateral decubitus" with either left or right. Therefore, left lateral decubitus is a side-lying position with the left side down. The head and neck should be supported by pillows or padding devices in a neutral position, neither markedly flexed nor extended. The overall alignment of the body from the head through the hips should be along the same linear plane if at all possible [4]. To alleviate pressure on the down arm and shoulder, an "axillary roll" should be placed under the down thorax, on the ribcage just slightly below the actual axilla [3].

The down arm should be placed on a padded arm board and extended perpendicularly to the torso, with the elbow flexed less than 90° [1]. It is acceptable in short procedures for the down arm to be flexed and placed on the bed under the pillow as in a natural sleeping position, if no patient discomfort results from this positioning. The up, or superior, arm can be secured to the down arm with adequate padding or pillows between the two arms, or the limb can be secured on a separate positioning device such as an elevated arm rest. If this is used, care should be taken that the suspended arm is in neutral position at the shoulder to avoid undue stretch on the neural plexus. It is recommended to place the cuff for monitoring non-invasive blood pressure (NIBP) on the up arm, as using the down arm can exacerbate any compression on vascular or neural tissue [4]. If the up arm is above the level of the patient's heart, the provider should realize that the NIBP readings may well be artificially low [2]. There should be padding provided between the legs to prevent pressure on bony prominences. Flexing either leg can help prevent pressure and stabilize the patient's position on the table [3]. Padding the lateral surface of the down leg which is in contact with the table, from the knee to the ankle, can protect vulnerable superficial nerve structures. Figures 8.2 and 8.3 show a patient in right lateral decubitus position, with axillary roll placed, and two options for arm positions depending upon needed exposure.

### 8.3.4 Lithotomy Position

The patient in lithotomy position is usually placed in this manner for access to the perineum and associated structures. In the lithotomy position, the patient is essentially supine, but the legs

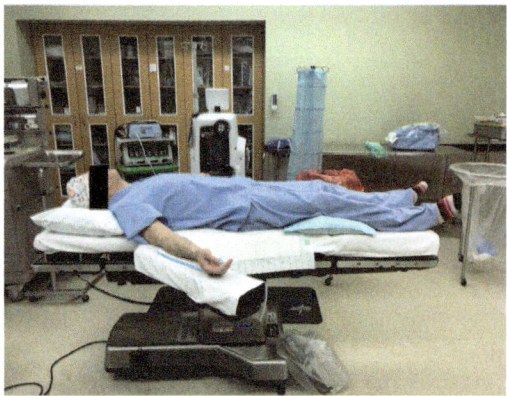

**Fig. 8.1** Supine position

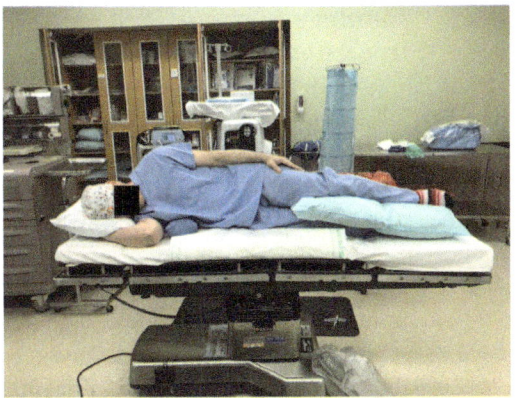

**Fig. 8.2** Lateral position. Up arm extended

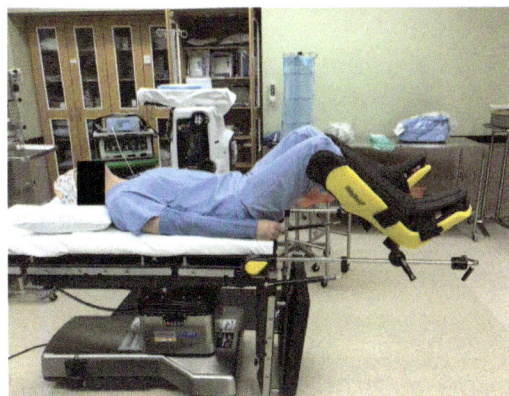

**Fig. 8.4** Lithotomy position

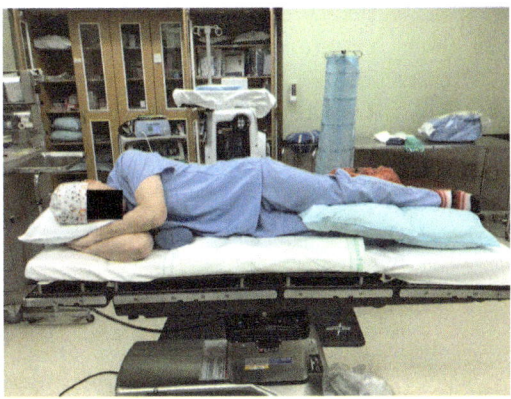

**Fig. 8.3** Lateral position. Up arm flexed

are positioned and secured above the torso, with hips and knees flexed and the hips abducted [3]. Legs are held in place with the use of stirrups, supports, or padded positioning boots [2]. With all leg positioning devices used, care should be taken to avoid pressure in the popliteal fossa and on the bony prominences of the tibia and fibula at the knee and ankle joints [4]. The extent of leg elevation differentiates low lithotomy from exaggerated lithotomy. In low lithotomy, the legs are suspended only slightly above the torso and hip/knee flexion is not extreme. With an exaggerated lithotomy position, the legs are high above the torso and hip/knee flexion is much more exaggerated. The more exaggerated the position is from neutral, the higher the risk of positioning injury. Exaggerated lithotomy positions should be utilized for the least amount of time possible, with positioning breaks occurring during longer cases.

Hips and knees should not be flexed greater than 90° to prevent neurovascular damage and undue joint stress [4]. When positioning the legs for lithotomy, the legs should be gently raised and lowered simultaneously to avoid undue stress on the hip joints. Controlled movements are very important, as sudden accidental movements of the legs in a sedated patient can cause injury or even joint dislocation [4]. The arms are often placed on padded arm boards or tucked as described in the supine position. If the arms are tucked and secured at the patient's sides, extreme caution must be taken when moving the patient or sections of the table, to avoid crush injuries to the hands and limbs [7]. Figure 8.4 shows a patient in low lithotomy position, using a positioning device sometimes called "bumblebee boots" to maintain the leg position necessary for the procedure.

In the following figure (Fig. 8.5) the angle of the hip joint is marked with red lines to show the area of concern for sustained or high degrees of hip flexion which can potentially lead to peripheral nerve or muscle injury.

### 8.3.5 Prone (Ventral Decubitus)

Prone positioning is used for access to the dorsal surfaces of the body, some intracranial procedures and for rectal procedures [4]. The patient in prone position is lying relatively flat, face downwards. For this reason, it is very important to know the patient's preexisting range of motion

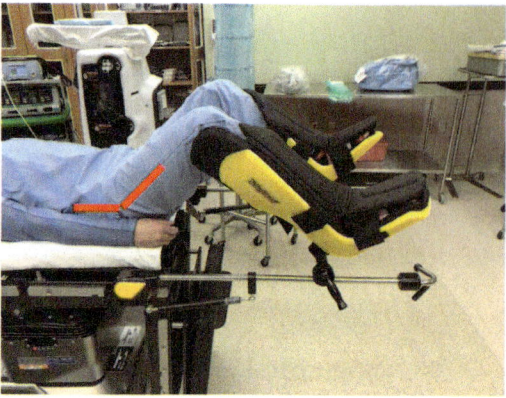

**Fig. 8.5** Angle of hip flexion in lithotomy position

in the arms and cervical spine [1]. For prone cases that strictly require little to zero patient movement, general anesthesia is recommended. Prone positioning for general anesthetics can involve several different positioning devices not necessary in sedation cases. For sedation in the prone position, it is common to allow the patient to assume the necessary position and adjust head, neck, arm, and leg position for optimal comfort prior to sedation. Nasal oxygen and monitors should be applied prior to the patient positioning, and free intravenous (IV) access should be assured. Comfort may be improved by the placement of a small pillow under the feet of the patient in prone position.

For short prone cases, it is acceptable for the patient's head to be rotated to the side if that is comfortable. This rotation is not acceptable if the case is prolonged, or the contralateral arm is abducted greater than 90°. Arms may be padded and tucked or may be placed at the sides of the patient's head, with less than 90° of shoulder abduction and elbow flexion. Alternatively, the arms may be differentially positioned, with one arm down by the patient's side and one arm at the side of the patient's head. The arms should never be on a horizontal plane higher than the torso. Breast and genitalia should be positioned to limit shear forces and pressure. If the sedated patient in prone position moves or shifts during the procedure, it is important to reassess the position prior to continuing, as visual inspection of many vulnerable areas is obscured.

## 8.3.6 Trendelenburg and Reverse Trendelenburg

The Trendelenburg position can be variation of any the base positions described above. However, it is most often associated with the flat supine position, with the patient lying recumbent and the foot of the bed inclined to varying degrees. Most often the angle of foot elevation is between 10 and 30°. This position may be assumed as a temporary hemodynamic intervention to treat hypotension by increasing venous return from the legs [3]. Brief periods of Trendelenburg positioning can often be used to facilitate central vascular access. Due to similar effects on other vascular or fluid beds, the position can increase central venous pressure, intracranial pressure, and intraocular pressures [4].

Trendelenburg positioning may also be assumed due to procedural requirements. If this is the case, often there is some device used to prevent continued slipping of the patient towards the declined head of the bed. This may involve the use of shoulder braces. Prolonged pressure from shoulder braces should be distributed across a wide surface area of each shoulder to minimize potential neurovascular compression or stretch injuries [1].

Reverse Trendelenburg positioning is the exact opposite of Trendelenburg, meaning that the head of the bed is inclined to varying degrees. This position may be assumed for patient comfort, especially for ease of breathing, in situations where the head of the bed (HOB) may not be singularly elevated. Otherwise, the position is usually only encountered when procedurally necessary. The same considerations for the base position apply in reverse Trendelenburg, but some cardiovascular effects may be revealed due to the change in gravity's effects from the elevation of the HOB.

Figures 8.6 and 8.7 show a patient model positioned in Trendelenburg and reverse Trendelenburg positions, respectively.

## 8.3.7 Specialized Positioning Equipment

Depending upon the needed procedure for which the patient requires sedation, there may be highly

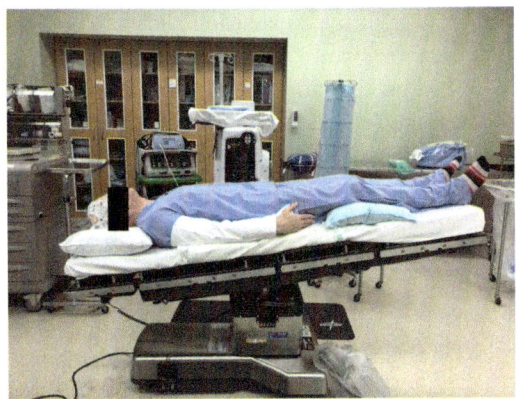

**Fig. 8.6** Trendelenburg position

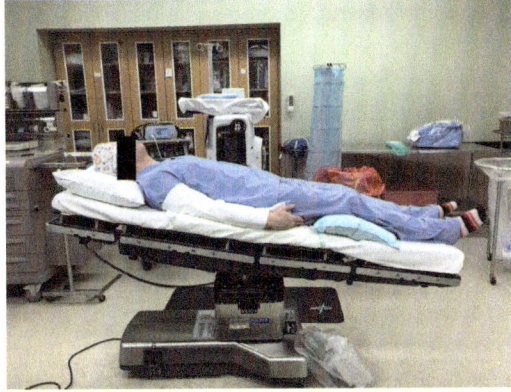

**Fig. 8.7** Reverse Trendelenburg position

specialized positioning equipment utilized. The wide array of these devices makes it impossible to include an exhaustive list of the same. However, one example would be devices made specifically to stabilize an extremity during a procedure, such as an arm rest which facilitates radial artery puncture and access.

## 8.4 Nerve Injuries Related to Procedural Positioning

Peripheral nerves are particularly vulnerable to positioning injury, especially if the patient is sedate enough that it allows the assumption of positions that would normally cause the patient discomfort or distress. The physiologic structure and function, as well as the anatomical positions of peripheral nerves, can lead to vulnerability to injury from various stressors due to positioning.

### 8.4.1 Physiology/Pathophysiology of Nerve Injury

Proper peripheral nerve function generally depends upon neuronal structural integrity, electrochemical homeostasis, and an adequate blood supply [3]. Peripheral nerves contain groupings of nerve fibers and supporting microvasculature, encased within protective connective tissue bundles. Individual fascicle groupings within a peripheral nerve are enclosed by the endoneurium and the perineurium [4]. Several of these fascicle groupings can be bound into a peripheral nerve that is structurally supported and housed by the epineurium [8]. The entire peripheral nerve is covered by other connective tissue that gives it protection and the ability to resist frictional forces encountered when moving across joints and tissue [4].

The primary mechanisms of peripheral nerve injuries are compression, stretch, and of course shearing or transection of the nerve bundle [8]. Compression can lead to nerve tissue injury due to direct neuronal trauma, arterial occlusion, or venous outflow obstruction. Any edema in peripheral nerves is poorly tolerated due to the fact that there is no lymphatic drainage available [4]. Neuronal compression may also result from improper placement or prolonged use of the NIBP cuff. The NIBP cuff should be placed high on the upper arm so that the area near the bony prominences of the elbow are not frequently compressed, which can lead to radial and ulnar nerve injury [8]. During a prolonged case, it is suggested to alternate arms for NIBP measurement if possible. Even though all nerve tissue has some elasticity, it is limited. Therefore, positions that impose either a large degree or prolonged amount of stretch upon peripheral nerves can also impose neuronal damage [6]. Stretch injuries can cause actual destruction of nerve fibers, alter electrochemical neuronal conduction pathways, or disrupt the vascularity supplying the nerve [4]. The common theme among these injury mechanisms is that each of them result in some manner of ischemia or hypoperfusion to the nerve tissue. Another cause of perioperative nerve dysfunction to consider is metabolic imbalance leading to an unfavorable electrochemical gradient for neuronal transmission [3, 9].

### 8.4.2 Patient and Procedural Risk Factors

There is a general consensus regarding risk factors intrinsic to the patient's condition that increase the risk of peripheral nerve injuries. These include preexisting peripheral neuropathy, diabetes mellitus, hypotension, hypovolemia, hypothermia, peripheral vascular disease, extremes of body habitus, malnutrition, tobacco use, alcoholism, liver disease, chronic and poorly controlled hypertension, anemia, atypical anatomical structure, age greater than 65 years, and male gender [2, 4, 6, 8]. Males are particularly more likely to develop perioperative ulnar neuropathy as compared to females [6]. Procedural risk factors include the specific position used, the length of the procedure, and specific positioning devices used [8, 9].

### 8.4.3 Recommendations

For the prevention of neurological injuries of the upper extremities related to positioning, the following general recommendations have been noted in the literature [2, 4, 6, 8–10]:

- Arm/shoulder abduction in the supine position should be limited to less than 90° on padded arm boards.
- The arm should be in supinated position (palm up) when abducted on padded arm boards; if this is not feasible, then neutral (thumbs up) is the next best option.
- Avoid pronation of the arms and hands in the supine position.
- Position the arms to avoid pressure on the ulnar groove of the elbow and the spiral groove of the humerus (posterior flat surface of the upper arm).
- Avoid both hyperextension and marked flexion of the elbows.
- When tucking arms at the sides, maintain the arms and hands in neutral position (thumbs up and palms inward).
- If using shoulder braces during prolonged Trendelenburg positioning, use a device that distributes the load across the width of the shoulder and avoid the supraclavicular fossa.
- Avoid placing the NIBP cuff near the elbow where it may compress neural structures within the cubital tunnel.

For the prevention of neurological injuries of the lower extremities related to positioning, the following general recommendations have been noted in the literature [2, 4, 6, 8–10]:

- Limit the amount of hip flexion and extension during positioning.
- In lithotomy position, use the least amount of hip and knee flexion that facilitates the procedure, and keep this flexion below 90°.
- Avoid compression against the fibular and tibial heads at the level of the knee during positioning, especially using devices to maintain lithotomy positioning.
- Provide positioning "breaks" for prolonged lithotomy position cases: one suggestion is a 10–15-min break every 3 h, or sooner if risk factors dictate [8].

## 8.5 Respiratory Compromise Related to Procedural Positioning

Every year there have been increases in the volume of sedation cases conducted outside the operating room, in various settings [11]. These can include, but are not limited to, radiology, endoscopy, diagnostic or interventional cardiology, and dental settings. The most common complications to be found in procedural sedation are hemodynamic compromise, respiratory compromise, and needed upgrade of care [2, 11]. The outcome most consistently associated with needed upgrade of care is prolonged respiratory compromise [3, 11]. Nearly all medications used to induce procedural sedation can lead to respiratory compromise. Of note, it has been found by some authors that the locations that have the highest number of respiratory complications are the radiology and cardiology settings [11]. So, vigilance in assessing respiratory function during the sedation procedure is key to patient outcomes.

### 8.5.1 Patient and Procedural Risk Factors

Patient risk factors for respiratory compromise include preexisting pulmonary or cardiac disease, history/risk factors for sleep apnea, obesity, abnormal airway anatomy, alteration in level of consciousness, elderly patients, concurrent medical regimen, and overall medical complexity. Many times, patients receiving procedural sedation for procedures outside of the OR have been disqualified for more definitive procedures under anesthesia, due to preexisting comorbidities [4, 11]. For these reasons, among others, it is imperative that standard monitoring requirements and due vigilance is exercised in procedural sedation. Supplemental oxygen and suctioning equipment should be immediately available and used as needed. Medications and airway equipment to facilitate emergent airway support or endotracheal intubation should be immediately available [2–4].

Positioning should facilitate not only the procedural needs but provide access to the patient by the sedation provider as necessary. This is especially true in order to maintain a patent airway, and to allow for vigilant re-assessment. The supine position leads to more airway obstruction than either the lateral, prone, or semi-recumbent positions [11]. When feasible, the flat supine position should be avoided to mitigate the risk of respiratory compromise from airway obstruction. The supine position should also be avoided if the patient cannot tolerate lying flat due to comorbidities. Although lateral positioning has been found to have a correlation with the incidence of hypotension [11], it should be noted that placing the NIBP on the non-dependent arm can provide artificially low BP readings.

## 8.6 Skin and Tissue Injuries Related to Procedural Positioning

Specific positioning needs during procedures requiring sedation can impart an increased risk of injury to skin and soft tissues. The necessary procedural sedation can impair the patient's own protective reflexes and functional discomfort [3]. Compression and shear forces imparted to the skin and soft tissues impose the risk of injury, including pressure injuries. Pressure injuries impart a large burden of cost to both the facility and the patient, and can confer significant morbidity as well [4, 7]. Therefore, mitigation of these injuries is most beneficial.

### 8.6.1 Patient and Procedural Risk Factors

Risk factors for skin and soft tissue injuries intrinsic to the patient include extremes of body habitus, poor nutritional status, cardiac disease, vascular disease, diabetes mellitus, renal disease, anemia, hypoproteinemia, age greater than 65 years, female vs. male gender, and overall medical complexity [3, 7]. Procedural or extrinsic risk factors include the total length of the procedure, total duration of sedation, total time with diastolic BP less than 50 mm Hg, positioning during the procedure, and incidences of sustained hypothermia [3, 7]. Positions that predisposed to skin or tissue injuries included prone > lateral > supine [7]. Studies have been equivocal in imparting increased risk according to gender. The use of general anesthesia has been confirmed as a specific risk factor for the development of pressure injuries, especially general anesthesia of a duration greater than 4 h [7]. Tissue areas at high risk of developing pressure injuries include the sacral area, flank, back, elbows, and cheeks [7].

### 8.6.2 Recommendations

Several recommendations can diminish the risk of skin and soft tissue injuries during procedural sedation. Careful pre-procedural assessment should guide the optimization of each patient's physical and nutritional status [4]. Vigilant, careful positioning and monitoring during the procedure is paramount. Maintaining hemodynamic stability, especially the avoidance of sustained hypotension, will guard against the development of pressure injuries [3, 7]. Monitoring of the patient's body temperature should be instituted, especially in elderly patients having procedures lasting greater than 1 h. Prevention of hypothermia, including the use of active warming therapies, is beneficial in guarding against soft tissue injury [7]. The use of standard mattresses is recommended over the use of specialized gel mattresses, but foam or gel padding of specific pressure areas is recommended [7]. Planning with the entire procedural team to expedite the time necessary for the procedure and sedation can diminish the time period the patient spends at risk for tissue injury.

## 8.7 Conclusion

Proper patient positioning for procedural sedation is a planned and proactive balancing act that weighs the need of procedural ease and efficiency against patient safety and comfort. As with many aspects of excellent and thoughtful care, individualized alterations upon basic tenets and procedures of safe positioning make it possible to have excellent patient outcomes. This planning of care requires collaboration and accurate communication within the procedural sedation team. The team includes pre-procedural staff, intra-procedural staff, and post-procedural staff and consists of technologists, ancillary staff, nurses, physicians, and advanced practice nurses/providers (Fig. 8.8). Important information relevant to position planning includes (but is not limited to) the preexisting physiological or pathophysiologic status of the patient, pertinent laboratory or imaging findings, assessment findings, knowledge of special operating factors needed for a successful procedure, likely duration of the sedation/procedure, necessary depth of sedation, and any specialized positioning aides to be used. Vigilant monitoring and assessment of the patient during all phases of care yield the best chance of an optimal outcome for both the patient and the procedural team.

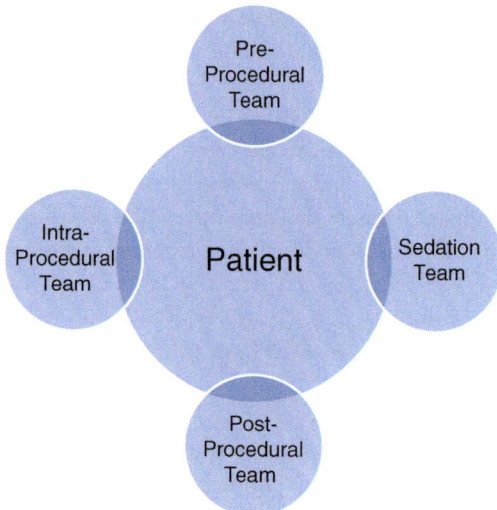

**Fig. 8.8** The interface of the phases of procedural sedation and team members

## References

1. Duffy BJ, Tubog TD. The prevention and recognition of ulnar nerve and brachial plexus injuries. J Perianesth Nurs. 2017;32(6):636–49.
2. Cassorla L, Lee J-W. Patient positioning and associated risks. In: Miller RD, editor. Miller's anesthesia. 8th ed. Philadelphia: Saunders; 2015. p. 1240-1265.
3. Butterworth JF, Mackey DC, Wasnick JD, editors. Morgan & Mikhail's clinical anesthesiology. 6th ed. New York: McGraw Hill; 2018.
4. Thompson JL. Positioning for anesthesia and surgery. In: Nagelhout JJ, Elisha S, editors. Nurse Anesthesia. 6th ed. St. Louis: Elsevier; 2018.
5. Klare P, Huth R, Haller B, Huth M, Weber A, Schlag C, Reindl W, Schmid RM, von Delius S. Patient position and hypoxemia during propofol sedation for colonoscopy: a randomized trial. Endoscopy. 2015;47(12):1159–66.
6. American Society of Anesthesiologists, Inc. Practice advisory for the prevention of perioperative peripheral neuropathies 2018: an updated report by the American Society of Anesthesiologists task force on prevention of perioperative peripheral neuropathies. Anesthesiology. 2018;128(1):11–26.

7. Bulfone G, Bressan V, Morandini A, Stevanin S. Perioperative pressure injuries: a systematic literature review. Adv Skin Wound Care. 2018;31(12):556–64.
8. Hewson DW, Bedforth NM, Hardman JG. Peripheral nerve injury arising in anaesthesia practice. Anaesthesia. 2018;73(Suppl 1):51–60.
9. World Federation of Societies of Anaesthesiologists. 2015 Jan 30. Anaesthesia tutorial of the week; Tutorial 311. https://www.wfsahq.org/components/com_virtual_library/media/a5da94469c304896052227a7b047c785-311-Patient-positioning-during-anaesthesia.pdf. Accessed 18 Mar 2019.
10. Welch MB, Brummett CM, Welch TD, Tremper KK, Shanks AM. Perioperative peripheral nerve injuries: a retrospective study of 380,680 cases during a 10-year period at a single institution. Anesthesiology. 2009;111:490–7.
11. Chang B, Kay A, Diaz JH, Westlake B, Dutton RP, Urman RD. Interventional procedures outside of the operating room: results from the national anesthesia clinical outcomes registry. J Patient Saf. 2018;14(1):9–16.

# Transradial Arterial Access

# 9

Paula Dixon

## 9.1 Introduction

Relatively new to the interventional radiology (IR) world, transradial artery access (TRA) is quickly becoming the preferred primary site for catheterization. TRA's minimally invasive technique, low complication rates, quicker patient recovery, and higher patient satisfaction all lend to this new approach. The superficial location of the radial artery makes it easily accessible regardless of a patient's body habitus and no major nerves or veins are located near common access points. Patent homeostasis is easily achieved due to the radial artery superior position to the radius. Misconceptions about the increased stroke risk, higher radiation doses, and lack of appropriate training have hindered TRA use until recently. Several newly published research articles and meta-analysis studies show that TRA has similar or even fewer complication rates as transfemoral artery access (TFA) and many advantages over the TFA approach. In addition, no increase of neurological complications or radiation exposure to the patient or the procedure room personnel is noted using TRA. These studies also emphasize that the use of TRA in obese patients and patients with a higher risk for bleeding have decreased hemorrhagic and vascular complications, and decreased mortality rates.

Another advantage mentioned frequently in the literature on TRA is the decrease in procedure delays to correct certain coagulopathies that are inherent to the IR patient population. Without the need of costly blood products, the time needed for safe infusion, and the wait while retesting of laboratory values, TRA can result in quicker and less costly interventions. In addition, anticoagulation may not need to be held or reversed. The use of commercial devices to achieve patent homeostasis within moments after sheath removal results often in significantly reduced recovery times and same day discharge. With shorter length of stay, patients spend more time at home and less in the hospital setting increasing patient satisfaction. Patient satisfaction is also higher because unlike TFA the patient can immediately sit up or even ambulate after a procedure instead of spending hours in a supine position with limited mobility. This translates into reduced costs to the institution and the ability to reduce labor costs.

## 9.2 Pre-procedural Planning and Radial Artery Evaluation

One of the most crucial aspects of procedure planning is obtaining safe and effective arterial access. Now with recent advancements in catheter and sheath technology, along with longer

P. Dixon, MSN, RN, CCRN, CEN (✉)
Department of Cardiology,
Medical University of South Carolina,
Charleston, SC, USA

© Springer Nature Switzerland AG 2020
K. A. Gross (ed.), *Advanced Practice and Leadership in Radiology Nursing*,
https://doi.org/10.1007/978-3-030-32679-1_9

rapid exchange systems and wires, IR procedures that were limited to TFA can now be considered for TRA. However, proper technique and equipment approved for use with the TRA approach are paramount to the safety and success of the procedure. Hands on learning workshops help the operator navigate through the common technical radial problems encountered. Before considering TRA as an alternative to TFA, institutions and operators need to ensure the proper training with learned skills and the availability of specialty equipment. Ideally the access site should be determined through the assessment of the individual patient's anticipated anatomical variants and pathologic conditions resulting in the safest approach. Selection of the correct vessel should be done before the patient arrives in the procedure suite. Pre-procedural evaluation plays an important role in determining the best treatment plan based on the individual patient's needs and preexisting factors. Previous procedures and surgeries, body habitus and obesity, concern for possible bleeding due to pharmacological therapies or organ dysfunction, and previous patient experience should all factor into initial access site consideration.

Whenever radial artery access is being considered, pre-procedural evaluation ensures a relatively low complication rate. Ensuring adequate collateral perfusion to the hand is critical before cannulation is achieved. The deep palmar arch is formed by the radial artery (laterally) and the deep palmar branch of the ulnar artery (medially) (Fig. 9.1a). The two most commonly used tests are the Allen and Barbeau. Using the Allen and/or Barbeau tests and measuring the diameter of the artery through sonographic evaluation ensures adequate circulation to the hand through the ulnar artery in case of radial artery spasming or other complications. Before proceeding with further testing ensuring a palpable radial pulse is mandatory.

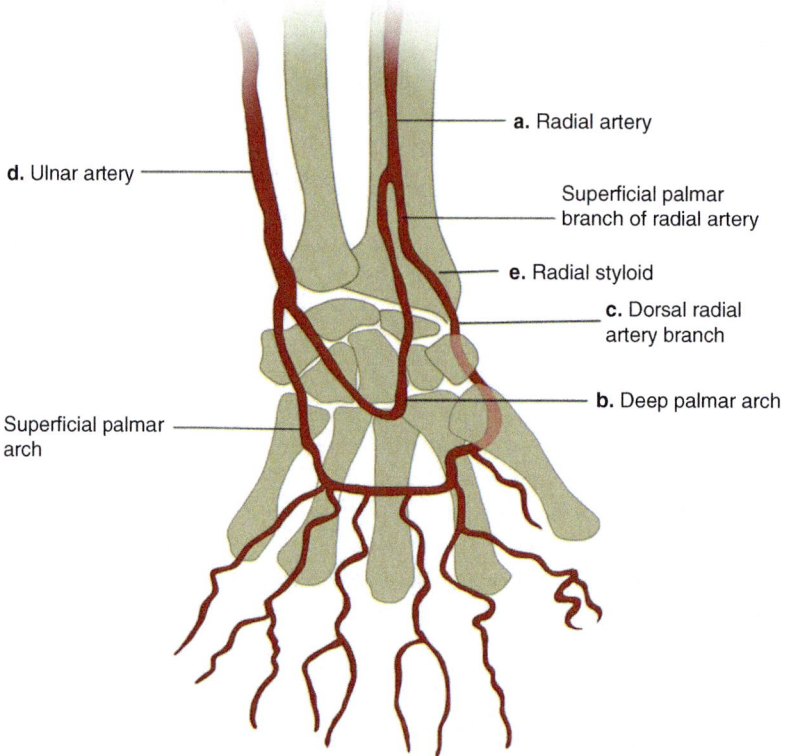

**Fig. 9.1** Anatomy of the hand with the (**a**) radial artery, (**b**) deep palmer arch, (**c**) dorsal radial artery branch (**d**) ulnar artery and (**e**) radial styloid. (Source: Marisa Dixon)

## 9.2.1 Allen Test

The Allen test is performed by first having the patient make a fist. The evaluator then occludes both the radial and ulnar arteries. The patient then opens the hand which should appear blanched with pallor at the fingernails. Release of the ulnar artery occlusion should result with the return of normal capillary refill within 3–10 s. This is considered a normal Allen's test, and ensures a complete palmar arch (Fig. 9.1a) confirming that radial access can be considered.

## 9.2.2 Barbeau Test

Unlike the Allen's test the Barbeau test involves the use of pulse oximetry and is considered a more sensitive test excluding only 1.5% of patients. A pulse oximetry probe is placed on either the thumb or index finger, the area of the hand supplied by the radial artery. After noting a waveform the ulnar and radial arteries are then occluded which causes the waveform to either dampen or flatline. The ulnar artery is released and a waveform should reappear or undampen. The Barbeau classifies the results as Barbeau type A, B, C, and D (Fig. 9.2). Patients with Barbeau type A, B, and C are considered candidates for radial access. In Barbeau type A, no change in waveform is seen. Barbeau type B occurs when the waveform is temporarily dampened but returns to normal amplitude after occlusion of the ulnar artery is released. Barbeau type C is defined as the flatline of the waveform during ulnar occlusion and a return of a dampened waveform after ulnar release. Barbeau type D is the flatline of the waveform after ulnar occlusion with a continued flatline after ulnar release for 2 min or longer. Barbeau type D is not recommended for radial access.

## 9.2.3 Ultrasonographic Evaluation

Once a patient is deemed eligible for radial access cannulation, the most appropriate sheath size can then be determined with the assistance of ultrasonography evaluation. The artery is visualized approximately 1 cm above the styloid process with the ultrasound machine setup to measure the anterior-posterior (AP) diameter. The artery is measured from inner wall to inner wall. Careful attention should be taken to

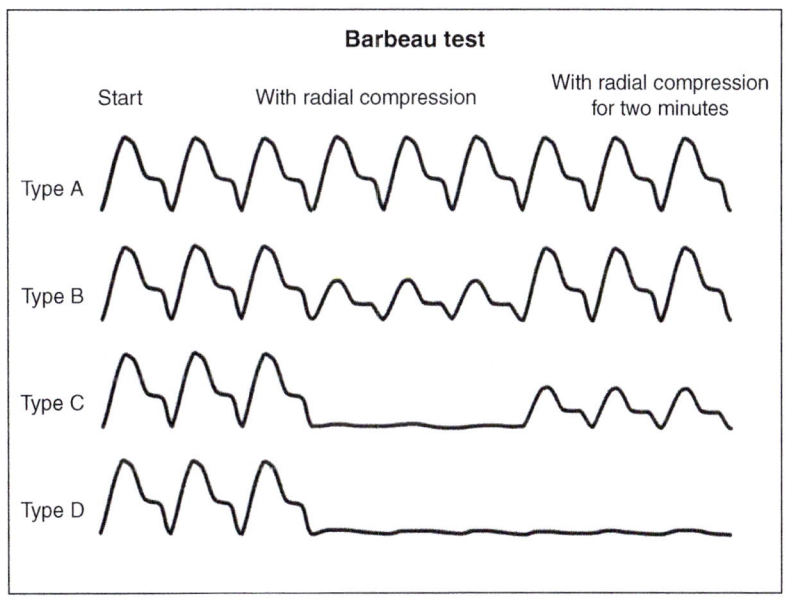

**Fig. 9.2** Barbeau Type A, B, C, D. (Source: Marisa Dixon)

avoid excessive compression while measuring which could result in an underestimate of the true AP diameter. A minimum of 1.8 mm is recommended; however, diameters as small as 1.6 have been successfully accessed. If prior radial access has been obtained scanning the artery to the brachial artery bifurcation is advised. The size of the inner diameter should either be printed from the machine or documented in the patient's record for future considerations.

### 9.2.4 Selection and Contraindications for Radial Access

Patients with a positive Allen test and/or Barbeau type A, B, or C with a radial artery diameter of 1.6 or greater are candidates for the radial approach. Sheath determination is based on the radial artery diameter and can range from 4 French to 7 French depending on the manufacturer's recommendations, with the most common access using a 5 or 6 French. The mean diameter of radial arteries measured by ultrasound is 2.6. Absolute contraindications for use of upper extremity access include same side dialysis graft, patient refusal, absence of radial pulses, and known asymptomatic radial stenosis calcification. Relative contraindications include abnormal tests for dual circulation, upper extremity vascular disease, patients with chronic renal failure that may require future permanent dialysis access and operator inexperience. Alternative upper extremity sites are discussed in Sect. 9.6.

### 9.3 Setup and Positioning

The patient's arm can be positioned in several different ways. The most common is to position the patient's arm next to their side mimicking groin access and allowing for equipment used to be placed on the sterile drape the same as TFA (Fig. 9.3). The use of a slide board can help in the positioning and securing of the arm. There are several commercial immobilization devices available specifically to help optimize access and stabilize the wrist throughout the procedure (Fig. 9.4a). Slight hyperextension of the wrist can also be achieved with the use of a rolled-up towel directly under the access site (Fig. 9.5a).

The arm can also be positioned and maintained abducted at a 70- to 90-degree angle (Fig. 9.5b)

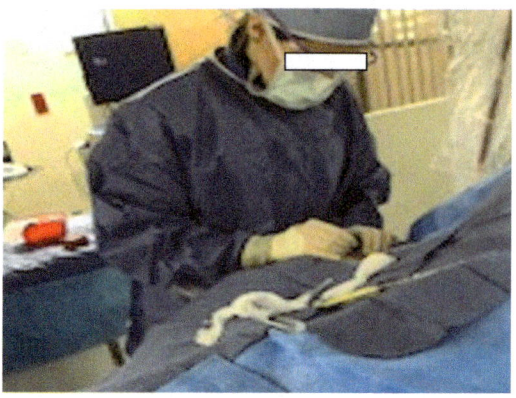

**Fig. 9.3** Right radial access. Right radial access with arm adjacent to groin, note the operator is in the same position as TFA

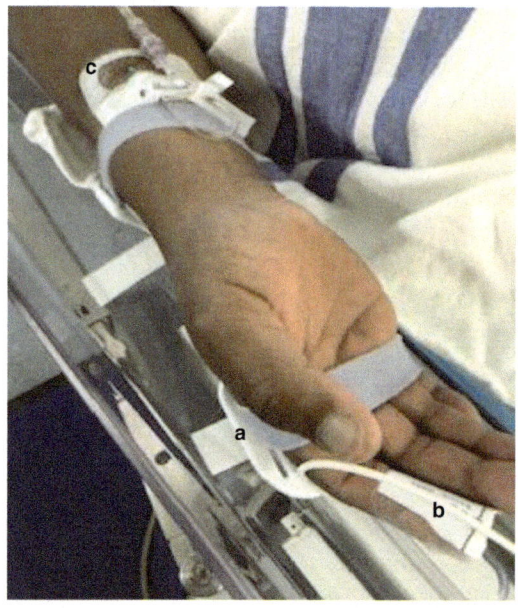

**Fig. 9.4** Use of wrist positioning device and arm board. (**a**) Use of a wrist positioning device. The device is hooked onto the arm board for stabilization and optimal wrist placement. (**b**) The pulse ox is placed on the index finger for monitoring radial artery patency during the procedure. (**c**) An IV is placed ipsilateral and out of the area where the procedure will occur

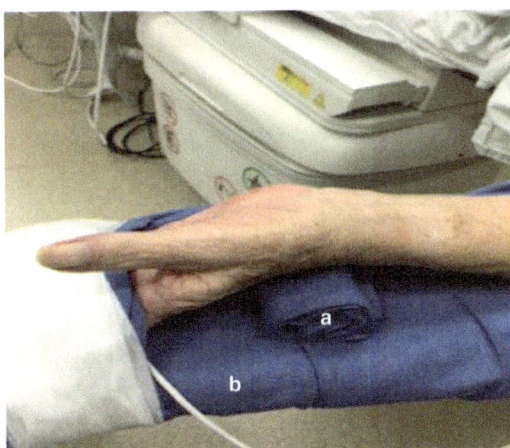

**Fig. 9.5** Left radial access. (**a**) Use of a rolled-up towel for hyperextension of the left wrist. Note the fingers are secured in a pocket made with towels and the pulse ox in place for monitoring. (**b**) A padded arm board is used to abduct the left arm to facilitate radial access insertion

with the use of an arm board. While this may initially help the operator gain access, it is more difficult to exchange devices and limits the movement of fluoroscopy equipment, requiring delays while the arm is repositioned closer to the body for certain fluoroscopy scans. If the left radial site is required, access can be obtained on the left side and the patient's hand can be positioned over the lower abdomen/groin area to facilitate working from the preferred right side. Determining left versus right radial access depends on the type of procedure and equipment available. For procedures below the diaphragm, left-sided access is recommended because of the shorter distance to the target area. Although the difference may only be several centimeters, this helps ensure that correct catheter lengths are available. Using left TRA also prevents the sheath or guiding catheters from being positioned over the great vessels in the aorta and theoretically decreases the chance of cerebral embolus or thrombus formation.

Avoidance of radial artery spasming is key to ensure access. Medications for sedation and utilization of lidocaine for infiltration help prevent radial spasming. Other techniques involve topical anesthetic cream applied to the wrist in the preprocedural setting. This helps reduce the amount of lidocaine used to infiltrate over the access site and decrease the chance of obscuring the radial pulse. Nitroglycerine (NTG) ointment can also be applied on the site to help with dilation and decrease radial artery spasming. Another strategy involves mixing NTG 200 micrograms in 1 mm with lidocaine 1% for infiltration. This not only helps reduce the chances of arterial spasming and but also helps predilate the artery.

Placing a pulse oximetry probe on the thumb or forefinger of the arm being accessed helps identify arterial spasming (Fig. 9.4b). Ideally intravenous (IV) access should be in the contralateral arm. If this is not possible, then an IV placed in the ipsilateral arm should be as far away as possible from the access site to ensure proper prepping and homeostasis can be achieved (Fig. 9.4c). A common place for blood pressure monitoring is on the patient's legs, as to not interfere with IV infusions.

## 9.4 Radial Access and Sheath Introduction

The wrist area is prepped following sterile technique with a standard antiseptic scrub solution. The area prepped extends from the upper palm to the right and left lateral points, and five-finger breadths above the radial artery pulsation. The drape is placed with the fenestrated area over where the radial pulse is palpable. The point of access is 1–2 cm proximal to the radial styloid (Fig. 9.1b). A sterile marker should be used to mark where the entry should take place. The most common method to obtain access is with ultrasound guidance and the Seldinger technique using a micropuncture needle (Fig. 9.6). Alternative methods include a modified Seldinger technique. Similar to the standard Seldinger technique the needle, catheter, guidewire, and sheath are all parts of a single radial access kit. Dilators included with the radial sheaths are tapered to 0.018 in. to allow sheath introduction without an incision or wire exchange. Access can also be obtained by the use of an angiocath needle. The angiocath technique differs in the Seldinger and modified Seldinger method because of the use of a through-and-through approach. The angiocath

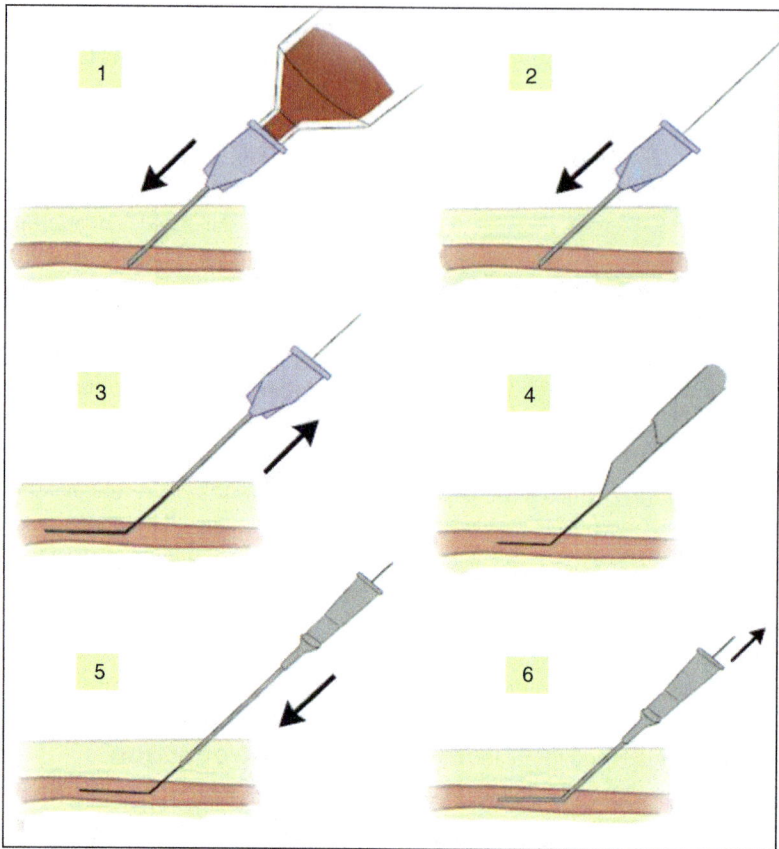

**Fig. 9.6** Seldinger technique. Step 1. After proper skin prep and sterile draping, the radial artery is palpated. The skin is entered at approximately a 30–45°. When the needle is through the skin, the operator begins pulling back on the plunger of the syringe. Needle advancement is stopped when blood (flash) starts to enter into the syringe. The needle is stabilized in place with the operator's non-dominant hand and then the syringe is removed. With the same hand that is stabilizing the needle in place, place the thumb over the hub to prevent both blood loss or to prevent air from entering the needle. (Air entering the needle can lead to an air embolism if negative pressure is created.) Step 2. The guide wire in then carefully inserted into the hub of the needle and advanced. There should be no resistance while advancing the guide wire. Resistance could mean the guide wire is no longer inside the lumen of the vessel, dissection of the vessel wall has occurred, thrombus is present, or vessel spasm is occurring. Step 3. When the guide wire is at the appropriate place, the operator should continue to hold onto the guide wire and retract the needle. While holding the guide wire in place, the operator removes the needle from the guide wire. Step 4. If enlargement of the insertion site is needed to place a larger catheter, a #11 blade scalpel is used. Care is needed to avoid touching the blood vessel. Step 5. While the operator holds the guide wire, the distal end of the catheter is placed over the tip of the guide wire and the catheter is advanced until the guide wire comes out of the catheter. The operator advances the catheter into the vessel while still maintaining a hold on the guide wire. Step 6. Once the catheter is in the vessel, the guide wire is very gently removed. After catheter placement is confirmed (blood return verified and then flushed per protocol) it is secured in place per routine. (Source: Marisa Dixon)

needle is sent through the posterior wall of the radial artery under direct palpation and then slowly pulled back until blood appears in the chamber. This method ensures access through the true lumen of the vessel. Preference of access should be determined by the operator skill and the equipment available.

Regardless of technique implemented, if any resistance while advancing the wire is met, fluoroscopy for direct visualization should be used. Once the wire is able to be advanced only a sheath with a hydrophilic coating is recommended. Research demonstrates the lubricating polymers of the coating, not the length or size of the sheath, reduce the likelihood of arterial wall irritation, spasming, and associated pain [1].

Once the sheath is introduced, a "radial cocktail" is utilized. Medications are given intra-arterially directly into the sheath and/or intravenously. These cocktails are used to help prevent arterial spasm, relax vascular tone, and reduce clotting. Nitrates and/or calcium channel blockers in combination with heparin or bivalirudin are used in various amounts and combinations and given at certain time intervals. This practice varies greatly in different institutions with no current consensus on an ideal amount or frequency in the interventional community.

If the sheath moves easily, advance it to the hub. If resistance is met during sheath introduction and placement has been verified through fluoroscopy, remove the wire and inject a vasodilator directly into the sheath (nitroglycerin 100–200 μg, verapamil 2.5–5 mg, and nicardipine hydrochloride 500–1000 μg). Reinsert the wire and the dilator and continue to advance under fluoroscopic guidance. Once the sheath is in place, flushed, and medications to reduce spasming are given, the sheath can be secured using a clear plastic covering or a suture.

Once the sheath is secured, the arm can be repositioned if needed to prepare for catheter insertion. A catheter is advanced with the use of a guidewire. A standard 0.035-in. J-wire is most commonly used with a small J-curve. A J-curve is recommended as it helps with steerability and prevents the wire from entering into small branches. Other wires can be used based on operator preference and experience. A coated hydrophilic wire may be used with caution because of the ability to easily travel into smaller vessels or become subintimal, thus increasing the potential of perforating a vessel. If any resistance of the wire and/or catheter is met while advancing up the arm fluoroscopy can be used with small "puffs" of contrast to ensure proper placement into central circulation. Fluoroscopy is always used when reaching the central circulation to ensure a safe passage through the aorta. Once the guiding catheter has passed into the aorta procedural catheters and wire selection will be based on the final destination and the procedure.

## 9.5 Patent Homeostasis in TRA

Patent homeostasis is the balance between applying just enough pressure to avoid bleeding or oozing but not so much pressure as to cause tissue necrosis or nerve damage and artery occlusion. This concept is demonstrated when manual pressure is held on the femoral artery and distal pulses are checked to ensure there is still blood flow. Patent homeostasis begins with preprocedural planning. The Allen and Barbeau test, anticoagulation, appropriate sheath size selection with ultrasonography, limiting the number of sheath and catheter exchanges, and patent homeostasis all play a vital role in minimizing the risk for radial artery occlusion. With a skilled operator and well-trained team these measures are instituted routinely. The goal of TRA is the maintenance of radial artery patency to ensure future use. Awareness to the importance of long-term patency should be a hallmark in all levels of training and education.

### 9.5.1 Sheath Removal and Post-procedure Care

A number of commercial devices are available for homeostasis. The more common designs involve a clear plastic bracelet that allows for visualization of the access site (Fig. 9.7a). These devices have some kind of bladder for air to be added into and then gradually removed after a certain amount of time. The device is placed on the wrist and over the sheath prior to sheath removal. Although instructions will greatly vary depending on the type of homeostasis device used. Regardless of the device there are several critical steps to follow. Place the devices around the wrist, ensuring the appropriate size based on the options and manufacturer recommendations. The compressing component of the device should be over the entire insertion site including any skin nicks and the sheath. A piece of gauze can also be placed under the sheath. This allows for any blood to be wicked onto the gauze (Fig. 9.7b). The device is then injected with a predetermined amount of air (usually 15–20 mL)

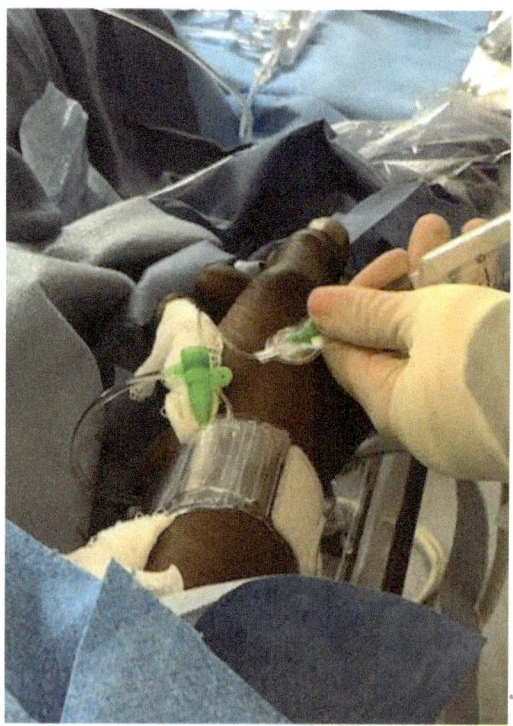 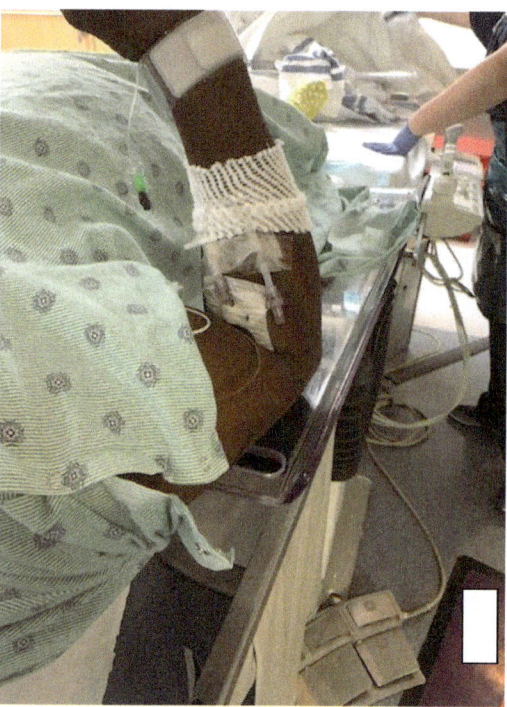

**Fig. 9.7** Wristband for homeostasis. A syringe with air being injected into the bladder of the wristband. A piece of gauze is used to wick away blood after proper amount of air is determined

**Fig. 9.8** Patient transfer technique. Patient using elbow to transfer back to stretcher immediately after placement of wristband

while the sheath is then slowly removed. Ideally the air should be injected as the sheath is slowly retracted. Patent homeostasis is accomplished once there is no active bleeding and the patient is free from pain or discomfort from overfilling of the device. After the device is applied patients are instructed to place no pressure on the hand or wrist and to continue to not use the wrist or hand while the device is still on. The patient is instructed to use their elbow to help transfer and reposition after the procedure (Figs. 9.8 and 9.9). If the patient is still sedated or having difficulty remembering instructions, the immobilization device used during the procedure can remain in place.

- To ensure there is no radial artery occlusion a reverse Barbeau test can be performed by occluding the ulnar artery and ensuring a waveform on the pulse oximetry reading. If type A, B, or C is seen with radial artery compression patent homeostasis is confirmed. If Barbeau type D occurs, air should be released; if bleeding occurs, reinsert the air and move the patient to the recovery area. Repeat the test after 15 min. Patent homeostasis can often be achieved after a short amount of compression time. Staff involved in the care of the patient while the compression device is utilized should be well versed in assessing for patent homeostasis and monitoring of the extremity to ensure there is no ischemia or hematoma formation. Until the practice of TRA access is well established in the institution, any findings suspicious of hematoma and/or hand pain, unrelieved with deflation of the device, requires *immediate* notification of the interventionalist. Mild hematoma formation can be treated with analgesics, an ice pack and/or the use of another compression device or blood pressure cuff. Frequent assessment and early detection of hematoma formation are crucial to avoiding complications. Ensuring that the same high standards of care occur in the post-procedure area as in the pre- and intra-

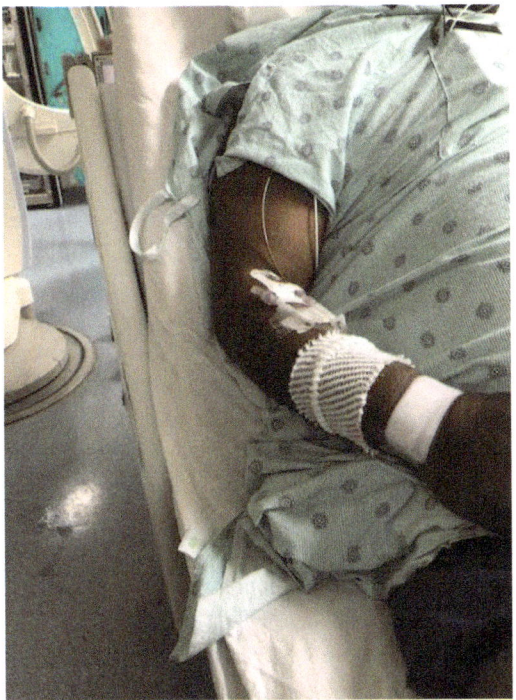

**Fig. 9.9** Patient transfer onto stretcher. Patient using elbow to sit up immediately after placement of homeostasis device and transfer onto stretcher

procedure setting is essential to ensure there is no radial artery occlusion and the artery is preserved for future use.

Protocols for the post-procedure area vary greatly but for most institutions standard site checks are done the same as for femoral access with no removal of air from the device for 60–90 min. Air removal standards also vary greatly but are usually done every 15 min and 1–4 mL of air or one-fourth of the initial total amount of air inserted into the device is removed. Most recovery areas start with a minimal amount of air removal and gradually increase the amount. If bleeding is noted after air removal, the air is reinserted for another 15 min, then removal can be attempted again withdrawing a smaller amount of volume. Usual deflation takes about an hour. Patient compliance with restricted wrist usage is critical to ensure deflation can occur in a timely manner. If noncompliance with wrist restrictions is observed, the securement device used during the procedure or other type of arm board device can be applied to help limit the movement of the wrist. Once the compression device is completely deflated it remains on the wrist for another 60 min in case reinsertion of air is necessary. A dressing is placed over the site for 24 h. The average time in from placement to removal of the hemostasis device is 3 h. After the device is removed the patient can be discharged or released to an area that is not familiar with post-radial access care. Patient discharge instructions focus mainly on limited use of the arm for 5–7 days and not lifting anything heavier than five pounds with the hand.

## 9.6 Alternate Sites to TRA Access

Good pre-procedural planning includes always determining and prepping a backup site. Although many institutions still use the TFA as backup if TRA access cannot be achieved, studies have shown that transulnar artery (TUA) access and dorsal transradial artery access (dTRA) or "snuffbox" access can also be acceptable backups or even primary sites if TRA is unsuccessful or contraindicated [2, 3]. Both sites have similar reduced major vascular and bleeding complications and offer the patient the same benefits of early patient ambulation, and reduced hospital stay when compared with TFA. All members of the health care team should anticipate a small amount of TRA complications regardless of the amount of preparation and testing when determining TRA eligibility. The majority of complications present themselves during initial TRA attempts. Artery spasming, smaller than expected inner artery diameter, radial stenosis calcification, tortuosity in any part of the artery, and other anatomic issues can all be causes to unsuccessful TRA.

### 9.6.1 Ulnar Artery Access

Since the ulnar artery is not as superficial as the radial artery, palpation is more difficult. To palpate the ulnar artery, hyperextend the hand and palpate at the fold of the wrist. Hyperextension of the wrist is critical for a successful procedure. Most common complications involve inability to advance the wire despite adequate blood flow.

TUA is not considered a primary site due to transulnar cannulation failure results and should only be attempted by highly skilled interventionalists [3]. After successful TUA access the intra- and post-procedure care is identical to that of TRA.

### 9.6.2 Distal Transradial Artery Access

Distal transradial artery access (dTRA or "snuffbox" access) involves the sheath insertion on the back of the hand in the anatomical location where the dorsal radial artery can be palpated, known as the "snuffbox." This access is preferable for patients who are unable to supinate their wrists due to orthopedic injuries and decreased range of motion. It can also be used instead of left TRA so the arm can be pronated towards the right side of the patient for right-sided procedures. The arm is placed in a neutral position with a rolled-up towel or rolled-up gauze placed in the hand to maintain neutrality. The dorsal radial artery is superficially located and may have one or two veins surrounding it. Ultrasound guidance is recommended for the same reasons as traditional TRA. Traditional TRA bands tend to move out of position too easily with the most subtle movements of the wrist in this area and are not recommended. Instead patent homeostasis is achieved with the use of a bulky pressure dressing using gauze and an elastic wrap. Staff are instructed to monitor the site with the same guidelines as TRA but since the dressing tends to loosen over time little manipulation of the area is required. Slow release of pressure usually occurs without assistance from the staff; however, the same attentiveness to site assessment is required.

### 9.7 Conclusion

TRA has been successfully performed by interventional cardiologists for three decades. In many practices cardiologists believe in the "radial first" approach, and it is quickly becoming the standard of care. In 2015, the European Society of Cardiology (ESC) gave the highest degree of recommendation for TRA over the TFA approach for coronary angiography and percutaneous coronary intervention in patients with acute coronary syndrome without persistent ST-segment elevations citing its superior results in fewer events concerning major bleeding, vascular complications, and on reducing all causes of mortality [4]. This endorsement also cautioned to ensure proficiency is maintained in both the TRA and the TFA approach, as both access sites are indispensable in the care of all heart disease patients. Many advocates for the TRA approach anticipate that following the recommendations of the ESC many other organizations will join in concluding that radial access is an equal and valuable approach. In 2018, the American Heart Association (AHA) published a scientific statement to affirm and recommend the "radial-first" strategy for patients with acute coronary syndrome in the United States [5]. With all the praise given to the TRA approach the benefits attributed emphasize there is a steep learning curve. To optimize procedural outcomes and success rates emphasis is attributed to expertise and skill of the operator and institution in the pre-, intra-, and post-procedure settings.

### References

1. Fischman AM, Swinburne NC, Patel RS. A technical guide describing the use of transradial access technique for endovascular interventions. Tech Vasc Interv Radiol. 2015;18(2):58–65. https://doi.org/10.1053/j.tvir.2015.04.002.
2. Zybulewski A, Edwards M, Nowakowski FS, Patel R, Tabori N, Lookstein R, Fischman A. Transulnar approach as an alternative to transradial approach in non-coronary intervention: safety, feasibility and technical factors. J Vasc Access. 2017;18(3):250–4. https://doi.org/10.5301/jva.5000691.2017.
3. Hahalis G, Deftereos S, Bertrand OF. Ulnar artery: the Ulysses ultimate resort for coronary procedures. Hell J Cardiol. 2016;57(4):238. https://doi.org/10.1016/j.hjc.2016.07.006.
4. Roffi M, et al. 2015 ESC guidelines for the management of acute coronary syndromes in patients presenting without persistent ST-segment elevation: task force for the management of acute coronary syndromes in patients presenting without persistent ST-segment elevation of the European society of cardiology (ESC). OUP Academic, Oxford University Press,

14 Jan 2016, https://academic.oup.com/eurheartj/article/37/3/267/2466099.

5. Mason BJ, Shah B, Tamis-Holland JE, Bittl JA, Cohen MG, Safirstein J, Drachman DE, Valle JA, Rhodes D, Gilchrist IC. An update on radial artery access and best practices for transradial coronary angiography and intervention in acute coronary syndrome: a scientific statement from the American Heart Association. Circ Cardiovasc Interv. 2018;11:e000035. https://doi.org/10.1161/HCV.0000000000000035.

# Section III

# Safety in Radiology

# Contrast Reactions

## 10

Alexandra Penzias and Gloria M. Salazar

## 10.1 Introduction

Contrast media is used to enhance visibility of soft tissue structures during computer axial tomography (CT), magnetic resonance imaging (MRI), ultrasound imaging (US), and diagnostic imaging (DI), as well as to enhance the vasculature in interventional radiology (IR). Contrast media are given orally, rectally, intracavitary, and intravascularly [1]. Approximately half of the 76 million CT scans and 34 million magnetic resonance imaging studies are performed with the use of intravenous contrast agents [2]. The goal of the administration of contrast media is a high concentration of contrast in body tissues with minimal systemic effects [3]. While contrast media are generally considered safe, they are not without risk, with reactions ranging from mild and self-limiting, to life threatening [2].

### 10.1.1 Staff Responsibility

Clinicians caring for patients undergoing contrast-enhanced imaging must be trained in early identification and management of acute contrast reactions. For leaders in the radiology setting, understanding the risks associated with contrast, development, and implementation of evidence-based protocols for screening patients prior to imaging, acute contrast reaction management, and a comprehensive plan for provision of team education are essential to ensuring the safe care of patients undergoing contrast-enhanced imaging. Routine refresher in-services, possibly including simulations, are needed.

## 10.2 Types of Intravascular Contrast Media

Iodine-based intravascular contrast agents can be divided according to osmolarity (high, low, or iso-), ionicity (ionic or nonionic), and the number of benzene rings (monomer or dimer) [2]. Currently nonionic low or iso-osmolar preparations are used almost exclusively for intravascular injections. Low-osmolar contrast agents are associated with significantly lower rates of acute reactions compared with high-osmolar agents. Gadolinium chelates, approved for intravascular use for MR imaging, are extremely well tolerated, with relatively few acute reactions and discomfort but the clinician should be aware reactions can occur. For more information on MR contrast agents, refer to the American College of Radiology Manual on

A. Penzias, DNP, MEd, APRN, ACNS-BC (✉)
Cooley Dickinson Hospital, Northampton, MA, USA

G. M. Salazar, MD
Department of Radiology, Massachusetts General Hospital, Boston, MA, USA

Contrast Media v10.3 (May 2018; Available on line at https://www.acr.org/Clinical-Resources/Contrast-Manual) and the manufacturer product inserts.

### 10.2.1 Physiological Effects of Intravascular Contrast Media Injection

Contrast media are known to cause certain physiological effects including peripheral vasodilation with temporary increase in heart rate, feeling of warmth, complement activation, osmotic diuresis, renal tubular effects, and vasoactive substance release, e.g., histamine. These are believed to be due to the chemical makeup and osmolar attributes of the contrast media. It is important to note that the low-osmolar and iso-osmolar agents have a lower incidence of these effects and have become the community standard for intravascular procedures as they are better tolerated by the patient. The amount of the contrast administered will affect the extent of some physiological effects. It is prudent to keep the amount of contrast to a minimum needed for the specific procedure image requirements and according to the patient assessment.

### 10.2.2 Contrast-Enhanced Ultrasound

Contrast-enhanced ultrasound (CEU) is an ultrasound study enhanced by the intravenous or intracavitary administration of microbubbles or microspheres. Ultrasound contrast agents have a similar safety profile to those used for CT and MR. There is insufficient evidence regarding the risk of ultrasound contrast media in pregnant women. Ultrasound contrast agents are contraindicated for intra-arterial administration, and in patients with previous hypersensitivity to microspheres. Unlike CT contrast, ultrasound contrast agents have no known renal toxicity when administered at approved doses [4].

## 10.3 Patient Safety

There are multiple elements to ensuring patient comfort and safety in the administration of contrast media. Having established protocols for the type and amount of contrast to be administered for imaging, who may administer contrast, and screening patients for conditions that identify patient conditions in which the administration of contrast media are contraindicated are essential. Contrast media are considered a medication, subsequently they should be stored in a secured, temperature-controlled environment. Warming contrast may facilitate ease of injection by reducing the viscosity and reducing injection discomfort during contrast injection in the patient [4]. Prior to injection, contrast should be inspected for expiration date, possible contamination, or particulate matter and administered through a large bore intravascular device or power-injectable centrally placed vascular catheter. Proper identification of a power-injectable device is mandatory prior to injection; patency should also be verified. Following administration, type of contrast, dose, and patient reaction should be documented in the patient medical record, and any observed patient reaction to contrast should be documented (and noted in the imaging report), reported in the hospital safety event reporting system, and communicated to the referring provider or team.

### 10.3.1 General Risks

For any procedure, clinicians must weigh the risk-to-benefit ratio for the patient. Patients have a right to make informed decisions about the care that they receive; subsequently ordering providers are obligated to communicate those risks to the patient prior to the test or intervention. For this reason, most institutions require a separate consent for the administration of contrast media; at some institutions the consent for contrast maybe implied or included in the procedure consent. Staff should adhere to the policies and procedures for contrast administration.

Children, the elderly, pregnant women, patients with heart disease, diabetes, sickle cell disease, or renal disease (or solo kidney), or those taking medications such as beta blockers, metformin, or nephrotoxic medications (e.g., chemotherapy or certain antibiotics) may require additional consideration prior to contrast-enhanced imaging [4]. All patients should be screened for previous allergic reaction to iodinated contrast and queried regarding the symptoms, extent of the reaction, and known treatment. Patients with an allergic history may be given a premedication with steroids or be advised to have a non-contrast study, have a study using another modality, e.g., ultrasound when feasible, or for a select group of interventional procedures, using carbon dioxide in place of contrast, as the best option.

### 10.3.2 Contrast-Associated Risks with Metformin

Metformin is a biguanide administered alone or in combination with other drugs for the treatment of type 2 diabetes mellitus, as well as polycystic ovarian syndrome. Metformin decreases production of glucose by the liver and enhances peripheral glucose uptake [4]. Metformin is excreted unchanged by the kidneys. Patients taking metformin with normal renal function are not at higher risk for post-contrast acute kidney injury (PC-AKI) [4]. Iodinated contrast is a potential risk for patients with renal impairment, and patients with acute or chronic impairment of renal function may be at greater risk of developing metformin-related lactic acidosis following the administration of contrast media [4, 5].

Proper screening of patients specific to renal function and medication use is essential to protecting patients from the risk of acute kidney injury following contrast administration (see Table 10.1 Guidelines for patients on metformin).

For guidance regarding the care of patients using metformin (and metformin combination medications) following contrast administration, refer to guidelines such as those published by

**Table 10.1** Guidelines for patients on metformin

*Category I*
In patients with no evidence of AKI and eGFR ≥30 mL/min/1.73 m$^2$—there is no need to hold metformin or recheck renal function following the administration of contrast [4, 6]

*Category II [4]*
In patients with known kidney dysfunction (stage IV or V), or eGFR<30 mL/min/1.73 m$^2$, or those undergoing arterial catheter studies associated with increased risk of emboli, metformin should be withheld at the time or prior to procedure and for 48 h following the study and reinstated only following reevaluation of renal function (ACR, 2018)

Source: ACR Manual on Contrast Media v 10.3

American College of Radiology, publish guidelines specific to the management of contrast-related emergencies (https://www.acr.org/Clinical-Resources/Contrast-Manual).

Department-specific protocols regarding metformin must be accessible by all staff and communicated both within the department and to referring providers requesting contrast-enhanced imaging of their patients taking metformin, in order that patients can be prescribed alternative agents for blood sugar management, as well as directions regarding the need for follow-up evaluation of creatinine. Additionally, patient education materials, specific to holding metformin, should be made available in radiology settings where contrast is administered.

### 10.3.3 Acute Kidney Injury

Post-contrast acute kidney injury (PC-AKI) is defined as deterioration in renal function which presents within 48 h of contrast administration [4]. Acute kidney injury (AKI) is poorly understood and may be caused in combination from contrast agent, dose and renal hemodynamic changes. It is a complication which can lead to increased morbidity and mortality [7]. Contrast-induced nephropathy (CIN) is a sudden deterioration in renal function following the intravenous injection of contrast and is therefore a subcategory of PC-AKI [4]. Routine testing of blood serum creatinine according to guidelines established by the American College of Radiology [4] should be considered in select patients, such as those with preexisting elevated serum creatinine clearance. A calculated estimated glomerular filtration rate (eGFR) may be the best index for evaluating renal dysfunction in those with risk of nephrotoxicity.

Volume expansion may reduce risk for PC-AKI. Only isotonic crystalloid hydration has been shown to reduce the incidence of kidney injury in at-risk populations although numerous other medications have been researched [4, 7]. Many other measures have been tested in the past, but none have proven to be of clinical value. Hydration should be done cautiously in certain patients, for example, those with cardiac disease.

Screening vulnerable populations for renal function, by calculating eGFR, prior to contrast injection, is essential in minimizing the possibility of PC-AKI [4, 7]. Guidelines for patient populations who should be screened prior to the administration of contrast should be established and based on existing recommendations available through societies such as the American College of Radiology (ACR), Royal Australian and New Zealand College of Radiologists (RANZCR), the Royal College of Radiologists (RCR), or the European Society of Urogenital Radiology (ESUR). Concern regarding risk for acute kidney injury(AKI) is a relative risk for future administration of contrast but does warrant careful risk-benefit analysis prior to subsequent contrast injection [4]. Gadolinium-based contrast media are not associated with post-contrast-induced nephropathy but may cause nephrogenic systemic fibrosis (NSF) in patients with preexisting renal compromise.

## 10.4 Extravasation of Contrast Media

Although extravasation is not considered a contrast reaction, providers may have to deal with a contrast media extravasation of varying severity. Extravasation occurs when contrast material infiltrates the interstitial tissue during injection. The reported incidence of contrast extravasation related to CT power injection of contrast media is 0.1–1.2% [4]. Extravasation of contrast media has been associated with skin ulceration, tissue necrosis, and compartment syndrome [8].

### 10.4.1 Prevention of Extravasation

Prior to the administration of contrast media, patients must be assessed for venous access capable of supporting power injection (1.5–3 mL/s). A peripheral intravenous, placed in a sufficient vein (antecubital) or a power-injectable implanted vascular access device (port-a-cath), power-injectable peripherally inserted central catheter (PICC), or small-bore tunneled catheter that is secured, position is verified, demonstrates good venous return, and flushes easily is optimal for the administration of intravenous contrast.

The most effective methods for identifying extravasation are (a) directly palpating the catheter venipuncture site during the initial seconds of injection, and (b) asking the patient to report any sensation of pain or swelling at the injection site [2]. Patients experiencing extravasation may be asymptomatic, or complain of burning, pain, tingling, redness, or swelling at the injection site [2, 4]. If extravasation is recognized during contrast injection, immediately halting injection is essential to minimizing tissue damage. There is no consensus regarding whether the application of warm or cold compresses is associated with minimizing tissue damage after an extravasation [4]. Patients who develop pain, swelling, decreased capillary refill, change in sensation, skin ulceration, or blistering should be referred for a surgical consult [4, 9]. The condition of the site should be assessed immediately and then on the following days as the initial injury may *not* be truly reflective of the extent of the damage [4, 9]. It is important that patients understand how to follow-up with an extravasation injury and have written instructions with contact numbers.

## 10.5 Special Populations

Some patients need additional consideration prior to contrast administration.

### 10.5.1 Children

There is limited research to examine the impact of low-osmolar contrast media or gadolinium-containing contrast media in children. Numerous factors distinguish contrast administration in children compared to administration to an adult: smaller volumes, smaller intravenous catheter sizes and vessels, and immature renal and immune system should be considered prior to contrast administration. Neonates and small children are particularly vulnerable to fluid shifts due to osmotic load; subsequently osmolarity of contrast media is an additional consideration. Children experiencing contrast reactions or those with an established history of contrast reactions should be premedicated using evidence-based, weight-specific dose guidelines [4, 10]. Calculated eGFR is an acceptable means of measuring renal function in children at risk of contrast-induced nephropathy or nephrogenic systemic fibrosis [4].

### 10.5.2 Pregnant Patients

Little research has been done on the impact of contrast media on pregnant women and the effects on the human embryo or fetus [4]. If contrast-enhanced imaging is needed, it is critical to review the risks and benefits of imaging and obtaining informed consent. Shortly after injection, contrast enters the fetal blood stream. The contrast will be excreted via the urine into the amniotic fluid and be subsequently swallowed by the fetus [4]. There is a small risk of thyroid suppression in the fetus of women who receive iodinated contrast during pregnancy [11]; however, to date, there have been no diagnosed cases of neonatal hypothyroidism in those who were exposed to low-osmolar contrast media in utero [4, 11]. A very small amount of iodinated contrast may be excreted in breast milk, though cessation of breastfeeding is not considered necessary, but may be left at the discretion of the mother [4, 11].

There is limited research specific to the administration of gadolinium-based contrast media to pregnant women [4, 11]. A retrospective review of Canadian provincial birth registries currently indicates that administration of gadolinium during the first trimester pregnancy is associated with increase in rheumatological, inflammatory, and infiltrative disorder, and administration of gadolinium at any point in pregnancy is associated with stillbirth and neonatal death [4].

Gadolinium should be avoided in pregnancy unless necessary, and nursing women who receive gadolinium are recommended to stop breastfeeding for 24 h following administration [11].

### 10.5.3 Older Patients

The terms "older" or "elderly" are quite often used to refer to patients 65 years of age and older. Aging refers to the inevitable and irreversible decline of organ function with age [12]. Kidney function is known to decline with age [13]. The kidney undergoes changes in both structure and function with age. Glomerular filtration rate (GFR) is known to slow with age, and this decline in renal function may predispose the older patient to acute kidney injury; subsequently, screening of older adults for kidney function prior to the administration of contrast media is recommended [2]. Additionally, due to age-related decline in renal and cardiovascular functioning, older patients are at greater risk of developing cardiovascular collapse during anaphylactic reactions to contrast media [14].

## 10.6 Premedication for Contrast-Enhanced Studies

Premedication using steroids and antihistamines may reduce the possibility of contrast-mediated hypersensitivity reactions in at-risk populations [4].

**Table 10.2** Premedication protocols

1. Prednisone-based protocol: 50 mg oral prednisone is administered by mouth 13, 7, and 1 h prior to contrast injection, with the addition of 50 mg diphenhydramine administered by mouth 1 h prior to contrast injection.
2. Methylprednisolone-based protocol: 32 mg by mouth administered 12 h and 2 h prior to contrast administration with the addition of 50 mg of diphenhydramine administered by mouth

Source: ACR, Manual on Contrast Media v10.3 [4]

Oral or intravenous pre-steroids and antihistamines may be used for premedication, with oral medications being more cost effective and convenient. Established protocols shared with referring providers can ensure that patients arrive to the radiology department with the protocol completed. However, despite premedication protocols, breakthrough reactions are possible. Subsequently, radiologists must have careful consideration to the risks and benefits of administering contrast media to patients with a history of prior allergic reactions to contrast media. Additionally, clinicians working in settings where contrast may be administered to patients with contrast allergies must receive education and training in the management of severe contrast reactions [15].

See Table 10.2 for premedication protocols.

## 10.7 Acute Contrast Reactions: Anaphylactic/Physiologic

Reactions to contrast media may be classified as mild, moderate, or severe [6]. Low-osmolar contrast agents are associated with significantly lower rates of acute reactions compared with high-osmolar agents. The rate of acute adverse events for low-osmolar iodinated contrast agents is 0.2–0.7% and for severe acute reactions, 0.04% [2, 4]. Allergic response to contrast media is often described as allergic or anaphylactic in nature. Anaphylaxis is a severe, immediate IgE-mediated immunologic response causing release of mediators from the mast cells and basophils. The term anaphylactoid has been used to describe a similar response, not mediated by IgE. Recently, the World Allergy Organization (WAO) has suggested that the term anaphylactoid be eliminated, and that all reactions presenting as clinically similar to anaphylaxis be treated as such [16].

Patients with a history of atopy, asthma, dermatitis, and urticaria have a threefold to sixfold increased risk of severe reactions to contrast media [2].

### 10.7.1 Types of Contrast Reaction

While the overwhelming majority of contrast-enhanced images are completed without negative effects on the patient, administration of contrast is not without risk. Adverse effects vary from minor physiologic and mild allergic-like reactions to rare but severe and life-threatening events [2, 4]. A third category, nonallergic reactions, encompasses adverse events to contrast media, such as CIN.

The American College of Radiology Manual on Contrast Media v10.3 (May 2018; Available on line at https://www.acr.org/Clinical-Resources/Contrast-Manual) provides explicit guidelines for the management of contrast reactions. The following provides information on the management of different types of contrast reactions, as well as those referenced therein.

1. *Urticaria* is a cutaneous, allergic-like response. Urticaria may be mild, moderate, or progressive.
    (a) Mild isolated urticaria may be self-resolving or respond to an oral antihistamine such as diphenhydramine or fexofenadine. Diphenhydramine, though inexpensive, is associated with drowsiness. Patients who have been administered diphenhydramine should avoid driving until the effects of the medication have resolved. Fexofenadine, though costlier than diphenhydramine, is often preferred by patients and clinicians, as it is not associated with drowsiness.
    (b) Moderate urticaria is a rash that is patchy, bothersome to the patient, and present in more than one area. Patients experiencing moderate urticaria should be monitored for progression of symptoms. It is recom-

mended to maintain intravenous access in this population, and that antihistamines be given intravenously.
   (c) If urticaria is progressive, and there are signs of respiratory compromise or hypoxemia, initiate the administration of oxygen and frequent vital signs. If the patient demonstrates signs of hypotension or multisystem compromise, initiate rapid fluid bolus and anticipate the administration of intramuscular epinephrine (1:1000) *in an age- and weight-appropriate dose.*

   If the patient demonstrates signs of profound shock or is hypotensive and unresponsive, anticipate intravenous (IV) epinephrine (1:10,000) *in an age- and weight-appropriate dose.* If epinephrine is to be administered, it is recommended that a second clinician verify the dose of epinephrine being given to the patient, as epinephrine dosing errors in the context of the treatment of acute contrast reactions have been associated with myocardial infarction, dysrhythmia, and death [8]. If budget permits, use of dose-controlled epinephrine auto-injectors, such as the Epi-Pen®, are available in adult and pediatric doses and help reduce risks associated with the administration of epinephrine during the treatment of moderate to severe allergic reactions to contrast.

   Clinicians should understand the differences in the strengths of epinephrine and usage for each. Education regarding dose calculation and administration of epinephrine should be included in team training specific to the management of acute contrast reactions.

2. *Sneezing, rhinorrhea, and scratchy throat* may present following contrast reaction. If vital signs are within normal limits, consider oral diphenhydramine and observe until symptoms resolve.
3. *Bronchospasm* is an anaphylactoid reaction and can be mild, moderate, or severe. The incidence of contrast-induced bronchospasm is rare and occurs most often in those with a prior history of atopy, allergies, and asthma. Patients who develop bronchospasm following the administration of contrast should be medically evaluated inclusive of vital signs, oxygen saturation, chest auscultation, and an evaluation of other potential signs of an acute contrast reaction. Patients with normal vital signs, oxygen saturation, and no additional symptoms of acute contrast reaction can be treated with a beta-agonist inhaler. Patients unresponsive to multiple doses of a beta-agonist or those demonstrating signs of hypoxia or shock may respond to intramuscular epinephrine and advanced cardiac life support guidelines for anaphylaxis.
4. *Hypotension with tachycardia* is an anaphylactoid reaction. Patients experiencing hypotension with tachycardia benefit from the administration of fluid volume expansion, and the administration of intramuscular (1:1000) or IV (1:10,000) epinephrine *in age- and weight-appropriate doses*. If the patient exhibits signs of hypoxia, administration of high flow oxygen is indicated.
5. *Laryngeal edema*: Laryngeal edema is an anaphylactoid reaction and a life-threatening emergency. Patient demonstrating signs of laryngeal edema (stridor, respiratory distress, and hypoxia) should be evaluated rapidly (for vital signs, oxygen saturation) and treated with intramuscular epinephrine (1:1000) or IV epinephrine (1:10,000) *in age- and weight-appropriate dose* and high flow oxygen. If the patient demonstrates signs of profound shock, intravenous epinephrine is preferable.
6. *Hypotension and bradycardia* is a physiologic reaction to contrast. Also known as a vasovagal reaction, patients with hypotension and bradycardia may experience dizziness, nausea, and/or syncope. Patients experiencing hypotension with bradycardia should have their intravenous site maintained, be positioned flat or in Trendelenburg position, and receive volume expansion using isotonic crystalloid. Where placing the patient in Trendelenburg position is not an option, raising the patient's legs may aid in volume return. Patients should have frequent evaluation of vital signs. Because hypotension with bradycardia is not an allergic-like reaction, these

patients do not need to be premedicated for future studies.
7. *Delayed reactions* to contrast media can also occur. In certain circumstances, e.g., cutaneous reactions, parotid swelling (iodine mumps), thrombophlebitis, hyperthyroidism, or acute polyarthralgia have occurred, but are rare.

## 10.8 Departmental Readiness

Care of the patient experiencing an acute contrast reaction should follow departmental care protocols. Department protocols should be specific, evidence-based [4], accessible, promote timely care and support compliance, and communicated to all members of the radiology team. The American College of Radiology Committee on Drugs and Contrast Media, the Royal College of Radiologists, and Royal Australian and New Zealand College of Radiologists publish guidelines, made widely available that are considered a standard of care for patients experiencing acute contrast reactions [4, 6, 11]. Institution and department-specific protocols, policies, and checklists that are based on the existing evidence should reflect available pharmacologic agents, composition of responding team, scope of practice limitations of responders, and a plan for sustainability.

A multimodal approach to communicating protocols ensures that all stakeholders will be aware of the standards of care surrounding the management of acute contrast reactions. Policies and protocols should always be accessible, and easily searchable. Institutions utilizing electronic medical records may link electronic policy and protocol folders, and order templates to support compliance with contrast reaction treatment algorithms. Where policies are housed electronically, team education must be inclusive of learning the pathway to locate the policy, protocol, order templates and documentation protocols specific to the management of acute contrast reactions. Institutions without websites must ensure availability of contrast reaction protocols, policies, and order sets at hand in each imaging or procedure suite, as well as in the workup and recovery areas where patients receiving or recovering from a contrast-enhanced image or procedure may be.

## 10.9 Contrast Reaction Kits

A consistent, well-communicated, sustainable plan for maintaining contrast reaction supplies is essential to ensuring ongoing readiness [4, 6, 11]. Pharmacy medication cabinets, such as Pyxis® or Omnicell®, allow for the creation of virtual kits, enabling clinicians to remove all required medications quickly. This method ensures medication security and inventory control but may create a delay in obtaining medications in departments without secured cabinets in each imaging or procedure suite. Supplemental emergency medication kits containing all the supplies needed to manage an acute contrast reaction should be located proximal to every area where intravascular contrast is administered. Kits should be distinguishable, consistently stocked across the department, approved by radiology and pharmacy leadership, with staff assigned to perform daily equipment checks, and/or restocking of supplies as needed. Professional organizations such as the American College of Radiology, the Royal College of Radiologists, and the European Society for Radiology regularly review and publish guidelines specific to achieving departmental readiness to manage patients with acute contrast reactions inclusive of recommendations regarding emergency equipment needs [17].

## 10.10 Training

Radiology nurses, radiologists, technologists, and any assistants in every environment where intravascular contrast agents are administered should be trained for rapid recognition and early intervention in the management of acute contrast reactions. This can be accomplished through online interactive learning [8, 18], simulation or drill training [19], or a mixture of modalities inclusive of online learning, online testing, simulation, and post-simulation testing [19]. Team training using high-fidelity simulation should balance clinical skills and nonclinical team skills necessary to ensure patient safety [20]. Online and live learning should be augmented through the dissemination of cognitive aids, such as identification (ID) badge cards or pocket cards [4] and posting of contrast reaction policies in imaging suites [4, 11]. In conjunction with team training, cognitive aids support the real-time knowledge resource needs of clinicians during emergencies.

In hospital settings where rapid response and code teams respond to severe contrast reactions, training specific to the management of contrast reactions reflecting both radiology practice standards [4, 6, 11] and emergency response activation may be necessary. Freestanding radiology centers without internal emergency response teams should be trained how to access outside emergency services.

## 10.11 Conclusion

Use of contrast media, though generally safe, carries potential risks for patients. A successful contrast reaction management program involves careful review of the evidence, investment in team education, training, procurement of safety equipment, and ongoing program evaluation. Advanced practice leaders who take comprehensive approach in creating an environment of safety for the populations that they serve can ensure positive outcomes and a high-quality patient experience.

## References

1. Radiological Society of North America. Patient safety: contrast materials. 2018. www.rsna.org/patientsafety. Accessed 16 Mar 2019.
2. Beckett K, Moriarty A, Langer J. Safe use of contrast media: what the radiologist needs to know. Radiographics. 2015;35(6):1738–50. https://doi.org/10.1148/rg.2015150033.
3. Pomara C, Pascale N, et al. Use of contrast media in diagnostic imaging: medicolegal implications. Radiol Med. 2015;120(9):802–9. https://doi.org/10.10007/s11547-015-0549-8.
4. American College of Radiologists. Manual on contrast media, Version 10.3. 2018. www.acr.org/clinicalresources/contrast-manual. Accessed 15 Mar 2019.
5. Baerlocher M, Asch M, Myers A. Metformin and intravenous contrast. Can Med J. 2013;185(1):E78. https://doi.org/10.1503/cmaj.090550.
6. Royal Australian and New Zealand College of Radiologists. Iodinated Contrast Media Guidelines:V2.3. 2017. https://www.google.com/search?source=hp&ei=RQORXKvaJemxggfzt5XYDw&q=contrast+reaction+management+european+society+of+radiology&btnK=Google+Search&oq=contrast+reaction+management+european+society+of+radiology&gs_l=psy-ab.3..33i299l3.561.13254..13619...4.0..0.141.4716.53j9......0....1..gws-wiz.....0..0i131j0j0i22i30j33i22i29i30j33i160.Hs4fqvm23wk. Accessed 15 Mar 2019.
7. Lambert P, Chaisson K, Horton S, Petrin C, Marshall E. Reducing acute kidney injury due to contrast material: how nurses can improve patient safety. Crit Care Nurse. 2017;37(1):13–25.
8. Wang CL, Cohan RH, Ellis JH, Adusumilli S, Dunnick NR. Frequency, management, and outcome of extravasation of nonionic iodinated contrast medium in 69,657 intravenous injections. Radiology. 2007;243(1):80–7.
9. Sbitany H, Koltz PF, Mays C, Girotto JA, Langstein HN. CT contrast extravasation in the upper extremity: strategies for management. Int J Surg. 2010;8(5):384–6.
10. American Heart Association. Handbook of emergency cardiovascular care for healthcare providers. Dallas, TX: American Heart Association; 2015.
11. Royal College of Radiologists. Standards for the intravascular administration of contrast administration to adult patients: Second edition. 2011. https://www.rcr.ac.uk/sites/default/files/docs/radiology/pdf/BFCR(10)4_Stand_contrast.pdf. Accessed 19 Mar 2019.
12. Besidine, R. Introduction to geriatrics. Merck manual: professional version. 2019. https://merckmanuals.com/professional/geriatrics/approach-to-the-geriatric-patient/introduction-to-geriatrics. Accessed 31 Jul 2019.
13. Denic, A; Grassock, R; Rule, A (2016). Structural and functional changes in the aging kidney. Adv Chronic Kidney Dis, 21(1), 19-28. https://www.ncbi.nlm.nih.gov/pmc/articles/PMC4693148/. Accessed 31 July 2019.
14. Kim SM, Ko BS, Kim JY, Ha SO, Ahn S, Sohn CH, et al. Clinical factors for developing shock in radiocontrast media induced anaphylaxis. Shock. 2016;45(3):315–9. https://doi.org/10.1097/SHK.0000000000000514.
15. Brokow K, Ring J. Anaphylaxis to radiographic contrast media. Curr Opin Allergy Clin Immunol. 2011;11:326–31.

16. World Allergy Organization. Ask the expert: anaphylaxis vs. anaphylactoid reactions. 2018. https://www.worldallergy.org/ask-the-expert/questions/anaphylaxis-vs-anaphylactoid-reactions. Accessed 12 Aug 2019.
17. European Society for Radiology. Review iodinated contrast media: classification, adverse reactions, interactions with other drugs and special situations. EPOS. 2017. https://posterng.netkey.at/esr/viewing/index.php?module=viewing_poster&task=&pi=137089. Accessed 19 Mar 2019.
18. Niell B, Vartanians V, Halpern E. Improving education for the management of contrast reactions: an online didactic model. J. Am. Coll. Radiol. 2014;11(2):185–92.
19. Niell B, Halperin E, Salazar G, Kattapuram T, Penzias A, et al. Prospective analysis of an interprofessional team training program using high-fidelity simulation of contrast reactions. AJR Am J Roentgenol. 2015;204(6):W670–6. https://doi.org/10.2214/AJR.14.13778.
20. Agency for Healthcare Research and Quality. TEAM STEPPS 2.0. 2015. www.ahrq.gov. Accessed 15 Mar 2019.

# Infection Prevention in Radiology

# 11

Caroline McDaniel, Sandra L. Schwaner, and Costi D. Sifri

## 11.1 Introduction

Advances in radiology benefit patients who now have many more minimally invasive diagnostic and treatment options. Higher volumes of patients, some of them critically ill, undergo complex procedures in radiology rooms. The potential to cause harm to patients through infection transmission exists in radiology departments whether the patient is undergoing noninvasive imaging or an invasive procedure. Although healthcare becomes ever safer, the Centers for Disease Control and Prevention (CDC) estimates that 5–10% of hospital patients suffer from hospital-acquired infections (HAIs) in US hospitals every year, resulting in nearly 100,000 deaths, and with an associated cost of $20 billion [1]. HAIs result from invasive procedures, contact with the contaminated hands of healthcare workers (HCWs) or equipment, and overuse or misuse of antibiotics [1].

Infection prevention and control has been practiced throughout history, even when medical knowledge was limited. In medieval times victims of bubonic plaque were isolated in their own homes and their belongings burned. If they died of the disease, their bodies were buried in mass graves away from town [2]. Over time, less drastic measures to prevent the transmission of infectious diseases have been developed: hand hygiene, standard precautions, contact precautions, and sterile techniques for invasive procedures. By the 1950s most operating suites worldwide had adopted surgical clothing and sterile drapes [3]. Unfortunately, the radiology procedural suite has been slower to adopt similar techniques. In 2007, less than 60% of practicing radiologists wore hats, masks, and sterile gowns, or used full sterile drapes during central line placement [4, 5]. Infection control has recently become a major focus in many radiology departments [6]. Proper practices have the ability to prevent transmission of nosocomial pathogens and to save lives. Infection preventionists and healthcare epidemiologists provide expertise in advising and educating staff [7]. This chapter provides the advance practice nurse and nurse manager with foundational knowledge in infection prevention and control for both general imaging and interventional radiology.

C. McDaniel, MSN, RN, CWON (✉)
University of Virginia Health System,
Charlottesville, VA, USA

S. L. Schwaner, MSN, RN, ACNP-BC
Department of Interventional Radiology, University of Virginia Health System, Charlottesville, VA, USA

C. D. Sifri, MD
Division of Infectious Diseases and International Health, Department of Medicine, University of Virginia Health System, Charlottesville, VA, USA

## 11.2 Standard Precautions

The radiology department is a potentially pathogen-rich environment. Almost every patient encounters radiology at some point, creating a unique level of risk. The CDC [8] defines standard precautions as a set of practices to be used whether or not the patient is diagnosed with an infection (Table 11.1). Radiology personnel must be vigilant in the use of personal protective equipment (PPE) to protect both themselves and the other patients they come into contact with on a daily basis [5]. Gloves should be worn for all interactions where there is potential for contact with blood or bodily fluids, mucous membranes, or non-intact skin. Gloves should fit well. Gloves that are too large may slip off and provide an incomplete barrier; gloves that are too small may tear more easily [5]. Gloves should never be used as a substitute for hand washing, as micro perforations can contaminate hands even when gloves are worn.

Use of non-sterile gowns as well as eye and mouth protection are needed when there is any chance of spray, splash, or splatter of blood or other body fluids. Some masks include eye protection. Eyeglasses are not considered complete protection against splash. Eye shields or goggles can be reused if they are disinfected in between patient encounters. Many radiology departments now opt for disposable eye shields. (This differs from lead eyewear to protect against radiation exposure though these can be used for both purposes). PPE should be removed when leaving the patient care area.

The use of sterile gowns is required for any personnel having direct contact with a sterile field (see "Surgical Attire" below). The CDC, the Institute for Healthcare Improvement (IHI), and American College of Radiology (ACR) all agree that sterile gowns are an essential infection prevention strategy when performing procedures such as abscess drainage or arterial puncture [6]. The CDC and the Association for Professionals in Infection Control and Prevention (APIC) also recommend that surgical masks be worn when performing spinal injection (e.g., myelography) or intracapsular procedures (e.g., arthrography) that include injection of material or insertion of a catheter [9, 10], as absence of mask use has been associated with iatrogenic bacterial meningitis and septic arthritis due to oropharyngeal microflora, presumably due to cross-contamination from respiratory droplets [11, 12].

## 11.3 Hand Hygiene

Hand hygiene provides the foundation for infection control. The earliest evidence of this dates backs to the 1840s when Semmelweiss and Holmes each observed that mortality rates decreased significantly when physicians washed their hands with antiseptic [13]. Unfortunately getting HCWs to perform hand hygiene remains a challenge in the modern era. The CDC [14] estimates that HCWs wash their hands about half the times they should.

The question of why HCWs miss opportunities to cleanse their hands is an interesting one. Transmission of bacteria is an invisible process, so there is no evidence "in the moment" when it occurs. Researchers have found that factors influencing compliance with hand hygiene can be divided into two categories: motivational factors and work environment [15]. Motivational factors include the actions of senior medical and nursing staff, the amount of self-perceived risk in a given patient care situation, the acuity of patient care, and the number of cues present to prompt hand hygiene. Work environment factors included availability of hand hygiene products, organizational commitment to compliance with hand hygiene, and educating HCWs [15]. Skin damage as a result of frequent washing has also been cited as a deterrent to frequent hand washing [16].

**Table 11.1** Standard precautions

| Standard precautions |
|---|
| • Hand hygiene |
| • Use of personal protective equipment |
| • Cough etiquette |
| • Sharps safety |
| • Safe injection practices |
| • Sterile instruments and devices |
| • Clean and disinfected environmental work surfaces |
| • Handle laundry carefully |

Source: https://www.cdc.gov/infectioncontrol/basics/standard-precautions.html

Alcohol-based hand rubs and soap and water are the two methods for hand hygiene available in the healthcare setting. A surgical scrub is done for sterile procedures. Alcohol-based hand rubs are the most effective at killing most fungi, viruses, and bacteria, including multidrug-resistant organisms (MDRO) such as methicillin-resistant *Staphylococcus aureus* (MRSA). These products are also less likely to cause skin irritation [16]. However, alcohol-based hand rubs are not the best choice when dealing with spore-forming bacteria such as *Clostridioides difficile* (formerly known as *Clostridium difficile*) and certain viruses such as noroviruses [17–19]. When performing hand hygiene for patients with infections due to alcohol-resistant pathogens or when hands are visibly soiled, handwashing with soap and water is recommended [18] (Table 11.2). For the emerging pathogen *Candida auris*, the CDC recommends adhering to standard guidelines (alcohol-based hand rubs unless hands are visibly soiled) [18]. As more information becomes available about *Candida auris* new guidelines may be developed [20]. Timely and effective communication between radiology personnel, infection prevention personnel, and primary clinicians that includes information about contact precautions needed and the recommended method of hand hygiene for a given patient are critical for optimal infection control practice in radiology departments.

Some studies show that even when HCWs perform hand hygiene, the correct technique may not be used. Common shortcomings include not cleaning for long enough and not cleaning all of the hand's surfaces (Table 11.3) [19, 21]. Alcohol-based hand rub dispensers and sinks for soap and water washing need to be readily available. Lotions compatible with the products used should be available to HCWs to prevent avoidance of hand hygiene caused by dermatitis. Nails should be no longer than a ¼" and artificial nail use is restricted as these have been shown to harbor bacteria [22].

**Table 11.2** Indications for when to perform hand hygiene and which product to use

| | Alcohol-based sanitizer | Soap and water | Surgical scrub |
|---|---|---|---|
| Before direct patient contact | ✓ | | |
| After contact with a patient's intact or non-intact skin, wounds, or dressings if patient does *not* have alcohol-resistant infection (e.g., *C. difficile*, norovirus) | ✓ | | |
| After contact with a patient's intact or non-intact skin, wounds, or dressings if patient *with* alcohol-resistant infection (e.g., *C. difficile*, norovirus) | | ✓ | |
| After removing gloves if patient does *not* have alcohol-resistant infection (e.g., *C. difficile*, norovirus) | ✓ | | |
| After removing gloves if patient with alcohol-resistant infection (e.g., *C. difficile*, norovirus) | | ✓ | |
| After touching items in the patient's environment, even if there was not contact with the patient if patient does not have alcohol-resistant infection (e.g., *C. difficile*, norovirus) | ✓ | | |
| After touching items in the patient's environment, even if there was not contact with the patient if patient with alcohol-resistant infection (e.g., *C. difficile*, norovirus) | | ✓ | |
| Prior to placing peripheral vascular catheters, indwelling urinary catheters, or any invasive device *not requiring surgery* | ✓ | | |
| Hands are visibly dirty | | ✓ | |
| Before invasive procedures requiring surgery (e.g., tunneled line placement) | | | ✓ |
| During patient care if moving from a contaminated body site to a clean body site | ✓ | | |

Source: https://www.cdc.gov/mmwr/PDF/rr/rr5116.pdf

**Table 11.3** Correct techniques for hand hygiene methods

| Type of hand hygiene | Correct technique |
|---|---|
| Alcohol-based hand rub | • Apply to palm of one hand, rub hands together covering all surfaces until dry<br>• Volume: Based on manufacturer (usually about 3 mls) |
| Surgical scrub | • Use either an antimicrobial soap or alcohol-based hand rub<br>• Antimicrobial soap: Scrub hands and forearms for length of time recommended by manufacturer<br>• Alcohol-based hand rub: Follow manufacturer's recommendations. Before applying, pre-wash hands and forearms with non-antimicrobial soap |

Source: https://www.cdc.gov/mmwr/PDF/rr/rr5116.pdf

The World Health Organization (WHO) has a wealth of slide set presentations, posters, and other teaching material available to assist in educating HCWs [23]. Another technique to educate staff about hand hygiene utilizes fluorescent gel products that mimic the way bacteria spread between healthcare workers' hands to patients or surfaces [24]. The fluorescent gel product is applied to hands and then the participants are led through different exercises such as shaking hands and handling equipment. A black light is used to illuminate fluorescent residue (representing "germs") on surfaces and hands. This exercise provides a powerful visual demonstration of how easy it is to spread organisms from dirty hands.

Observational audits are the most common way of measuring compliance with hand hygiene [16, 19]. HCWs are observed to see if they perform hand hygiene when entering or exiting a patient room, as proxy measures of hand hygiene opportunities before or after touching a patient and/or their surroundings, respectively. The audits can be performed by infection preventionists or by unit personnel. The advantage to this method is that the quality of hand hygiene can be assessed as well. The main disadvantage is that staff may be aware that they are being audited and this can skew the results. Change in behavior due to an awareness of being observed is termed the Hawthorne effect [25]. Another important limitation of observational audits performed outside a patient room is that opportunities for hand hygiene that occur in the room during patient care may not be assessed. Examples include before performing a clean or aseptic procedure or after a potential body fluid exposure. Hand hygiene compliance can be posted on units and used as educational and quality improvement tools. Sample audit tool templates are available on the WHO website [23].

Recently electronic monitoring devices have been brought to market as an alternative to traditional, observer-based auditing programs. These technologies have the potential to measure compliance with hand hygiene opportunities that occur throughout the workday, including nights, weekends, holidays, and other times that are challenging to audit using traditional methods. Moreover, these products have the ability to markedly increase the frequency of audits without the expense of personnel to perform manual audits. Finally, these systems also may have an advantage of minimizing the Hawthorn effect. However, installation of these devices is expensive and may be tied to certain products, making it difficult for organizations to switch products [16]. Some studies have also reported that HCWs and patients may not regard the technology positively, and it remains to be determined whether these systems improve hand hygiene compliance or help reduce HAIs [26, 27]. A final option to assess hand hygiene is measuring product usage. Although this method doesn't provide any data on how well the hand hygiene was performed, it has been more accurately associated with HAI trends than observational audits and is less time-consuming [16].

## 11.4 Environmental Cleaning and Disinfection

It has been well established that patients can acquire infections from the hospital environment [28, 29]. Organisms such as MRSA, vancomycin-resistant *Enterococcus* (VRE), and *C. difficile* can

**Table 11.4** Classification system for disinfection and sterilization

| Classification | Definition | Examples | Type of disinfection needed |
|---|---|---|---|
| Critical | Enter sterile tissue or vascular system | Surgical instruments<br>Implants<br>Cardiac and urinary catheters<br>Ultrasound probes used in sterile body cavities | Sterilization with steam—Destroys all organisms including bacterial spores. Implants and catheters should be bought packaged sterilely. |
| Semicritical | Contacts mucous membranes or non-intact skin | Endoscopes<br>Laryngoscope blades<br>Cystoscopes<br>Respiratory therapy and anesthesia equipment | High level disinfection—Destroys all organisms except some bacterial spores |
| Noncritical | Contacts intact skin (but not mucous membranes) | Blood pressure cuffs<br>Pulse oximeter probes<br>Bedside tables | Low level disinfection—Destroys vegetative bacteria, some fungi, some viruses but not mycobacteria or spores |

Source: Adapted from Rutala WA, Weber DJ. Disinfection and sterilization: An overview. Am J Infect Control 2013; 41(5, Supplement): S2–S5

remain viable on surfaces for days to months [28, 30]. Items that come into physical contact with patients need to be either disinfected or sterilized based on their use (Table 11.4). All equipment cleaning should take into account the manufacturer's instructions. This chapter will include low-level disinfection only as it applies to all areas of radiology. It should be noted that ultrasound probes that contact body cavities and non-intact skin require high-level disinfection, even when a sterile sleeve is used to cover the probe. This includes probes used for ultrasound guided punctures. For more information on sterilization and high-level disinfection, please refer to CDC guidelines.

Equipment and surfaces in radiology rooms need disinfection in between patients. This includes mattresses, control panels, tables, carts, positioning devices, and pillows. For interventional cases, planning ahead to have necessary devices, wires, and equipment on hand helps to prevent frequent room entry and exit and thereby avoids contaminating items unnecessarily. Items such as radiographic markers and lead aprons may be overlooked. Cleaning protocols for these items should be understood and practiced by HCWs, including clinicians and environmental service personnel [31, 32]. Use of keyboards and computers in radiology for documentation in electronic medical records is now commonplace. These items should be included in room turnovers [33].

Knowing how to use disinfectants is essential knowledge for radiology teams. Chlorine-based products, quaternary ammonium compounds, or phenolics are examples of liquids used for low-level disinfection [28]. These products are usually packaged as wipes. The manufacturer of each product will have a contact time listed on the packaging to instruct how long the liquid must remain in contact with the surface in order for successful disinfection to occur. Chlorine-based products are often used for point-of-care cleaning in areas occupied by patients with *C. difficile* or other pathogens intrinsically resistant to quaternary ammonium disinfectants, such as non-enveloped viruses (e.g., norovirus). HCWs should be well acquainted with different products available to them and be aware of the contact time for each product. HCWs should also be educated to make sure lids on wipe canisters are shut to avoid drying them out. Environmental cleaning staff play an integral role in patient safety and should be acknowledged for their work.

No-touch decontamination of patient care areas is a more recent development in environmental cleaning. Ultraviolet light or hydrogen peroxide mist can be used as an adjunct to regular cleaning for patients with *C. difficile,* MRSA, or other resistant infections. The devices are programmed according to the size of the room and have proven effective in eliminating pathogenic bacteria from the environment. However, since these technologies are expensive and can take several hours to complete, they are not a viable option for routine room turnovers but can be considered for terminal cleaning at the end of the day [28].

Surfaces can appear perfectly clean but still harbor pathogenic organisms. How do we know that surfaces are truly disinfected? How can we quantify cleanliness? ATP (adenosine triphosphate) bioluminescence testing was developed in the food industry and is now used in the healthcare environment [34]. ATP identifies organic material on surfaces although it does not specifically identify what organic material is present. A commercial swab is used on surfaces to be tested and the swab is placed in a machine (luminometer) which detects the presence of ATP (Fig. 11.1). ATP is the energy source for all organic materials and remains stable in the environment over time, making this a reliable indicator of cleanliness [35]. Different brands of luminometers have different ranges for cleanliness thresholds. Results can be posted in a graph format and discussed with staff (Fig. 11.2). Fluorescent gels, discussed

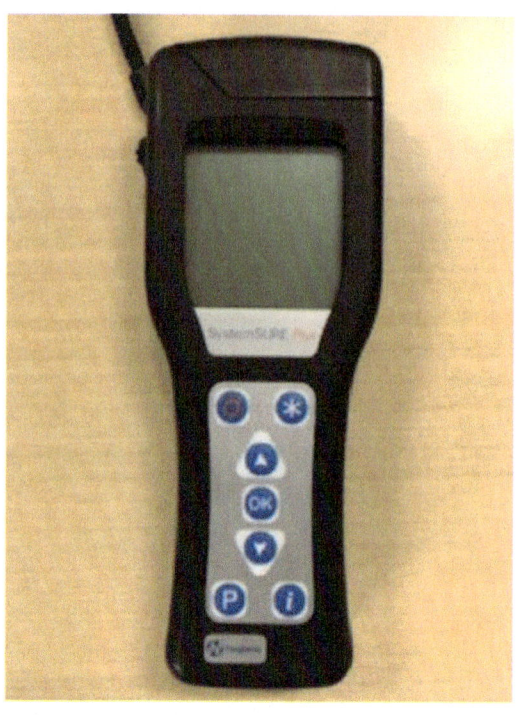

**Fig. 11.1** Sample ATP luminometer (photo credit: Caroline McDaniel)

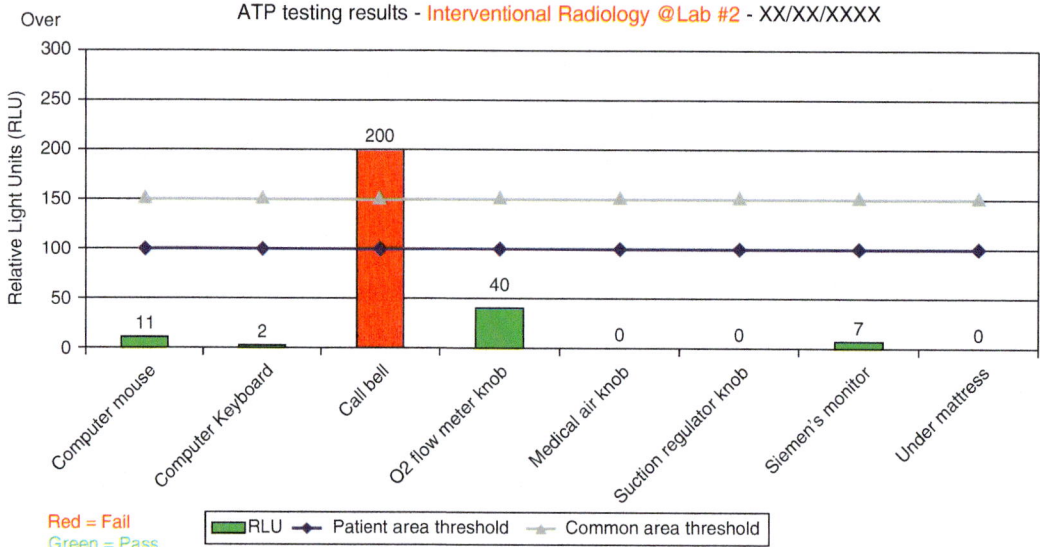

**Fig. 11.2** Sample of graph showing ATP testing results

earlier, can also be used to audit cleaning practices between room turnovers. The CDC provides guidance on what surfaces should be tested in patient care areas [36].

## 11.5 Transmission-Based Isolation Precautions

Transmission-based precautions are used for any communicable disease. Multidrug-resistant organisms (MDROs) have been on the rise all over the world. These organisms cause infections that can be difficult and potentially impossible to treat. Although identifying these patients is important so that staff can practice the appropriate precautions, it is important to remember that patients may not yet be identified as having been colonized or infected with an MDRO; consequently, standard precautions should always be used to protect both patients and staff. There should be clear communication about isolation precautions needed for patients traveling to the radiology setting. Patients undergoing procedures should also be clearly identified while in the radiology suite to avoid an accidental break in precautions. Posting signs on doorways can alert staff that isolation precautions apply and make clear the preferred method of hand hygiene.

Modes of transmission are contact (direct or indirect), droplets, or airborne (Table 11.5). Some diseases can be transmitted in more than one way. Airborne isolation requires not only the use of PPE, but also a special air handling system to prevent infectious respiratory particles from traveling to other areas of the hospital [37]. For patients requiring airborne isolation their case should be delayed until treatment has been completed if this does not pose a threat to the patient. If the case cannot be delayed, a negative pressure room should be used. High-efficiency particulate air (HEPA) filters do *not* take the place of negative pressure rooms but are sometimes used to mitigate the risk in locations without negative pressure [38]. Some organizations try to schedule isolation cases at the end of the day. The number of patients on isolation precautions is on the rise, so this may not always be a practical strategy.

## 11.6 Surgical Attire

The use of surgical scrubs in the operating room dates back to the 1930s and 1940s. Prior to this, street clothing was covered by a sterile gown [3]. The purpose of specialized surgical garments is twofold: prevention of surgical site infection from extra procedural bacteria and reduction in contamination of clothing worn outside the surgical suite [3, 5, 6]. As recently as 2008, many interventional radiology departments did not require scrub attire in the procedural suite [4].

**Table 11.5** Methods of transmission of infectious diseases

| Mode of transmission | Definition | Precautions needed | Example |
|---|---|---|---|
| Contact (direct) | Microorganisms are transferred from infected person to another without an intermediate object or person | Gown and gloves | MRSA VRE *C. difficile* |
| Contact (indirect) | Transmission occurs from a contaminated object or person (surfaces, toys, etc.) | Gown and gloves | MRSA VRE *C. difficile* |
| Droplet | Respiratory droplets travel from infected person to mucous membranes of another person, usually over short distances (3–6 feet) | Mask | Pertussis Influenza virus Rhinovirus |
| Airborne | Respiratory particles are carried over long distances and is inhaled by a susceptible person | Particulate respirators (N95 masks) OR powered air purifying respirators (PAPRs) Negative pressure rooms | Mycobacterium tuberculosis Measles Varicella zoster (chicken pox) |

Source: https://www.cdc.gov/infectioncontrol/basics/transmission-based-precautions.html

This practice is changing, as the IR suite more closely resembles an operating suite in terms of infection prevention practices and with the advent of hybrid interventional/OR rooms. Indeed, this is the recommendation of the Society of Interventional Radiology (SIR), the Association of perioperative Registered Nurses (AORN), and the Association for Radiologic and Imaging Nursing (ARIN) [6]. Hospitals should provide and launder specific garb for wearing in surgical suites; this garb is *not* to be worn outside the hospital or laundered at home. Some hospitals identify these scrubs with a distinctive color.

Maximum barrier precautions are recommended when performing any sterile procedure such as thoracentesis, central line insertion, or percutaneous endovascular aneurysm repair. This includes the use of hats and masks, sterile gowns, sterile gloves, and full sterile draping of the patient. Sterile gloves and masks should be worn during joint injection or lumbar punctures as oral flora can cause septic arthritis and other infections [12]. There is little data currently to support the use of shoe covers as an infection prevention tool; shoe covers are recommended to prevent splash contamination for shoes that will be worn outside of a procedure area [6]. Traffic in the room during the procedure should be minimized, and others in the room should also be wearing hats and masks [6].

## 11.7 Preparing the Patient's Skin

The patient's skin provides a natural barrier to infection. Skin preparation is done with an antimicrobial agent for invasive procedures. If necessary, hair removal should be done with clippers prior to applying the antimicrobial agent. Chlorhexidine gluconate is most commonly used because of its broad range of antimicrobial activity, ease of application, and proven efficacy in preventing surgical site infections [6]. If the patient has an allergy to chlorhexidine gluconate, other agents, such as povidone-iodine, can be used as a substitute.

## 11.8 Antibiotic Prophylaxis

The Society of Interventional Radiology (SIR) separates procedures performed in the interventional radiology area into categories from clean (such as diagnostic arteriogram) to dirty (such as abscess drainage or placement of gastrostomy tubes). Recommendations for antibiotic prophylaxis from the SIR continue to evolve as new data becomes available. The accompanying table is accurate as of 2018 (Table 11.6). While antibiotics are no longer recommended for most procedures, pre-procedural antimicrobial prophylaxis still has a place in management. Prolonged antibiotic therapy is no longer recommended. Procedures listed

**Table 11.6** Recommendations for antibiotic prophylaxis

| Procedure type | Potential organisms | Suggested antibiotic | Comments |
| --- | --- | --- | --- |
| **Dirty procedures** | | | |
| Abscess drainage | Polymicrobial | Single agent regimen for intra-abdominal sources; piperacillin/tazobactam, meropenem, imipenem | Only needed if patient not already on antibiotics |
| Percutaneous transhepatic biliary drain or cholecystostomy tube placement | *Enterococcus, Candida, Viridans streptococci, E. coli, Klebsiella* | Ceftriaxone, ampicillin/sulbactam, gentamicin | Vancomycin or clindamycin for penicillin allergic patients |
| Percutaneous nephrostomy tube | *E. coli*, Proteus, *Klebsiella, Enterococcus* | Ceftriaxone, ampicillin/sulbactam; gentamicin | Patients with indwelling catheters or ureteroileal anastomoses at higher risk |
| **Clean, clean contaminated procedures** | | | |
| Gastrostomy tube placement | *S. aureus, S. epidermidis* (oropharyngeal flora for pull type) | Cefazolin | Oral cephalexin or clindamycin for 5 days for pull type placement |

**Table 11.6** (continued)

| Procedure type | Potential organisms | Suggested antibiotic | Comments |
|---|---|---|---|
| Transjugular intrahepatic Portosystemic shunt (TIPS) | S. aureus, Enterococcus, E. coli, Klebsiella, Lactobacillus, Gemella morbillorum, Acinetobacter | Ceftriaxone; ampicillin/sulbactam | Vancomycin or clindamycin for penicillin allergic patients |
| Tumor ablation | S. aureus, S. epidermidis, E. coli, clostridium, Enterococcus | Cefazolin, ceftriaxone | 5–14 days of ciprofloxacin or levofloxacin with metronidazole when sphincter of Oddi is compromised. |
| Vascular malformation | S. aureus, S. epidermidis | Cefazolin, clindamycin for oral lesions | |
| Tunneled dialysis catheters | S. aureus, S. epidermidis | Cefazolin | Vancomycin for penicillin allergic patients |
| Partial splenic embolization | Streptococci, Staphylococcus | Gentamicin, cefoxitin "soaking of embolic spheres with 1,000,000 U penicillin and 40 mg gentamicin also recommended) | If 70% of spleen expected to be embolized, continue antibiotics for 5–7 days after |
| Hepatic embolization and Chemoembolization | S. aureus, S. epidermidis, enteric flora and anaerobes | Ampicillin/sulbactam; Cefazolin and metronidazole; ampicillin and gentamicin | Continue antibiotics for a total of 20 days, starting 3 days prior to procedure when sphincter of Oddi compromised |
| Uterine artery embolization | S. aureus, S. epidermidis, streptococcus, E. coli, vaginal flora | Cefazolin, clindamycin | One week doxycycline following if Hydrosalpinx present |
| Arterial endografts | S. aureus, S. epidermidis | Cefazolin | Vancomycin if penicillin allergic |

Source: JVascIntervRadiol 2018; 29:1483-1501 https://doi.org/10.1016/j.jvir.2018.06.007

in the table are the only procedures for which antibiotic prophylaxis is recommended. Prophylaxis for routine angiography, closure device deployment, routine biopsy (except transrectal biopsy), radioembolization, and fistulography is no longer recommended [39]. Timing of the administration of any antibiotic should be per current guidelines and institutional policy.

## 11.9 Summary

The modern-day radiology suite typically sees a large volume of patients ranging from the ambulatory to the critically ill. This is a likely environment for the potential transmission of pathogenic organisms. Factors that play a role in decreasing the occurrence of HAIs in radiology include having clear infection prevention and control guidelines and easy access to disinfectants, alcohol hand rubs, sinks, and PPE. On the organizational level, having senior clinicians demonstrate best practices and promoting a culture of teamwork creates an environment that emphasizes safety for both patients and HCWs. Advanced practice nurses can partner with infection preventionists and hospital epidemiologists, as well as other clinicians and administration to provide leadership regarding implementation of guidelines from the CDC, the Association for Radiologic and Imaging Nursing (ARIN), and SIR and have these embraced by staff.

# References

1. Centers for Disease Control and Prevention. Healthcare-associated infections. https://www.cdc.gov/hai/index.html. 2018. Accessed 1 Mar 2019.
2. Smith PW, Watkin K, Hewlett A. Infection control through the ages. Am J Infect Control. 2012;40:35–42.https://ajicjournal.org. https://doi.org/10.1016/j.ajjic.2011.02.019.
3. Adams LW, Aschenbrenner CA, Houle TT, Roy RC. Uncovering the history of operating room attire through photographs. Anesthesiology. 2016;124(1):19–24. https://doi.org/10.1097/ALN.0000000000000932.
4. Reddy P, Liebovitz D, Chrisman H, Nemcek AA, Noskin GA. Infection control practices among interventional radiologists: results of an online survey. J Vasc Interv Radiol. 2009;20:1070–4.
5. Mizra SK, Tragon TR, Fukui MB, Hartman MS, Hartman AL. Microbiology for radiologists: how to minimize infection transmission in the radiology department. Radiographics. 2015;35:1231–44. https://radiographics.rsna.org. https://doi.org/10.1148/rg.2015140034.
6. Chan D, Downing D, Keough CE, Saad WA, Annamalai G, Janned'Othee B, et al. Joint practice guideline for sterile technique during vascular and interventional radiology procedures: from the Society of Interventional Radiology, Association of periOperative Registered Nurses, and Association for Radiologic and Imaging Nursing, for the Society of Interventional Radiology (Wael Saad, MD, Chair), Standards of Practice Committee, and Endorsed by the Cardiovascular Interventional Radiological Society of Europe and the Canadian Interventional Radiology Association. J Radiol Nurs. 2012;31(4):130–43.
7. Kok HK, Torreggiani WC, Nihill DM. Imaging services and radiation oncology. In: Text of infection control and epidemiology. Association for Professionals in Infection Control and Epidemiology. 2014. http://text.apic.org/toc/infection-prevention-for-practice-settings-and-service-specific-patient-care-areas/imaging-services-and-radiation-oncology. Accessed 1 Mar 2019.
8. Centers for Disease Control and Prevention. Standard precautions for all patient care. https://www.cdc.gov/infectioncontrol/basics/standard-precautions.html 2018. Accessed 1 Mar 2019.
9. Dolan SA, Arias KM, Felizardo G, Barnes S, Kraska S, Patric M, et al. APIC position paper: safe injection, infusion, and medication vial practices in health care. Am J Infect Control. 2016;44:750–7.
10. Siegel JD, Rhinehart E, Jackson M, Chiarello L, Health Care Infection Control Practices Advisory Committee. 2007 Guideline for isolation precautions: preventing transmission of infectious agents in health care settings. Am J Infect Control. 2007;35(Suppl 2):S65–164.
11. Veringa E, van Belkum A, Scheliekens H. Iatrogenic meningitis by Streptococcus salivarius following lumbar puncture. J Hosp Infect. 1995;29(4):316–8.
12. Cain SM, Enfield KB, Giannetta ET, Sifri CD, Lewis JD. Septic arthritis due to oral streptococci following intra-articular injection: a case series. Am J Infect Control. 2018;46(11):1301–3.
13. Lane HJ, Blum N, Fee E. Oliver Wendell Holmes (1809–1894) and Ignaz Philipp Semmelweis (1818–1865): preventing the transmission of puerperal fever. Am J Public Health. 2010;100(6):1008–9.
14. Centers for Disease Control and Prevention. Hand hygiene in health care settings. 2018. https://www.cdc.gov/handhygiene/science/index.html. Accessed 15 Mar 2019.
15. Smiddy MP, O'Connell R, Creedon SA. Systematic qualitative literature review of health care workers' compliance with hand hygiene guidelines. Am J Infect Control. 2015;43(3):269–74.
16. Gould D. Auditing hand hygiene practice. Nurs Stand. 2010;25(2):50–6.
17. Lawson PA, Citron DM, Tyrrell KL, Finegold SM. Reclassification of Clostridium difficile as Clostridioides difficile (Hall and O'Toole 1935) Prévot 1938. Anaerobe. 2016;40:95–9.
18. Cohen SH, Gerding DN, Johnson S, Kelly CP, Loo VG, McDonald LC, et al. Clinical practice guidelines for *Clostridium difficile* infection in adults: 2010 update by the Society for Healthcare Epidemiology of America (SHEA) and the Infectious Diseases Society of America (IDSA). Infect Control Hosp Epidemiol. 2010;31(5):431–55.
19. Centers for Disease Control and Prevention. Guidelines for hand hygiene in healthcare. 2018. https://www.cdc.gov/mmwr/PDF/rr/rr5116.pdf. Accessed 15 Mar 2019.
20. Ku TS, Walraven CJ, Lee SA. Candida auris: disinfectants and implications for infection control. Front Microbiol. 2018;9:1–12.
21. Hass J. Hand hygiene. In: Text of infection control and epidemiology. Association for Professionals in Infection Control and Epidemiology. 2014. http://text.apic.org/toc/basic-principles-of-infection-prevention-practice/hand-hygiene. Accessed 1 Mar 2019.
22. Hedderwick SA, McNeil SA, Lyons MJ, Kauffman CA. Pathogenic organisms associated with artificial fingernails worn by healthcare workers. Infect Control Hosp Epidemiol. 2000;21(8):505–9.
23. World Health Organization. https://www.who.int/gpsc/5may/tools/training_education/en/. 2019. Accessed 1 Mar 2019.
24. Fishbein A, Tellez I, Lin H, Sullivan C, Groll M. Glow gel hand washing in the waiting room: a novel approach to improving hand hygiene education. Infect Control Hosp Epidemiol. 2011;32(7):661–6.
25. Hagel S, Reischke J, Kesselmeier M, Winning J, Gastmeier P, Brunkhorst FM, et al. Quantifying the

Hawthorne effect in hand hygiene compliance through comparing direct observation with automated hand hygiene monitoring. Infect Control Hosp Epidemiol. 2015;36(8):957–62.
26. Ellingson K, Polgreen PM, Schneider A, Kaldjian LC, Wright D, Thomas GW, et al. Healthcare personnel perceptions of hand hygiene monitoring technology. Infect Control Hosp Epidemiol. 2011;32(11):1091–6.
27. McGuckin M, Govednik J. A review of electronic hand hygiene monitoring:considerations for hospital management in data collection, healthcare worker supervision, and patient perception. J Health Manag. 2015;60(5):348–61.
28. Rutala WA, Weber DJ. Disinfection and sterilization: an overview. Am J Infect Control. 2013;41(Supp 5):S2–5.
29. Weber DJ, Anderson D, Rutala WA. The role of the surface environment in healthcare-associated infections. CurrOpin Infect Dis. 2013;26(4):338–44.
30. Shelly MJ, Scanlon TG, Ruddy R, Hannan MM, Murray JG. Methicillin-resistant *Staphylococcus aureus* (MRSA) environmental contamination in a radiology department. Clin Radiol. 2011;66:861–4.
31. Boyle H, Strudwick RM. Do lead aprons pose an infection risk? Radiography. 2010;16:297–303.
32. Tugwell J, Maddison A. Radiographic markers – a reservoir for bacteria? Radiography. 2010;17:115–20.
33. Rutala WA, White MS, Gergen MF, Weber DJ. Bacterial contamination of keyboards: efficacy and functional impact of disinfectants. Infect Control Hosp Epidemiol. 2006;27(4):372–7.
34. Amodio E, Dino C. Use of ATP bioluminescence for assessing the cleanliness of hospital surfaces: a review of the published literature (1990–2012). J Infect Public Health. 2014;7(2):92–8.
35. Alfa MJ, Olson N, Murray B. Adenosine tri-phosphate (ATP)-based cleaning monitoring in health care: how rapidly does environmental ATP deteriorate? J Hosp Infect. 2015;90(1):59–65.
36. Centers for Disease Control and Prevention. Options for evaluating environmental cleaning. 2018. https://www.cdc.gov/hai/toolkits/appendices-evaluating-environ-cleaning.html. Accessed Mar 1 2019.
37. Fiutem C. Risk factors facilitating transmission of infectious agents. In: Text of infection control and epidemiology. Association for Professionals in Infection Control and Epidemiology. 2014. http://text.apic.org/toc/microbiology-and-risk-factors-for-transmission/risk-factors-facilitat. Accessed 1 March 2019.
38. Lee JY. Tuberculosis infection control in health-care facilities: environmental control and personal protection. Tuberc Respir Dis. 2016;79:234–40.
39. Monzer AC, Thakor AS, Tulin-Silver S, Connolly BL, Cahill AM, Ward TJ, et al. Adult and pediatric antibiotic prophylaxis during vascular and IR procedures: A Society of Interventional Radiology practice parameter update endorsed by the Cardiovascular and Interventional Radiological Society of Europe and the Canadian Association for Interventional Radiology. JVIR. 2018;29(11):1483–501.

# Radiation Safety Considerations in Interventional Fluoroscopy

**12**

Michael C. Talmadge

## 12.1 Introduction

Interventional fluoroscopy presents special radiation safety concerns for both patients and staff due to the potential for exposure to ionizing radiation in the form of X-rays [1]. While a patient undergoing a fluoroscopic procedure is exposed at a much higher level than the attending staff due to the nature of radiological imaging, the radiation exposure to the staff must be viewed from a different perspective that takes into account the repetitive nature of this occupational hazard to a presumably healthy working population. Additionally, the exposure to the patient is counterbalanced by the medical benefit or necessity of the procedure whereas the rationale for the exposure to the staff is much simpler in that it should be minimized as much as practically possible. Although occupational radiation exposure in many countries is specifically limited by regulation and/or international standards, many health care professionals that are involved in interventional fluoroscopic services are not necessarily exposed at such a level that they are likely to approach these limits. Therefore, it is prudent to continually examine and act on measures, within reason, to minimize the exposure of staff in the interventional suite.

---

M. C. Talmadge, DABR, CHP (✉)
Radiation Oncology, Massachusetts General Hospital (MGH)/Newton Wellesley Hospital,
Newton, MA, USA

## 12.2 Radiation Health

Ionizing radiation is often conceptualized as "energy moving through space" and in some respects behaves similarly to visible light; however, ionizing radiation is classified as such because it has enough energy to remove electrons that are bound to an atom, thus ionizing the atom. This property is unique to ionizing radiation and is significant because of the way in which it can produce chemical changes in a material, which, in turn, can produce unique biological effects. While most of our knowledge of ionizing radiation came about during the last century roughly, our environment has exposed us to it throughout our existence in the form of naturally occurring radiation originating from the earth, atmosphere, and outer space. With this perspective it is perhaps fair to say that exposure to ionizing radiation is not an entirely foreign or unnatural occurrence as it has always been an unavoidable condition. Nevertheless the hazards presented by ionizing radiation became evident soon after it was discovered because humans began to find ways to produce sources of ionizing radiation that could result in substantially more exposure to those nearby than the naturally occurring sources. This is noteworthy as it underscores a fundamental concept that applies to the biological effects from ionizing radiation as it does may substances: the magnitude of the exposure is the key determinant in terms of potential for harm.

The health effects associated with exposure to ionizing radiation have been studied extensively. At very high levels, such as those a patient could potentially experience while undergoing interventional fluoroscopy, ionizing radiation can produce clinically observable affects that are largely unique to ionizing radiation, such as skin injuries among many others. At such levels, there are fairly well-defined thresholds at which these injuries or effects have been observed, and generally once that threshold is exceeded the severity of the affect worsens with the magnitude of the exposure (deterministic effect). At lower levels of exposure, such as those that a properly protected health care worker might experience, these types of effects do not occur. However, because ionizing radiation can damage cellular DNA, it can also increase the occurrence of cancers and genetic effects within a population that is exposed. Genetic effects, meaning those that are observed in the offspring of an exposed individual, have not been observed in human populations, whereas an increased occurrence of cancer has been clearly seen in populations that have been exposed to significant levels of ionizing radiation, such as survivors from the use of atomic weapons in Japan in 1945.

At high levels, it is well-established science that exposure to ionizing radiation increases the occurrence of cancer within a population in a proportional fashion (stochastic effect). At lower levels, such as those permitted occupationally in the United States, the relationship between radiation exposure and cancer risk is not as well understood because the cancer risk at these levels is, if it exists, so small that it is very difficult to observe statistically. This knowledge gap is, however, not for lack of trying but instead a consequence of the fact that cancer is a relatively common disease within the general population and there is no definitive way to discriminate radiation-induced cancers from all cancer occurrences aside from statistical methods. While this area continues to be studied, it is clear that low levels of radiation exposure, such as those considered acceptable in an occupational setting, pose a very small risk if at all. As a matter of course, radiation protection standards have largely been developed assuming that this risk, however small, does exist and it therefore follows that good radiation safety practices must always seek to reduce exposure in the workplace to the lowest levels that are reasonably achievable. In the United States, this is codified into regulatory standards and it is often referred to using the acronym ALARA (as low as reasonably achievable).

Radiation exposure is quantified in terms of *absorbed dose* which is a measure of energy deposition in a material by ionizing radiation. When X-rays, for example, pass through the body during imaging, some of the individual X-rays interact with the material they encounter while others do not. These interactions tend to lead to a transfer of energy from the radiation to the material and often produce ionization while deflecting or stopping the individual X-ray. *Absorbed dose* is the basis for measuring radiation exposure as the energy deposition is associated with the amount of ionization that occurs which is the primary mechanism by which ionizing radiation affects material.

## 12.3 Principles of Fluoroscopy

Fluoroscopy is essentially on-demand X-ray imaging that is typically operated by or at the direction of the proceduralist and used for real-time image guidance and evaluation. A fluoroscopy system is usually operated by a button or foot pedal such that when the controlling mechanism is depressed X-rays are being generated continuously to provide real-time imaging. When the system is imaging, a beam of X-rays is emitted from the X-ray tube. The beam passes through the patient and is received by the image receptor in the form of a cylindrical image intensifier or, on later equipment, a flat panel detector. The beam of X-rays comprises a very large number of individual X-rays some of which are stopped within the patient and others pass through and make it to the image receptor. The type of tissue or material encountered by an X-ray as it passes through the body influences the probability that the X-ray will be stopped. The resulting image results from the variable attenuation of X-rays which is dependent on the patient's anatomy. Additionally, contrast can be introduced into the bloodstream, gastrointestinal tract, or cavity in order to allow for improved visualization or to evaluate flow.

There are many operating parameters that a fluoroscopy user can modulate that affect both the image quality and radiation exposure to the patient and the attending staff. The diligent fluoroscopy operator must be judicious to provide the necessary imaging for the procedure at-hand while minimizing the radiation dose to the patient and staff. There are many strategies and techniques that can be used to achieve this; however, the most important factor is generally the amount of the time the X-ray beam is on during a given procedure as this relates directly to the quantity of X-rays produced and the potential for the dose to the patient and staff.

Modern fluoroscopy systems make use of automation to help the operator achieve an appropriate balance between image quality and radiation dose. One very common feature that is widely used is referred to as "automatic brightness control." This feature essentially adjusts the X-ray output in an attempt to provide a given level of image brightness. In practice, this feature will increase the X-ray output if the X-ray beam is required to traverse more tissue or denser materials, such as bone or metal implants. While this is a very useful feature in practice, it is important to understand how it works because if any unneeded material is introduced into the X-ray beam, such as a shield, instrument, or even the patient's arm, the X-ray tube output will increase as it attempts to maintain comparable imaging. For this reason, shielding, leaded gloves, or aprons, for instance, should never be placed into the X-ray beam when such automatic controls are enabled. It is also important to recognize that the patient habitus will affect the radiation output of the fluoroscopy system in the same way; a larger habitus will require a more intense beam of X-rays with possibly a higher average energy to form a useful image. In turn, this will elevate the radiation exposure potential posed by the scattered X-rays.

If there is nothing in between the X-ray tube and image receptor, then the beam of X-rays is largely unchanged as it traverses the intervening air; however, when a patient is present, many of the X-rays interact within the patient such that they are deflected off course. This is referred to as *scatter* and scattered X-rays are generally the primary source of radiation exposure to staff in a fluoroscopy suite. These scattered X-rays effectively originate from the part of the patient being imaged as this is where the X-rays are deflected from their original course. When an X-ray is scattered, it could be deflected any way, but with the type of X-rays used in medical imaging it is most likely that the X-rays are backscattered, meaning that they are deflected by more than 90° such that they are heading back toward the X-ray tube roughly. This results in higher rates of exposure for anyone that is located near the part of the patient at which the X-ray beam is entering the patient.

Many fluoroscopy systems can also be set up to operate to perform high-intensity imaging in a pre-programmed fashion in which many images are created and recorded in rapid succession. This is often times done in conjunction with intravenous contrast and is referred to as "*cine*." Some fluoroscopy systems also can perform a type of three-dimensional image comparable to a computed tomography (CT) scan. It should be noted that when a fluoroscopy system is used in this way it has the potential to produce significantly higher X-ray output than is used during normal operation. For this reason, staff should exit the suite or be in shielded location whenever possible when the fluoroscopy system is used in this way.

## 12.4 Radiation Protection

Fluoroscopic procedures generally represent one of the greatest sources of occupational exposure in the health care setting in terms of both the number of staff that may be present during use and the potential for exposure to individual members of the staff.

### 12.4.1 Time

Certain procedural areas such as interventional cardiology and interventional radiology often employ much greater use of the fluoroscopic techniques and it follows that these areas are often associated with higher levels of staff exposure than those that may use fluoroscopy on a more limited basis, such as orthopedics or urology.

### 12.4.2 Distance

Typically, the practitioner performing a fluoroscopically guided procedure (and possibly an assistant) has the greatest exposure potential largely due to their need to be near the patient while the imaging is being performed whereas much of the staff is further afield during imaging and thereby is exposed at a markedly lower level. This trend underscores one of the primary means in which staff can minimize their exposure during fluoroscopy: by increasing the distance between themselves and the part of the patient that is being imaged (the source of scattered radiation). This technique is particularly effective due to the fact that the rate at which one would be exposed during fluoroscopy tends to be highly dependent on the distance from the radiation source. This can be approximated by applying what is commonly referred to as the *inverse square law*, which essentially relates the rate of exposure to the inverse of the square of the distance from the source. Practically this means that if you double the distance between yourself and the source of radiation, you reduce the rate at which you are being exposed when the beam is on by approximately 75%. For this reason, distance can play a significant role in reducing one's exposure and while one may not be able to remain stationary throughout a procedure there should be an ongoing awareness of this such that one can back away from the patient when possible during imaging.

### 12.4.3 Shielding

The use of shielding is the other primary means of protection in the fluoroscopy suite. Due to the fact that the X-rays used for imaging are relatively low in energy, it is relatively easy to make use of shielding materials that can be readily worn or positioned. Historically, lead was the most widely used material for this purpose; however, in many applications lead has been replaced by other materials. Regardless, protective apparel and equipment is generally rated in terms of lead equivalent thicknesses, meaning that the item in question provides shielding equal to that of a given thickness of lead. Only 0.5 mm of lead or lead equivalence will generally attenuate at least 90% of the X-rays that attempt to pass through it, which in turn reduces the exposure roughly tenfold. For this reason, protective apparel in addition to mobile shields, such as those on wheels or adjustable screens mounted to the ceiling, can be used to great effect in the fluoroscopy suite. Many of these devices are transparent as well and can be easily moved and positioned within the suite.

It is generally a good practice to ensure that all staff in the fluoroscopy suite are wearing protective apparel in the form of one- or two-piece aprons of 0.5 mm lead equivalence that is designed to provide coverage from above the knee to the shoulders. While the added weight of such apparel is certainly not negligible, it is generally not overly burdensome for staff. Thyroid collars are also often used to extend the protection of the apron though not necessarily required to the same extent. Proceduralists and perhaps other dedicated staff may have their own fitted apparel whereas circulating staff or those that are only involved in fluoroscopic work occasionally may use shared apparel. Protective apparel can degrade with time and use and will become damaged if it is not stored properly on hangers. As such, apparel is typically checked on a routine basis such as yearly, which is typically performed by fluoroscopically imaging the apparel to look for cracks, holes, or shifting in the shielding material.

Beyond such protective apparel, there are a variety of shields that can be used as well, though these are generally seen as a supplement to the use of apparel. Most shields that are in use now tend to be transparent and come either on wheels or are ceiling mounted on adjustable arms. The latter type tends to be designed such that the shield can be positioned right up against the patient so that it is in between the part of the patient being imaged and the proceduralist (who is generally the closest member of the staff). The advantage to employing these shields, in addition to supplementing the protection afforded by the apparel, is that they can provide shielding to parts of the body that are not protected by an apron.

### 12.4.4 Cataracts

The eye lens is radiosensitive and the formation of cataracts in the lens of the eye is known to be influenced by exposure to ionizing radiation. This has fueled concern and even serious debate over lowering occupational exposure limits as they apply to the lens of the eye. The International Commission on Radiological Protection (ICRP) publishes recommended dose limits to the eye lens and in 2011 recommended a substantially lower dose limit than previously recommended [2]. While these recommendations have not been uniformly adopted by regulatory agencies worldwide at this time, there is reason to consider increasing radiation protection efforts as they pertain to radiation exposure to the eyes. In response, the use of protective eyewear has become more prevalent in interventional fluoroscopy with some regulatory bodies making them a requirement for certain staff. This eyewear is typically of 0.75 mm lead equivalence which has been shown to provide a substantial reduction in the exposure to the lens of the eye. Many styles and frames including prescriptions as well as larger framed models that can fit over prescription glasses have become available. Proceduralists that perform extensive interventional fluoroscopy may be well advised to have a pair of their own whereas the use of such eyewear among other members of the staff may be more discretionary based on the level of exposure.

### 12.4.5 Pregnancy and Radiation Protection

Pregnancy among staff often heightens radiation protection concerns and rightly so as the developing fetus is known to be at increased sensitivity to radiation exposure. In the United States, a pregnant worker has the option to formally declare a pregnancy for radiation protection purposes which then requires the employer to observe fetal dose limit of 5 mSv, which in most cases effectively reduces the mother's allowable occupational dose limit tenfold during the pregnancy. As such, it is possible for some staff, such as an interventionalist, that this may require a change in work assignments or case load; however, for many no significant changes are needed as their exposure is already well within the fetal dose limitations. Staff should be aware of their rights as they pertain to pregnancies as well as any applicable institutional policies but should also be encouraged to consult with the facilities radiation safety officer (RSO) on a confidential basis in relation to radiation safety during a pregnancy.

It is not uncommon for a pregnant staff member to consider wearing a second protective apron during pregnancy. While this can be done it is worth bearing in mind that the use of second apron only provides a fraction of the protection afforded by a single apron since it is likely that 90% or more of the incoming X-rays that could contribute to fetal dose would be removed by a single apron assuming 0.5 mm lead equivalence. Therefore, the second apron comes at the expense of additional weight while providing diminished protective benefit.

### 12.4.6 Radiation Exposure Measurement

Radiation exposure or dose is generally measured using a dosimeter which is a monitoring device worn by individual working in a radiation environment. There are several forms of monitoring, which are often referred to as badges, ranging from radiation-sensitive materials to electronic devices that record and transmit exposure information wirelessly. Generally, these monitors are fairly unobtrusive to wear and are managed by the facilities RSO, although the consistent wearing and exchange practices are necessary in order to provide accurate and timely exposure information. In the United States there are regulatory requirements that define when an employer must provide radiation monitoring to employees based in part on exposure levels that individual workers could be expected to receive. In a typical hospital setting many employees that work with or near sources of ionizing radiation, such as fluoroscopic systems, do not meet the regulatory threshold at which monitoring is required; however, it is not uncommon for many of these workers to be monitored such that a conservative approach to radiation monitoring exists, which not only monitors the individual employees but also monitors the overall radiation profile of the workplace. The disadvantage to this approach though, which should be noted, is that it can be difficult to manage, and rather than focusing the monitoring program on those that have a higher potential for exposure, a much wider net is cast that likely includes staff that receive little to no substantial radiation exposure. Balancing these trade-offs is an important consideration in a large monitoring program, and in the author's experience a two-tiered approach to staff monitoring can be a good option as it allows for a broad monitoring program while intentionally directing oversight and management energy to a subset of the monitored staff who are likely to incur more occupational exposure.

For the individual staff member, one of the most important practices when it comes to radiation monitoring is the placement of the monitor or badge on the body. There are different approaches that can be used here but it is vital that the facilities radiation safety program provide staff with clear instructions as to how monitors should be worn. At a minimum, staff involved in fluoroscopy (if they are monitored) should wear a dosimeter outside all protective apparel generally between the waist and collar. This allows the dosimeter to measure the exposure to unprotected parts of the body such as uncovered skin of the face and extremities as well the eyes. At times a second dosimeter is also worn under the protective apparel which allows for the use a weighted-sum between the two badges to estimate the dose to organs and tissues deep within the body. A second dosimeter under the protective apparel is often used in the case of a pregnancy as well to provide a more meaningful measure of fetal exposure.

### 12.4.7 Measuring and Reporting Patient Radiation Dose

There are multiple ways in which the exposure to a patient that has undergone fluoroscopy can be described or quantified. Generally, these efforts are aimed at providing an estimate of the dose to the skin through which the X-ray beam enters the patient because this tissue typically receives the most exposure and is at the highest risk for injury during a procedure that requires high levels of fluoroscopic output. Estimating the dose to the skin, though readily achievable, is not entirely straightforward but the greater problem lies in identifying the parts of the skin that were exposed during a fluoroscopy procedure as these are areas on the skin that one may attempt to avoid re-exposing during a subsequent procedure. At a minimum, modern fluoroscopy systems record both "fluoro time" which captures the amount of time in which the X-ray beam was on and an "air kerma" value given in units of absorbed dose (often mGy) which is used as a surrogate for the dose to the skin at the beam entry point. These, as well as details pertaining to the procedure itself and the equipment used, can be used to describe the radiation exposure that the patient received. Additionally, many regulatory and accreditation agencies and institutions have implemented reporting and follow-up thresholds for fluoroscopy dose. The radiation safety officer (RSO) or a medical physicist should be able to advise staff on the institutional policies and procedures regarding dose thresholds and their implementation.

In recent years, there has been efforts to develop methods and systems to quantify and document radiation exposure to patients from medical procedures such that an individual's medical radiation exposure can be tracked internally as well as between multiple facilities. While no one system has been widely implemented to facilitate this on a large scale in the United States, many institutions have implemented systems to accomplish this within their own facilities with the intention of reducing medical exposure by avoiding unnecessary or duplicate procedures and improving accountability [3]. Discussion of radiation exposure is one part of the consent process that should take place between the patient and provider. The American College of Radiology has launched initiatives such as Image Wisely® and Image Gently®, which provide educational resources for pediatric and adult patients (see https://www.imagewisely.org/) [4]. The Image Gently® Alliance similarly provides educational information for parents of children and young people [5] (see https://www.imagegently.org/). International programs include AFROSAFE[RAD], Arab Safe, Canada Safe Imaging, EuroSafe Imaging, and LATIN SAFE; information about these can be found at https://www.imagewisely.org/International-Safety-Initiatives [6].

## 12.5 Regulatory Standards

In the United States, occupational exposure to X-rays is generally regulated at the state level though many important standards are largely consistent across the country. The applicable regulatory authority should be clear and generally there are postings issued by the regulator that are to be displayed conspicuously in the facility. The regulator may also require that all equipment and sometimes staff be registered. In many states there are also regulatory requirements that come into play when new X-ray equipment is acquired. While the specifics of these requirements are beyond the scope of this chapter, it is vital that physics and radiation safety expertise is available and engaged both operationally and in planning for new equipment.

As previously mentioned, occupational exposure is limited by regulation. Additionally, institutions generally establish investigational thresholds well below the regulatory limits that allow them to effectively monitor and respond to exposure trends. The regulatory limits themselves are not intended to reflect levels at which any injuries or other biological changes could be observed but rather they are intended to establish limits such that the risk posed by occupational exposure to ionizing radiation is comparable to that posed by other occupational hazards that exists within a workplace that could be considered safe. Though somewhat nuanced, this statement brings into focus the relationship between the concept of the safety and its relationship with real-life risk. In any workplace or any setting or circumstance it is fair to say that risk cannot be eliminated altogether and yet we both individually and collectively need to make judgments as to whether or not something can be considered safe. It follows logically then that safety is not the absence of risk but rather an assessment that the risks are acceptable. For example, one could decide that a given car is safe to drive or that a roadway is safe to use even though the risk of an accident still exists. Of course if there existed a practical way to eliminate the chance of an accident altogether that still allowed us to enjoy the many benefits afforded by modern transit by road, then our assessment of roadway safety could change; though in the meantime the risks cannot be removed so instead we take a variety of steps to mitigate that risk (driver education, seatbelts, speed limits, licensure, insurance). The same philosophy applies to occupational hazards as is the case with ionizing radiation: it would be unreasonably difficult to completely eliminate occupational exposure to ionizing radiation so, though we acknowledge the possibility (however small) of the risk posed by this, we accept it within certain bounds because we acknowledge the benefits that its use can provide. Although we would also be prudent to continually seek to minimize risks in working with radiation, just as a driver may not only wear a seatbelt and observe traffic laws but also drive defensively to reduce the chance of accident. This is analogous to the ALARA philosophy applied to occupational radiation exposure.

In practice, this means that an entity that uses ionizing radiation must not only observe regulatory exposure limits but also continually evaluate and take steps to minimize radiation exposure within reason. Industry standards and best practices shared within a profession can often help to define acceptable practices, technologies, and techniques; however, the ALARA philosophy is intended to be applied in a local sense by individuals as well. For example, a nurse who works in an interventional radiology setting may have enough experience to know that their current practices are sufficient to maintain their exposure levels below regulatory or institutional standards; however, they should also evaluate what practical steps could be taken to further reduce this exposure, such as standing further away from the patient during imaging when possible. In these efforts staff should be educated and empowered.

## 12.6 Training

Radiation safety knowledge and competency among health care staff can vary widely. In the fluoroscopy setting, extensive training in this subject is not necessary for all staff. While fluoroscopy operators, such as physicians, should have a much more extensive knowledge of not only radiation safety but also on the use of the equipment and fundamentals of radiological imaging, the supporting staff often require a basic training that can be obtained easily upon hiring and renewed (e.g., by online module with posttest or other) with some regularity, preferably annually. This training should provide a basic understanding of radiation, the risk involved, effective radiation safety practices, and programmatic information some of which may be specific to the institution such as who to contact for radiation safety or physics expertise. The RSO will play an important role in staff education.

## 12.7 Radiology Nurse Responsibilities

The radiology nurse should be aware of not only the risks of radiation exposure but also how to be an effective member of the radiology team when considering medical radiation and its implications for the staff and patient. Observance of radiology safety procedures and patient education are new roles for the nurse in the imaging setting. A better understanding of radiation exposure issues will lead to better quality patient care.

## 12.8 Conclusion

An understanding of the risks posed by ionizing radiation, as well as the practical means by which these risks can be mitigated, should be fostered within the diagnostic imaging and interventional setting such that staff have an educated and empowered approach to radiation protection and are able to appropriately prioritize radiation safety.

## References

1. NCRP Report No. 168, Radiation Dose Management for Fluoroscopically-Guided Interventional Medical Procedures.
2. Boal TJ, Pinak M. Dose limits to the lens of the eye: International Basic Safety Standards and related guidance. ICRP. 2013;44:112–7. Proceedings
3. Rehani MM. Patient radiation exposure and dose tracking: a perspective. J Med Imaging. 2017;4(3) https://doi.org/10.1117/1.JMI.4.3.0321206.
4. Brink JA, Amis ES Jr. Image wisely: a campaign to increase awareness about adult radiation protection. Radiology. 2010;257(3):601–2. https://doi.org/10.1148/radiol:10101335.
5. Image Gently Alliance® Available at https://www.imagegently.org/
6. International Safety Initiatives. Available at https://www.imagewisely.org/International-Safety-Initiatives

# Waste Anesthetic Gases (WAGs): Minimizing Health Risks and Increasing Awareness

**13**

John E. Moenning Jr., Dina A. Krenzischek, and James D. McGlothlin

## 13.1 Introduction

The scavenging of waste anesthetic gases (WAGs) is recommended by every professional organization and government agency involved with anesthesia to reduce occupational exposure to healthcare personnel [1]. WAGs in healthcare environments have been associated with adverse health outcomes in unscavenged situations [2–13]. Methods to decrease occupational exposure by scavenging WAGs and minimizing potential health problems is important in both the operating room (OR) and in the postanesthetic care unit (PACU) [14, 15]. By extension this also means it is important to discuss WAG in relation to any imaging environment where anesthesia is used as well as the imaging procedure recovery area.

J. E. Moenning Jr, DDS, MSD
Indiana Oral & Maxillofacial Surgery Associates, Fishers, IN, USA

D. A. Krenzischek, PhD, RN, CPAN, FAAN (✉)
Patient Care Service, Mercy Medical Center, Baltimore, MD, USA

J. D. McGlothlin, PhD, MPH, CPE, FAIHA
Emeritus Purdue University, West Lafayette, IN, USA

## 13.2 Standards and Guidelines for WAG

Assuring that employers provide safe working conditions for employees was the purpose of the Occupational Safety and Health Act of 1970, Public Law 91-596 [16]. This act created the Occupational Safety and Health Administration (OSHA) under the US Department of Labor, and the National Institute for Occupational Safety and Health (NIOSH) under the Department of Health and Human Services. OSHA and NIOSH are federal agencies concerned with possible health hazards to employees associated with exposure to WAGs. Other recommending bodies that publish occupational exposure information are the American Conference of Government Industrial Hygienists (ACGIH), the American Society of Anesthesiology (ASA), the American Dental Association (ADA), and the Joint Commission (TJC), also known as the Joint Commission on Accreditation of Healthcare Organizations (JCAHO).

In 1977, NIOSH promoted research on the effects of occupational exposure to WAGs, the means for preventing occupational injuries, and recommended occupational safety standards [17]. It made recommendations to four areas of occupational health: (1) scavenging and exposure to trace WAG concentrations; (2) work practices to minimize WAG concentrations; (3) medical surveillance for possible occupational exposure in the healthcare environment, and (4) monitoring WAGs. NIOSH recommended that workers should not be exposed to halogenated agents at concentrations of >2 parts per million (ppm) when used alone or >0.5 ppm when used in combination with nitrous oxide over a sampling period not to exceed 1 h. NIOSH also recommended that occupational exposure to nitrous oxide, when used as the sole anesthetic agent, should not exceed a time-weighted average of 25 ppm during the time of anesthetic administration. In addition, this federal agency recommended that all anesthetic gas machines, non-rebreathing systems, and t-tube devices have an effective scavenging device that collects all WAGs. Within these recommendations, the agency provided a thorough discussion of other work-practice techniques, such as turning on the scavenging system before administering anesthetic gases to the patient to minimize WAG exposure to medical staff.

In 1989, the ACGIH assigned a threshold-level limit value time-weighted average for nitrous oxide of 50 ppm for an 8-h work day [18]. ASA, in its Guidelines for Non-Operating Room Anesthesia Locations, approved by its House of Delegates in 1994, stated that in any location that inhalation agents are administered, there should be adequate and reliable systems for scavenging WAGs [1]. The ADA recommends the scavenging of all WAGs for all procedures involving anesthetic gases in the dental office [15]. Finally, in 1997, JCAHO recommended that educational programs and orientation should be established for all personnel who have contact with hazardous materials and waste.

Other countries around the world have also established standard guidelines to occupational exposure for nitrous oxide. These can range anywhere from 25 ppm (the Netherlands) to 100 ppm (Italy, Sweden, Norway, Denmark, and Great Britain) [19, 20]. While some of these government agencies and healthcare associations have different occupational exposure standards in regard to ppm, all unanimously agree that scavenging WAGs should be utilized.

OSHA's responsibilities are to adopt and mandate job safety and health standards, establish the rights and responsibilities of employers and employees for safe occupational conditions, establish recordkeeping and reporting procedures of injuries, and evaluate work-related safety practices (Table 13.1). OSHA is also responsible for carrying out NIOSH recommendations [21]. Currently, OSHA recognizes NIOSH-recommended exposure limits (RELs) to WAG exposure, but to date, it has not set its own standards for WAGs. However, OSHA can cite under the General Duty Clause 5a(1), which states, "each employer shall furnish to each of his employees employment and a place of employment which are free from recognized hazards that are causing or are likely to cause death or serious physical harm to his employees" [22].

To minimize and create an environment as safe as possible for healthcare workers, NIOSH recommends a well-designed scavenging system as part of an anesthetic delivery system for collecting WAGs. These recommendations apply to any place where anesthetic agents are delivered, as well as to the PACU. Patients may out-gas (i.e., exhale) anesthetic agents following their surgical procedures; NIOSH recognizes that close proximity to patients can result in exposure to quantifiable concentrations of WAGs. It also indicates that while random room samples may indicate relatively low levels of WAGs, the breathing zone of the nurse in close proximity to the recovering patient may expose that nurse

**Table 13.1** OSHA guidelines to manage WAG risks in the OR and PACU

| |
|---|
| *Facility design and engineering* |
| WAG scavenging systems in the OR |
| Room air changes (OR: 15 with 3 fresh/h; PACU: 6 with 2 fresh/h) |
| Isolated fresh air intakes |
| *Administrative* |
| Work practices, training, hazard communication |
| Professional organization guidelines (e.g., ASA, ADA) |
| *Maintenance and proper use of equipment* |
| Installation of proper equipment, calibration, and maintenance |
| Periodic leak checks |

Source: Occupational Safety and Health Administration, U.S. Department of Labor. (Revised 2000, May). Anesthetic Gases: Guidelines for Workplace Exposures. Retrieved from http://www.osha.gov/dts/osta/anesthetic-gases/index.html

to levels of anesthetic gases that are above the NIOSH RELs. In 2007, NIOSH Publication No. 2007-151 reemphasized these recommendations in regard to WAGs [23]. This publication intended to increase awareness of the adverse health effects of these gases, describe how workers are exposed to WAGs, and recommend work practices to reduce these exposures and identify methods to minimize leakage of WAGs into the work environment. Steege et al., in their 2014 NIOSH-sponsored survey, found that 56% of workers dealing with anesthetic gases were unaware whether their employer had standard procedures for handling/minimizing exposure to these gases [24].

## 13.3 WAG Risks: Toxicology and Mechanisms

Lassen et al., in a 1956 Lancet article, found that severe bone marrow depression could occur after prolonged nitrous oxide anesthesia in some patients who were being treated for tetanus [25]. Later in 1967, the first indication that anesthetic gases could be a problem for humans was reported by Russian scientist Vaisman [26], who reported that female anesthesiologists had had problems with fatigue, nausea, and headaches, and that 18 of 31 pregnancies ended in spontaneous abortion. In 1968, additional articles with regard to nitrous oxide and its effects on bone marrow were reported. Banks et al. and Amess et al. reported that nitrous oxide can inactivate vitamin B12 and thus cause biochemical derangements similar to those seen in pernicious anemia [27, 28]. In 1974, Bruce et al. published their studies dealing with nitrous oxide and audiovisual impairment [29]. In 1977, NIOSH reported that levels of 50 ppm for nitrous oxide were the lowest level at which human effects had been reported [17]. NIOSH quoted audiovisual impairments that Bruce et al. illustrated.

In 1980, Cohen et al. published an article reporting on health problems experienced by dentists and chairside assistants who had been exposed to nitrous oxide in their jobs [6]. They considered dentists as having light exposure if they used nitrous 1–8 h a week, or heavy exposure if used >8 h a week. They found the following information: nitrous oxide use doubled the likelihood for congenital abnormalities or spontaneous abortions; nitrous oxide was shown to have an increased effect on neurologic problems, as well as liver and renal problems for male dentists and assistants; and nitrous oxide use doubled the likelihood for cervical CA in the female study group.

In 1992, Rowland et al. reported that fertility problems occurred in women exposed to high levels of unscavenged nitrous oxide [12]. They also found a 2.5-fold increase in spontaneous abortions experienced by women who worked in dental operatories that did not scavenge nitrous oxide and found no increase in infertility or spontaneous abortion in women who worked in dental operatories that scavenged waste nitrous oxide.

In a government technical report, McGlothlin et al. (1994) reported similar findings from the literature, where the effects of acute and chronic occupational exposure had been shown to cause bone marrow depression (primary granulocytopenia), paraesthesia, difficulty concentrating, equilibrium disturbances, and impaired visual effects [30].

As a result of numerous epidemiological evaluations, the ASA commissioned a group of epidemiologists and biostatisticians to evaluate the significance of these studies with regard to possible health hazards resulting from exposure to WAGs. Buring et al. reviewed 17 published studies, and after evaluating these studies for the best statistical controls they concluded that there was a 30% increased risk of spontaneous abortion for women working in operating rooms and a similar, but less consistent increase in congenital abnormities among offspring of exposed physicians [31]. They also concluded that all of the studies reviewed had weaknesses in their response rates and other confounding variables, making it difficult to draw specific conclusions.

A study by Krajewski looked at alterations in the vitamin B12 metabolic status of 95 operating room nurses with a history of exposure to nitrous oxide and compared them to 90 nurses who were not exposed to nitrous oxide [32]. They found significantly lower vitamin B12 status in personnel exposed to nitrous oxide with higher total homocysteine levels. The changes in vitamin B12 status were found to be primarily in subjects who were exposed to nitrous oxide in concentrations substantially exceeding occupational exposure limits.

In 2008, Sanders et al. published a thorough review of the biological effects of nitrous oxide, including how nitrous oxide affects methionine synthase function [33]. They discussed as a result of the interaction of vitamin B12 with nitrous oxide, methionine synthase is inactivated, resulting in alterations to one carbon and a methyl group transferred, which is important for DNA, purine, and thymidylate synthesis. These alterations potentially may result in the increased risk for reproductive consequences, megaloblastic bone marrow depression, neurologic symptoms, and increased levels of homocysteine, which can cause cardiovascular changes.

While the anesthetic use of nitrous oxide with halogenated agents may be decreasing, the use of halogenated agents has not gone down. The agents, sevoflurane, isoflurane, and desflurane, make up the vast majority of inhalation anesthetic gases. Fodale reviewed 54 articles on the health effects of nitrous oxide and halogenated gases and found that these agents were associated with general health and genotoxic risks and stressed the need for further studies [34]. Recently, studies on humans and rodents have shown that low-dose anesthetic gases can cause changes in liver blood chemistry, DNA damage, and antioxidant status [35–38].These reviews create significant debate about the long-term effects of anesthetic agents. These possible health changes become even more concerning in the developing brains of children and the elderly, and these neurocognitive issues are being investigated by the Federal Food and Drug Administration (FDA) in the USA [39]. As a result, all organizations have concluded that good scavenger systems are needed to decrease these possible health consequences from exposure to WAGs with halogenated agents and/or nitrous oxide gas.

## 13.4 WAGs in the PACU

In 1996, the American Society of Perianesthesia Nurses (ASPAN) issued a position statement in regard to air safety in the postanesthesia environment [40]. It stated that necessary, appropriate, and protective engineering controls, technologies, work practices, and personal protective equipment be utilized in the perianesthesia environment. ASPAN recommended that occupational exposure to WAGs, and blood-borne and respiratory pathogens, be controlled by adherence to regulations and guidelines set forth by nationally recognized agencies, such as NIOSH, the Centers for Disease Control and Prevention (CDC), and OSHA's hierarchy of controls based on principles of good industrial hygiene.

In 1997, an article by Badgwell discussed air safety source control technology for the PACU [41]. In addition, Brodsky concluded his review of the literature by stating, "Why risk potential health and reproductive problems while waiting for definitive proof, when this is not likely to be forthcoming. Even without direct proof of cause, we should reduce levels of WAG to their lowest possible concentration by careful use of efficient control measures" [42]. Badgwell also stated that as a result of the body of research and careful analysis, the inclusion of source-control scavenging has become the de facto standard for anesthetic machines in all operating rooms in the USA since 1980 [41].Badgwell also reviewed literature related to exposure of PACU personnel to WAGs and concluded that WAG levels in the breathing zone of personnel in the PACU appeared to exceed NIOSH RELs. Over the last 10 years, articles have begun to appear with regard to WAG levels in the PACU. Prospective studies have looked at exposure levels in the PACU. Sessler et al. recently summarized several papers on healthcare personnel exposed to WAGs and possible health concerns from this exposure [43]. He reported that the majority of these studies concluded that there is a correlation between reproductive toxicity and exposure to WAGs. The majority of these health concerns involve spontaneous abortions and infertility; neurobehavioral effects; megaloblastic anemia; neuropathies; psychophysiological effects of impaired cognitive, perceptual, and/or motor function; and more recently vitamin B12 deficiencies and homocysteine elevations.

Sessler and Badgwell [43] found that postoperative nurses were frequently exposed to exhaled anesthetic gas concentrations exceeding NIOSH-recommended exposure levels. Interestingly, they found that volatile anesthetic curves did not demonstrate the expected exponential decrease over time. They found that one-fourth of the nurses demonstrated time-weighted average (TWA) that exceeded the 25 ppm NIOSH recommendations, even though they had been caring for patients who had received nitrous oxide-free anesthesia. Sessler points out that this could have been due to limitations in ventilation air exchanges in the PACU design. The data suggested that PACU nurses were exposed to exhaled anesthetic gases exceeding the NIOSH RELs.

Krenzischek found that concentrations of nitrous oxide were close to 300 ppm in a patient's breathing zone [44]. This pilot study identified the potential for staff exposure to WAGs in the PACU setting. A simulated PACU environment was constructed to obtain an understanding of how the concentration of nitrous oxide varies with distance from the patient. Austin found that the concentration of nitrous oxide decreases with distance from the patient and the patient's respiration increases the level of nitrous oxide based on the location of the nurse. Also, the respiration of the nurses pulls the nitrous oxide plume toward them, increasing their exposure to the gas [45]. Austin questioned the inadequacy of attempting to measure levels of gas exposure at random points in a room. There are other articles that have looked at breath analysis to determine whether PACU personnel or operating room personnel are inhaling the gases and then exhaling them at a measurable limit. Cope et al. and Summer et al. have found that exhaled anesthetic agents are present in the breath of personnel [46, 47]. In 2015, Cheung et al. found that WAG concentrations are higher in the patients' breathing zone when patients' airway devices are removed in the PACU vs. in the OR [48].

As stated earlier, it can be surmised that PACU personnel may be exposed to WAGs that are above NIOSH REL standards; this could have health consequences from exposure to WAGs. In addition, the potential for neurocognitive problems can result from chronic exposure. When nursing personnel are exposed to a large number of PACU patients throughout an 8-h day, the potential for cognitive problems may increase. This is important, considering that the Institute of Medicine (IOM) states that as many as 44,000 to 98,000 people die in US hospitals every year as a result of medical errors [49]. Furthermore, nonfatal adverse events related to medication errors can increase hospital costs by as much as $2 billion a year. IOM also states that higher error rates may be more common in emergency departments, operating rooms, or intensive care units (ICUs). Helmreich, in analyzing errors in aviation, found that multiple physiological and psychological factors impact attention spans and make medical errors more likely [50]. Some of the causes include increased workload, fatigue, cognitive overload, ineffective interpersonal communication, and faulty information processing. If cognitive problems are known to increase secondary to exposure to WAGs above NIOSH limits, it seems reasonable to conclude that minimizing exposure to WAGs would help prevent possible adverse health consequences to personnel, as well as decrease the potential for human error during the times patients are in the PACU.

## 13.5 Exposure Assessment Methods for Detecting WAGs

Evaluation of WAGs, particularly nitrous oxide, is typically done through three traditional methods. The first utilizes nitrous oxide dosimetry badges. These sampling monitors are very similar to radiology monitors, where the nitrous oxide gas is absorbed by a zeolite molecular sieve with a pore size of 5 angstroms. These sampling badges are opened at the beginning of a sampling period. Upon completion of the sampling phase, the badge is double-sealed in a bag and then sent to a lab for analysis.

A second method utilizes a small handheld infrared spectrophotometer. An example of one used in PACUs is the Medigas PM 3010 developed by the Bacharach Company in Pittsburgh, PA, USA. This handheld device pulls in the nitrous oxide to be analyzed by a small port and reads nitrous oxide concentrations by infrared analysis spectrophotometry. However, the device that has been used the longest for WAG monitoring has been the Miran 1B SapphIRE Ambient Air Analyzer (Thermo Fisher, Waltham, MA, USA). NIOSH RELs were all established by using the Miran infrared spectrophotometer. Recently, the use of Fourier transform infrared spectroscopy (FTIR) (Gasmet Technologies Oy, Finland) has become the standard for measuring gases. FTIR works by being able to measure the entire IR spectrum and thus measure multiple gases at the same time. While all of these devices measure WAGs as a part per million (ppm), none of these measuring devices can visualize gases.

By utilizing infrared thermography, a new way to visualize WAGs, especially nitrous oxide, has been established. An infrared camera (Merlin Mid-INSB Midwave FLIR infrared camera, FLIR Systems Inc., Boston, MA, USA) uses the infrared light through a special lens to capture the nitrous oxide molecule absorbing the infrared image in a spectrum of 45 to 50 nanometers. Using this technology has made it possible to visualize nitrous oxide, and most recently halogenated agents, and thus develop ways to minimize occupational exposure to personnel not previously possible. Specifically, this allows researchers to "see" where the WAGs may be escaping into the environment (Fig. 13.1).

This technology was utilized in a study that appeared in the February 2009 issue of the Journal of the American Dental Association (JADA) [51]. Two nitrous oxide scavenging systems were evaluated to determine their ability to control waste gas emissions. As a result of this study, it was discovered that nitrous oxide is present in the postoperative respirations of individuals long after discontinuation of the gas. The use of this technology was then taken to the PACU as a proof-of-concept to determine if WAG occurs in the breathing zone of recovering patients and exposes nurses to these exhaled WAGs.

To visualize possible WAGs in the PACU, identical instrumentation used in the JADA February 2009 issue was utilized. Preliminary data were collected using three types of instrumentation. These were infrared thermography by means of an infrared camera (Merlin Mid-INSB Midwave infrared camera, National Instruments Corporation, Austin, TX, USA), digital videography by means of a camcorder (Handicam, DCR-SR100, Sony, Tokyo, Japan), and real-time nitrous oxide and sevoflurane air concentration levels parts per million (ppm) by means of an infrared spectrophotometer (Miran 1B SapphIRE Ambient Air Analyzer, Thermo Fisher Scientific, Waltham, MA, USA) [52]. By using all three methods to measure WAGs, McGlothlin et al. proved that sevoflurane and nitrous are present in the PACU, are present in the patient's and nurse's breathing zones, are above the NIOSH RELs for extended periods of time, and can be controlled (Fig. 13.2).

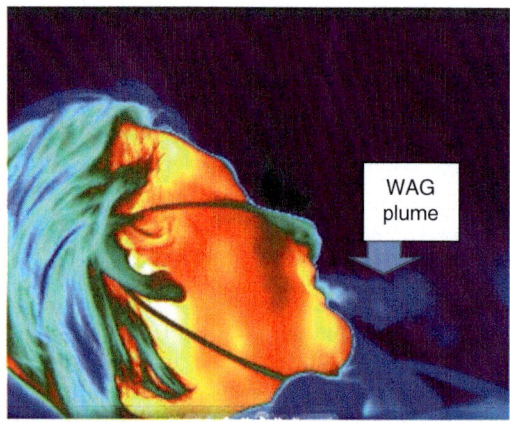

**Fig. 13.1** New patient admitted to PACU following general anesthesia. The Infrared allows the visualization of the WAG as seen by the WAG plume from the mouth (Permission to re-print Dr. John Moenning Source)

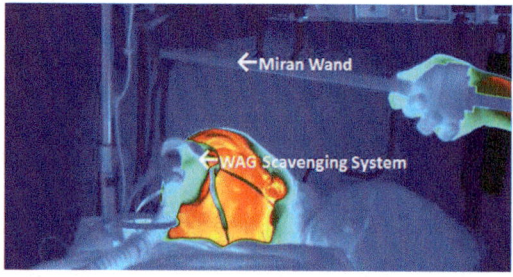

**Fig. 13.2** WAG Scavenging System in place capturing the WAG's following general anesthesia (Permission to re-print Dr. John Moenning Source)

Hillar et al. also evaluated WAGs in the PACU and showed that the rate of washout of sevoflurane was dependent solely on the duration of the anesthetic exposure. They found that when their patients were extubated at 0.2% (2000 ppm) and assuming a constant cardiac output, even after 25 min (92% elimination), the concentrations would still be 184 ppm. To get to the current NIOSH RELs of 2 ppm would require a 98.998% reduction of the inhaled anesthetic gas and could take more than an hour [53]. In 2018, Tallent et al. also documented PACU WAGs in 120 patients after tracheal extubation in the patient breathing zone and nurse work zone. More importantly, they were able to document the reduction of elevated WAGs (exhaled Sevoflurane and Desflurane) in the PACU to concentrations below the NIOSH RELs in greater than 85% of extubated patients within 20 s of applying the ISO-Gard® scavenger mask [54].

Utilizing techniques to measure and visualize WAGs in the PACU has proven the existence of occupational exposure (Fig. 13.3) [52–54]. A review of the literature in regard to possible health concerns from postanesthetic gases and the conclusions from governing bodies and professional organizations indicate a general agreement that control of WAGs should be considered. Utilizing engineering controls, best-work practices, and personal protective equipment (such as a mask) should be used in the PACU environment. Developing methods and practices to minimize these WAGs is important. In fact, OSHA has stated, "the preferred and most effective means of protecting workers is to prevent hazards entering their breathing zone in the first place" [55].

The American Society of PeriAnesthesia Nurses (ASPAN), at its National Meeting in 2016, identified the following issues pertinent to perianesthesia occupational hazard exposure prevention:

1. Exposure to waste anesthetic gases above NIOSH RELs exhaled by patients in the breathing zone of nurses providing care at the bedside and cross contamination to other PACU patients, including immune suppressed patients
2. Lack of sufficient monitoring within the breathing zone of PACU patients following general anesthesia
3. Lack of engineering control interventions to reduce the level of waste anesthetic gas exposure to healthcare workers (HCWs) and other patients
4. High risk of exposure for HCWs and patients to respiratory pathogens in the perianesthesia environment; open architectural designs including lack of air exchanges of perianesthesia care areas increase the risk of transmission of respiratory pathogens among patients and between patients and HCWs
5. Increased risk of exposure to droplet and airborne infectious diseases (e.g., M. tuberculosis [TB] and rubella virus [measles], and viral illnesses, such as norovirus, Ebola virus, and Zika virus) [56, 57]

As a result of all of the research, new techniques in monitoring and the visualization of WAGs ASPAN updated its position statement in 2016 [40] (Table 13.2).

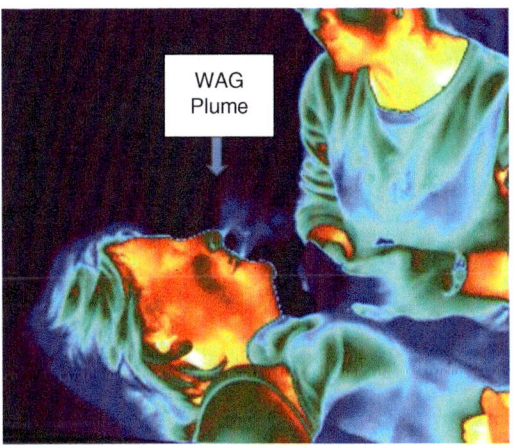

**Fig. 13.3** Nursing personal in the breathing zone being exposed to the WAG (WAG plume) following general anesthesia (Permission to re-print Dr., John Moenning Source)

**Table 13.2** ASPAN's position states that "necessary, appropriate, and evidence-based protective engineering controls, technologies, work practices, and personal protective equipment be utilized in the perianesthesia environment" [40]. Key points of ASPAN's recommendations are to

- Promote a safe environment for nurses and patients
- Adhere to national regulations and guidelines to establish a hierarchy of controls based on principles of good industrial hygiene including waste anesthetic gases
- Protect healthcare workers and patients based on national regulations and evidence-based guidelines
- Support the development of healthcare policies, research collaborative projects that improves quality and safe environment including air quality and reduction of occupational exposure hazards

Source: 2019–2020 ASPAN Perianesthesia Nursing Standards, Practice Recommendations and Interpretive Statements: A Position Statement on Air Quality and Occupational Hazard Exposure Prevention (Permission to print by ASPAN)

## 13.6 Use of Scavenging Systems to Reduce and Prevent WAGs and Airborne Pathogens in the PACU

As discussed above, engineering controls, including scavenging systems in the PACU, are one of the most effective means to reduce and prevent exposure to WAGs. However, there are mounting concerns that nurses and related healthcare personnel in the PACU are also exposed to harmful airborne pathogens from patients' expired breath and nurses breathing this contaminated air during the patient's recovery. In fact, when a patient indicates that he or she has had a respiratory illness that could be harmful to PACU nurses, these patients are typically protected from exposing other patients by isolating them in a corner of the PACU. In addition, the nurses will wear additional respiratory protection (face shields, along with N-95 respirators). In some instances, the additional cost for these precautions are added to the patient's bill and/or is passed on to their provider. Because of this, many patients may not be forthcoming about their current or previous illnesses or may not even know that their airborne infectious diseases could harm the health of nurses in the PACU.

To address this issue, researchers at Purdue University have conducted preliminary research on the utility of market-available scavenging systems (e.g., ISO-Gard® [58]) to not only remove WAGs in the PACU, but also harmful airborne pathogens. As a proof of concept, the initial research was conducted in a Purdue University laboratory using a market-available scavenging system using state-of-the-art bioluminescence techniques [59]. The initial study showed a significant reduction in pathogens compared to not using the market-available scavenging system [60]. A follow-up study was conducted to better understand how well this market-available scavenging system worked to capture the bacteria, and where it deposited most of the bacteria in the scavenging system. Results showed that the bacteria were mostly concentrated in the patient's scavenging mask, then all along the exhaust tubing. Because of the success of both research studies (now pending publication) it was reasoned that this scavenging system could also benefit nurses in the PACU from airborne pathogens.

## 13.7 Translation of Evidence to Practice

There is increased attention to patient and workplace safety in healthcare facilities, which is driven by regulatory agencies, advocacy groups, litigators, and most importantly the patients or healthcare staff themselves. The most common challenge is not only the translation of evidence, but also the time it takes to drive change to practice despite published guidelines, policies, and evidence recommendations. Behavior change among organizations and/or individuals (providers, patients) is inherent in the translation process, engagement of stakeholder organizations, healthcare delivery systems, and individuals. This is important to achieving effective translation and sustained improvements [61].

## 13.8 Conclusion

Most PACU/recovery room (RR) nurses may not be aware of the WAG risks in their workplace environment. Understanding the evidence and putting it into practice is a start, especially toward increasing awareness. However, evidence and awareness are only meaningful when translated into practice. The assessment of potential risk in the clinical area and collaboration with appropriate resources (clinical chain of command and clinical engineering) are necessary steps in the implementation process. The clinical engineering department is responsible for monitoring potential WAGs in the OR/theater. In the PACU/RR, WAG assessment within the breathing zone of the patient can be monitored by clinical engineering health and safety professionals using appropriate monitoring devices. Monitoring of WAGs in the PACU has to be done on a routine basis whenever patients with anesthetic gas are admitted into the unit. Controlling the source of WAGs (typically from patients' exhalation in the PACU) protects not only the nurses but also other health-compromised patients. As a perianesthesia nurse in the PACU/RR or radiology post-recovery phase, the nurse's role is to provide safe and quality care to patients and be an advocate for a safe workplace environment. Protecting nurses and other healthcare staff from any risk of exposure, be it WAGs, airborne pathogens, infection, or any adverse outcome, is the responsibility of the entire healthcare team. So, extending the assessment, monitoring, and implementation of engineering control also means it is important to discuss WAG in relation to any imaging/interventional radiology environment where anesthesia is used as well as the imaging/interventional procedure recovery area.

## References

1. McGregor D. Task force on trace anesthetic gases, committee on occupational health. Waste anesthetic gases: an update on information for management in anesthetizing areas and the postanesthesia care unit. ASA Newsl. 1999;63:7.
2. Cohen EN, Bellville JW, Brown BW. Anesthesia, pregnancy, and miscarriage: a study of operating room nurses and anesthetists. Anesthesiology. 1971;35:343–7.
3. Rosenberg P, Kirves A. Miscarriages among operating theater staff. Acta Anaesthesiol Scand. 1973;53:37–42.
4. Cohen EN, Brown BW, Bruce DL, et al. Occupational disease among operating roompersonnel: a national study. Anesthesiology. 1974;41:321–40.
5. Corbett TH, Cornell RG, Endres JL, Lieding K. Birth defects among children of nurse-anesthetists. Anesthesiology. 1974;41:341–4.
6. Cohen EN, Brown BW, Wu ML, Whitcher CE, Brodsky JB, Gift HC, et al. Occupational disease in dentistry and chronic exposure to trace anesthetic gases. J Am Dent Assoc. 1980;101:21–31.
7. Ericson A, Kallen B. Survey of infants born in 1973 or 1975 to Swedish women working in operating rooms during their pregnancies. Anesth Analg. 1979;58:302–5.
8. Rosenberg PH, Vanttinen H. Occupational hazards to reproduction and health in anesthetists and pediatricians. Acta Anaesthesiol Scand. 1978;22:202–7.
9. Axelsson G, Rylander R. Exposure to anaesthetic gases and spontaneous abortion: responsebias in a postal questionnaire study. Int J Epidemiol. 1982;11:250–6.
10. Guirguis SS, Pelmear PL, Roy ML, Wong L. Health effects associated with exposure to anaesthetic gases in Ontario hospital personnel. Br J Ind Med. 1990;47:490–7.
11. Rowland AS, Baird DD, Shore DL, Weinberg CR, Savitz DA, Wilcox AJ. Nitrous oxide and spontaneous abortion in female dental assistants. Am J Epidemiol. 1995;141:531–8.
12. Roland AS, Baird DD, Weinberg CR, Shore DL, Shy CM, Wilcox AJ. Reduced fertility among women employed as dental assistants exposed to high levels of nitrous oxide. N Engl J Med. 1992;327:993–7.
13. Tannenbaum TN, Goldberg RJ. Exposure to anesthetic gases and reproductive outcome: are view of the epidemiologic literature. J Occup Med. 1985;27:659–68.
14. American Society of Anesthesiologists. Waste anesthetic gases in operating room air: a suggested program to reduce personnel exposure. Park Ridge, IL: American Society of Anesthesiologists; 1981.
15. ADA Council on Scientific Affairs, ADA Council on Dental Practice. Nitrous oxide in the dental office. JADA. 1997;128:364–5.
16. Occupational Safety and Health Act of 1970. Public Law 91-596. 5.2193. 1970.
17. National Institute for Occupational Safety and Health: Criteria for a Recommended Standard: Occupational Exposure to Waste Anesthetic Gases and Vapors. DHEW (NIOSH) Publication No. 77-140. U.S. Department of Health, Education and Welfare, Public Health Service, Center for Disease Control, National Institute for Occupational Safety and Health, Cincinnati, OH. 1977.
18. ACGIH. Threshold limit values for chemical substances and physical agents and biologicalexposure indices. Cincinnati, OH: American Conference of Governmental Hygienists; 2001.

19. Health Services Advisory Committee: anaesthetic agents: controlling exposure under COSHH. Suffolk, Health and Safety Executive. 1995.
20. Gardner RJ. Inhalation anaesthetics–exposure and control; a statistical comparison of personal exposures in operating theatres with and without anaesthetic gas scavenging. Ann Occup Hyg. 1989;33:159–73.
21. Waste Anesthetic Gases. OSHA Fact Sheet. 91-38. U.S. Department of Labor, Washington, DC. 1991.
22. Public Law 91-596,84 STAT. 1590, 91st Congress, S. 2193 Occupational Safety and Health Act of December 29, 1970. 1970.
23. National Institute for Occupational Safety and Health: Waste anesthetic gases–occupation hazards in hospitals: NIOSH Publication No. 2007-151.
24. Steege AL, Boiano JM, Sweeney MH. NIOSH health and safety practices survey of healthcare workers: training and awareness of employer safety procedures. Am J Ind Med. 2014;57(6):640–52.
25. Lassen HAC, Henriksen E, Neurich F, Kristensenn HS. Treatment of tetanus: severe bone marrow depression after prolonged nitrous oxide anesthesia. Lancet. 1956;270:527–30.
26. Vaisman AI. Working conditions in surgery and their effect on the health of anesthesiologists. Anesthesiology. 1968;29:565.
27. Banks RGS, Henderson JR, Pratt JM. Reactions of gases in solution. III. Some reactions of nitrous oxide with transition-metal complexes. J Chem Soc A. 1968;3:2886–90.
28. Amess JAL, Burman JF, Rees GM, Nancekievill DG, Mollin DL. Megaloblastic haemopoiesis in patients receiving nitrous oxide. Lancet. 1978;2:339–42.
29. Bruce DL, Bach MJ, Arbit J. Trace anesthetic effects on perceptual, cognitive, and motor skills. Anesthesiology. 1974;40:453–8.
30. McGlothlin JD, Crouch KG, Mickelsen RL. Control of nitrous oxide in dental operatories. Cincinnati National Institute for Occupational Safety and Health: 1994. U.S. Department of Health and Human Services (NIOSH) publication 94-129.
31. Buring JE, Hennekens CH, Mayrent SL, Rosner B, Greenberg ER, Colton T. Health experiences of operating room personnel. Anesthesiology. 1985;62:325–30.
32. Krajewski W, Kucharska M, Pliacik B, Fobker M, Stetkiewicz J, Nofer J-R, et al. Impaired vitamin B12 metabolic status in healthcare workers occupationally exposed to nitrous oxide. Br J Anaesth. 2007;99(6):812–8.
33. Sanders RD, Weimann J, Maze M. Biologic effects of nitrous oxide: a mechanistic and toxicologic review. Anesthesiology. 2008;109:707–22.
34. Fodale V, Mondello S, Aloisi C, Schifilliti D, Santamaria LB. Genotoxic effects of anesthetic agents. Expert Opin Drug Saf. 2008;7(4):447–58.
35. Casale T, Caciari T, Rosati MV, Gioffre PA, Capozella A, Pimpinella B, et al. Anesthetic gasses and occupationally exposed workers. Environ Toxicol Pharmacol. 2014;37(1):267–74.
36. Paes ERC, Braz MG, Lima JT, Silva MRG, Sousa LB, Lima ES, et al. DNA damage and antioxidant status in medical residents occupationally exposed to waste anesthetic gases. Acta Cir Bras. 2014;20(4):280–6.
37. Rocha TLA, Dias-Junior CA, Possomato-Vieira JS, Gonçalves-Rizzi VH, Nogueira FR, de Souza KM, et al. Sevoflurane induces DNA damage whereas isoflurane leads to higher antioxitative status in anesthetized rats. Biomed Res Int. 2015;4:1–6.
38. Deng H-B, Feng-Xian L, Cai Y-H, Xu S-Y. Waste anesthetic gas exposure and strategies for solution. J Anesth. 2018;32(8):269–82.
39. Flick RF, Ing CH. Anesthetic-related neurotoxicity in children–ASA works in close cooperation with FDA and others to advance research. Am Soc Anesthesiol. 2015;79(3). https://smarttots.org.
40. American Society of Perianesthesia Nurses. A position statement on air safety in the Peri Anesthesia environment. J Perianesth Nurs. 1996;4:204–5. and 2019-2020.
41. Badgewell JM. A clinical evaluation of an operational PACU source control system. J Perianesth Nurs. 1997;12:73–81.
42. Brodsky J. Exposure to anesthetic gases: a controversy. AORN J. 1983;38:132–44.
43. Sessler D, Badgwell J. Exposure of postoperative nurses to exhaled anesthetic gases. Anesth Analg. 1998;87:1083–8.
44. Krenzischek D, Schaefer J, Nolan M, Bukowski J, Twilley M, Bernacki E, et al. Waste anesthetic gas levels in the PACU. J Perianesth Nurs. 2002;4:227–39.
45. Austin PR, Austin PJ. Measurement of nitrous oxide concentration in a simulated PACU environment. J Perianesth Nurs. 1996;11:259–66.
46. Cope KA, Merritt WT, Krenzischek DA, Schaefer J, Bukowski J, Foster WM, et al. Phase II collaborative pilot study: preliminary analysis of central neural effects from exposure to volatile anesthetics in the PACU. J Perianesth Nurs. 2002;17(4):240–50.
47. Summer G, Lirk P, Hoerauf K, Riccabona U, Bodrogi F, Raifer H, et al. Sevoflurane in exhaled air of operating room personnel. Anesth Analg. 2003;97:1070–3.
48. Cheung SK, Özesel T, Rashiq S, Tsui BC. Postoperative environmental anesthetic vapour concentrations following removal of the airway device in the operating room versus the postanesthesia care unit. Can J Anaesth. 2016;63:1016–21.
49. Institute of Medicine. To err is human: building a safer health system. 2000. http://www.nap.edu/catalog.php?record_id=9728. Accessed 13 Mar 2013.
50. Helmreich RL. On error management: lessons from aviation. BMJ. 2000;320:781–5.
51. Rademaker AM, McGlothlin JD, Moenning JE, Bagnoli M, Carlson G, Griffin C. Evaluation of two nitrous oxide scavenging systems using infrared thermography to visualize and control emissions. JADA. 2009;140:190–9.
52. McGlothlin JD, Moenning JE, Cole SS. Evaluation and control of waste anesthetic gases in the

postanesthesia care unit. J Perianesth Nurs. 2014;29(4):298–312.
53. Hiller KN, Altamirano AV, Cai C, Tran SF, Williams GW. Evaluation of waste anesthetic gas in the postanesthesia care unit within the patient breathing zone. Anesthesiol Res Pract. 2015;2015:354184. https://doi.org/10.1155/2015/354184.
54. Tallent R, Corcoran J, Sebastian J. Evaluation of a novel waste anesthetic gas scavenger device for use during recovery from anesthesia. Anesthesia. 2018;73:59–64.
55. National Institute for Occupational Safety and Health (NIOSH). Respiratory protective devices. Code of Federal Regulations. 1995. Title 42, Part 84.
56. Centers for Disease Control and Prevention. Infection prevention and control recommendations for hospitalized patients under investigation for Ebola virus disease in US hospitals. 2010. Available at http:/www.cdc.gov/vhf/ebola/healthcare-us/hospitals/infection-control.htm. Accessed 11 July 2018.
57. Centers for Disease Control and Prevention. Interim guidelines for pregnant women during a Zika virus outbreak-United States, 2016. Available at http://www.cdc.gov/mmwr/volumes/65wr/mm6502e1.htm. Accessed 11 July 2018.
58. https://www.theinsiblerisk.org. Accessed 27 March 2019.
59. Sedgley C, Applegate B, Nagel A, Hall D. Real-time imaging and quantification of bioluminescent bacteria in root canals in vitro. J Endod. 2004;30(12):893–8.
60. Horton JL. Laboratory study of a scavenging mask system to evaluate and control airborne pathogens for healthcare workers in the Post Anesthesia Care Unit (PACU) and Intensive Care Unit (ICU). Purdue University. Masters Thesis. 2014.
61. Gonzales R, Handley MA, Ackerman S, O'Sullivan PS. Increasing the translation of evidence into practice, policy, and public health improvements: a framework for training health professionals in implementation and dissemination science. Acad Med. 2012;87(3):271–8. https://www.ncbi.nlm.nih.gov/pmc/articles/PMC3307591/. Accessed 9Feb 2019

# Medical Laser Safety

Vangie Dennis

## 14.1 Introduction

When lasers are introduced into a healthcare environment, whether in a hospital, surgery center, or a physician's office, healthcare professionals must be prepared to address issues of safety for both the staff and the patient. All lasers present hazards to patients and to the individuals utilizing them as well as anyone present in the area in which they are being activated. This equipment should be utilized in accordance with established regulations, standards and recommended practices, manufacturer's recommendations, and institutional policies. Laser safety is based on knowledge of the specific laser being utilized, its instrumentation, mode of operation, power densities, action in tissues, and risks. Key terms to understand include the following:

*Controlled area*: An area where the occupancy and activity of those within is subject to control and supervision for the purpose of protection from laser radiation hazards.

*Laser*: A device, which produces an intense, coherent, directional beam of light by stimulating electronic or molecular transitions to lower energy levels.

*LASER*: An acronym for light amplification by stimulated emission of radiation.

*Laser safety officer (LSO)*: One who has authority to monitor and enforce the control of laser hazards and effect the knowledgeable evaluation and control of laser hazards.

*Laser operator*: A person responsible for setting up the laser prior to use or who operates the console to control the laser parameters under the supervision of the user. The person who handles the laser equipment and in general controls the application of the laser radiation at the working area.

*Laser user*: One who uses the laser for its intended purpose within the user's scope of practice, training, and experience (i.e., the laser surgeon).

*Maximum permissible exposure (MPE)*: The level of laser radiation to which a person may be exposed without hazardous effects of adverse biologic changes in his or her eyes or skin.

*Nominal hazard zone (NHZ)*: The space within which the level of the direct, reflected, or scattered radiation during normal operation exceeds the applicable MPE. Exposure levels beyond the boundary of the NHZ are below the appropriate MPE level.

*Reflectance*: The ratio of total reflected radiant power to total incident power. Also called reflectivity.

*Wavelength*: The distance between two successive points on a periodic wave which have the same phase.

V. Dennis, MSN, RN, CNOR, CMLSO (✉)
WellStar Atlanta Medical Center,
Atlanta, GA, USA

*Optical density (O.D.)*: The ability of a lens to filter out a specific wavelength or wavelength range.

Before discussing safety it is important to understand what is laser, its effect on biological tissue, characteristics of laser light, and operating parameters.

### 14.1.1 Definition of Laser

Laser is a device, which produces an intense, coherent, directional beam of light by stimulating electronic or molecular transitions to lower energy levels. Laser is an acronym for light amplification by stimulated emission of radiation.

### 14.1.2 Laser Effects on Biological Tissue

Laser surgery is primarily a more accurate and efficient method of performing thermal surgery. The actual surgery results from the conversion of the electromagnetic energy into heat. In tissue, protein denaturation occurs at and above 60 °C, which also corresponds roughly to the temperature resulting in irreversible tissue injury. At 100 °C, water converts into steam. At some point between 300° and 400 °C, skin will begin to carbonize, and then to smoke. At approximately 530 °C and in the presence of oxygen, skin will burn and evaporate. Although these temperature-related effects are similar for all medical lasers once the energy is converted to heat, the differences in absorption of the various wavelengths by the various components of tissue makes a great difference in the actual heat conversion process during laser surgery.

The latent heat of vaporization of water acts as a tremendous energy drop and maintains the temperature at 100 °C at the tissue surface as long as water or steam is present. Any heat energy inputted into water-containing tissue above that required raising the temperature of the water to 100 °C is spent in the conversion of water to steam. Even if the conditions were just right for superheating of the cellular water just prior to steam formation, the expansion of the steam would result in an immediate cooling of the tissue surface to 100 °C. Thus, the formation of steam from cell water acts as a 100 °C thermostat for the surface of the tissue and helps to prevent any high temperature damage from occurring below the surgical surface.

### 14.1.3 Characteristics of Laser Light

Laser light produced by stimulated emission possesses three properties that distinguish it from ordinary light produced by spontaneous emission. The three properties are monochromaticity, coherence and collimation (5).

*Monochromaticity* means that all of the photons of light emitted by the laser are at one frequency and are moving in the same space and time. However, laser light is as close to being at one frequency as is physically possible. White light produced by spontaneous emission consists of light of all visible frequencies (all colors) mixed. Even visible light that is a single color can consist of a broader spectrum of frequencies than light which is produced by stimulated emission. Therefore, laser light is one color of light.

*Coherence* is a term referring to the wave nature of light and describes the fact that all of the peaks of the sinusoidal waves representing each photon are precisely in phase with each other, both in the same space and time. White light produced by spontaneous emission consists of all different wavelengths or colors of the light spectrum. Therefore, it is impossible for the waves of the individual photons to sum up consistently as does monochromatic light, since each frequency has its unique wavelength, and the difference in wavelength will ensure that the photons of different frequencies will be out of phase the majority of the time. The many colors of the light spectrum that compose white light will cancel each other out unlike the laser light due to the coherency causing it to become in sync. The result is the brilliance often seen with a visible laser beam.

*Collimation* describes the fact that all of the photons, or waves, produced by the stimulated emission process are going in the same direction, parallel to each other. This property allows the stimulated emission photons to remain in phase for a long distance away from the laser source. Light produced by spontaneous emission tends to spread in all directions, as does the light produced by a light bulb. Although spontaneous emission light can be "collimated" using special optical lenses or mirrors to form a beam, it can never be as well collimated as light produced by stimulated emission.

### 14.1.4 Operating Parameters

There are three operating parameters that determine precisely what the laser beam will do when exposed to tissue during surgery. These parameters are power, spot size, and exposure time.

*Power* is an operating parameter given in watts and is proportional to the force of the beam in surgery. When the laser is turned on, the laser surgeon must decide what power setting he will be using for the procedure. This parameter should be dictated by that surgeon's own experience. There is no such thing as a definitive power setting for a given procedure. The power setting that should be used is always the highest setting that a given laser surgeon feels comfortable using. In this way, the laser surgeon will always be using his laser as efficiently as possible, getting the surgery done as rapidly as possible.

*Spot size* is the second operating parameter and describes the diameter of the minimum spot achievable with a given lens. This parameter is typically given in millimeters. It is important to remember that spot size specifications are usually given for the spot size diameter, and not the spot size radius, which is typically used in power density calculations. The spot size determines how concentrated the beam's power will be at the focal point of the laser. For a given laser, the minimum spot size is fixed by the focal length of the focusing lens; changing the focal length by changing the lens will also change the spot size.

*Exposure time*, generally given in seconds but also occasionally in milliseconds ($1 \text{ ms} = 1 \times 10^3 \text{ s}$), is the feedback parameter during laser use. The longer the beam stays on tissue with a given power and spot size, the deeper that beam will cut. A laser surgeon must use the feeling of time as feedback in the same manner that one would use the feeling of pressure as feedback when cutting with the scalpel. There is also a similar learning curve that must be mastered when first using the laser. Learning to use the scalpel took time and experience to master just how much pressure was necessary to make a cut that was not too shallow and not too deep. Learning to use the laser also necessitates the accumulation of experience to master how much time on tissue is required to cut or ablate tissue to the depth desired.

## 14.2 U.S. Federal Regulatory Agencies and State Regulations

Lasers are classified as medical devices and are subject to regulation. The Code of Federal Regulations' Performance Standards for Light Emitting Products (https://www.accessdata.fda.gov/scripts/cdrh/cfdocs/cfcfr/cfrsearch.cfm?FR=1040.10) provides specifications for manufacturers of medical laser systems. Becoming acquainted with the organizations, laws, and standards regulating or affecting the use of lasers in a medical setting familiarizes the healthcare professional with the information necessary to develop and implement an appropriate laser safety program.

### 14.2.1 National Center for Devices and Radiological Health

All medical lasers are regulated by the U.S. Food and Drug Administration (FDA) under the Medical Device Amendments to the Food and Drug act and apply primarily to laser manufacturers. These regulations are enforced by the National Center for Devices and Radiological Health (NCDRH). The FDA regulates more than 250 types of lasers including those intended for medical and surgical use. The federal guidelines require manufacturers to classify the medical laser systems based on its ability to cause damage to the eye and skin. Medical lasers are catego-

**Table 14.1** Medical device regulations

**FDA Classification of medical devices**
Medical devices were classified in 1976 by the FDA according to their safety factors
*Class I*
Subject to general controls
*Class II*
Devices for which general controls are not enough
*Class III*
Implant and life support devices
**Classification of lasers**
Lasers are classified according to potential hazard of exposure
*Class 1*
Enclosed system, considered safe based on current medical knowledge. NO light emission escapes the enclosure
*Class 2*
Limited to visible light (400–780 nm). Output power is 1 mW or less. Momentary viewing (0.25-s maximum permissible exposure) is not considered hazardous. Staring into the beam is not recommended. Protective eyewear of the correct optical density should be worn
*Class 3A*
Emitted laser viewed directly through collecting optics would cause permanent eye damage. Output power is 0.5 mW or less. Protective eyewear of the correct optical density should be worn
*Class 3B*
Continuous laser light with 0.5 mW or less output can cause permanent eye damage. Exposure to the beam should be avoided. Protective eyewear of the correct optical density should be worn
*Class 4*
Laser light produced is hazardous to skin and eyes. Strict control measures are enforced. Protective eyewear of the correct optical density should be worn

Adapted from the ANSI 136.32018 Guidelines

rized under FDA classification of medical devices as class III, subdivision class 4, due to the potential hazards (Table 14.1). Manufacturers must conform to all safety requirements of the federal standard. They must also be approved by the NCDRH prior to any marketing or testing a laser for a particular clinical application or use, and comply with the labeling requirements.

### 14.2.2 American National Standards Institute

The American National Standards Institute (ANSI) is a voluntary organization of experts, including manufacturers, consumers, and scientific technical and professional organizations and government agencies who determine industry consensus standards in technical fields (https://www.ansi.org). ANSI's mission is to provide a guide for the safe use of lasers and laser systems for diagnostic and therapeutic use in healthcare facilities. The first cohesive blueprint for building safe clinical laser services was the "American National Standard for the Safe Use of Lasers in Health Care Facilities" or ANSI Z136.3. ANSI implies that an adequate program for control of laser hazards be established in every healthcare facility that utilizes surgical lasers. The program must include provisions for a laser safety officer, education of users, protective measures, and management of accidents. ANSI Z136.3 covers many areas of lasers and their safe use including terminology, hazard evaluation, classification, control measures, and administrative controls. Federal legislation and state laser safety regulations, as well as professional and advisory standards, are based on the ANSI standard.

### 14.2.3 Occupational Safety and Health Administration

The Occupational Safety and Health Administration (OSHA) is concerned primarily with the safety of healthcare workers. OSHA is the agency that can enforce the ANSI standards despite the fact that there is not any specific legislated regulations governing laser safety in healthcare facilities. OSHA can cite violations under the General Duty clause if the level of compliance is not satisfactory.

### 14.2.4 State Regulations

State regulations, including the FDA, are the only guidelines for laser safety that are backed by legislative action. The concern over laser safety is reflected in the increasing number of states that are enacting medical laser safety legislation. Regulations governing the safe use of lasers present healthcare personnel with a complex set of guidelines. Only FDA and individual state enactments are supported by legislation. All other guidelines are recommended practices or standards, and are based on the ANSI Z136.3 practices.

## 14.3 Nongovernmental Agencies

### 14.3.1 American Society for Lasers in Medicine and Surgery

The American Society for Lasers in Medicine and Surgery (ASLMS), in 1980, issued reports that were adopted as recommendations by the society's members (see https://www.aslms.org).

In 1990, the board of directors released nine recommended perioperative practices relating to patients undergoing laser procedures. These included assessment, nursing diagnosis, planning, implementation, and evaluation of nursing care.

### 14.3.2 Association of PeriOperative Registered Nurses (AORN)

AORN's "Recommended Practices for Laser Safety in the Practice Setting" was first published in 1989. These are currently being updated. These broad recommended practices provide guidelines to support perioperative nurses in developing policies and procedures for the safe use of lasers in their practice setting. These practices represent an acceptable level of practice.

### 14.3.3 The Joint Commission on Accreditation of Health Organizations (TJC)

TJC does not currently recommend specific guidelines for laser use; however criteria may be based on ANSI recommendations.

## 14.4 Standards and Practice

Control of potential health hazards associated with the use of surgical laser systems requires adoption of appropriate safety standards and policies that are relevant to the specific laser situation. It is imperative that, for the safety of patients, physicians, nurses, and other medical personnel, everyone involved with medical lasers understands how to safely manage each type of laser in a medical setting. Before a laser is utilized clinically, a laser program should be established with written policies and procedures to establish authority, responsibility, and accountability.

The Laser Safety Officer (LSO) is a person appointed by the administration that has attained the training and education to administer a laser safety program. This does not mean the LSO must be present during every laser procedure. The Laser Safety Officer is responsible for appropriate classification of lasers within the facility, hazard evaluation, control measures, procedural approval, protective equipment, maintenance of equipment, training to all personnel associated with lasers, and medical surveillance [1].

## 14.5 Hazard Evaluation and Control Measures

Hazard evaluation is influenced by various factors of the laser system being utilized. The classification of the laser and the wavelength of the laser may also assist in defining the necessary control measures to be incorporated into the safety program. These factors affect which control measures need to be incorporated into the laser safety program and implemented into practice. Control measures are those procedures or methods implemented to minimize hazards associated with a particular laser when it is in the operational mode. Control measures may be influenced by the ability of the laser energy to injure, the environment in which the laser will be activated, personnel that may use or be exposed within the nominal hazard zone, the delivery systems, and the non-beam hazards associated with the specific laser. Ancillary hazards create the potential for significant injuries to occur. Injuries, including death, may occur during testing of laser equipment, during electrical servicing, from fires, explosions, and even embolisms.

### 14.5.1 Administrative Controls

Administrative controls are those methods or procedures specifying explicit criteria that determine the implementation of engineering controls or work practices for personnel protection. Standard operating procedures (SOPs) are established from institutional policies and procedures. Safety controls, maintenance and service, as well as the function of the laser should be incorporated into the facility's SOPs. SOPs may also include documentation requirements for pre-procedure safety checklists, intra-procedural laser operation, and safety. The LSO is responsible for the execution of the SOPs.

### 14.5.2 Procedural and Equipment Controls

Engineering and procedural controls are determined by the LSO and must be implemented when appropriate to circumvent potential hazards. Procedural controls require adherence to written SOPs to ensure the safety of all personnel working in the region of lasers. SOPs should provide for operational guidelines, emergency shut-off mechanisms, stand-by functions, use of low reflective materials near the laser beam path, and storage.

Operational guidelines should require switches, whether foot-pedal or finger trigger, which control the laser energy, to be guarded to prevent accidental activation. This may necessitate one foot-pedal access for the individual controlling the delivery device to prevent inadvertent activation of the laser [2]. Accessory attachments to lasers must also be compatible with the laser safety guidelines. This includes laser filters on operating microscopes that protect the operator at the binocular viewing tube and through the accessory viewing tubes.

Lasers should be placed in the *"stand-by" mode* when then laser is on but not being fired, or when the user in no longer in control of the delivery device to prevent accidental discharge. When not in use, storage of the laser and/or disabling of the laser is necessary to prevent inadvertent activation of the laser by non-authorized personnel. Lasers should be stored in areas of low traffic.

Nonreflective instruments (dull, anodized, or matte-finished) should be used in or near the laser beam to defocus or disperse the laser beam [3]. Appropriate backstops or guards should be used to prevent the laser beam from striking normal tissue or non-targeted tissues.

## 14.6 Laser Treatment Controlled Area

The nominal hazard zone (NHZ) is the space in which the level of the direct, reflected, or scattered radiation used during the normal laser operation exceeds the applicable maximum permissible exposure (MPE) [4]. A nominal hazard zone should be identified by the LSO to prevent unintentional exposure to the laser beam. Determination of the NHZ should take into consideration information gathered from the manufacturer's labeling, by analysis, to radiation transmission of the beam and the potential for equipment failure. The nominal hazard zone is usually contained within the room but may extend through open doors or transparent windows, depending on the type of laser used. It is the LSO's responsibility to define the NHZ and ensure that the proper safety practices are adhered to in the NHZ.

The appropriate warning signs posted at every entryway into the laser treatment controlled area should define the NHZ. *The symbols and wording on the warning sign should be specific for the type of laser in use and designed according to the information described in the ANSI standard for the Safe Use of Lasers in Health Care Facilities.*

Windows and viewing areas should be limited because the NHZ may reach beyond the room in which the laser is in use. Additional safety controls, such as closing doors and covering windows with applicable filters or barriers or restricting traffic, may need to be implemented depending on the laser used. Screens, curtains, or a blocking barrier may be placed near entryways to avert laser radiation.

Only authorized persons (including patient), approved by the laser safety officer, should be in the vicinity of the nominal hazard zone. Only authorized laser operators (that have been delegated specific responsibilities by the laser safety officer) may operate a laser. An authorized laser operator is a person trained in laser safety and approved by the facility to operate the laser. This person is responsible for the safety of the equipment and the treatment environment in the nominal hazard zone. They must remain at the laser control while the laser is in use. Their responsibilities include:

- Assessing procedure needs including anesthesia needs, type of laser, and accessory equipment.
- Performing equipment checks prior to use including accessories, operation, and safety equipment to ensure safe working conditions.
- Ensuring safety controls for all personnel (including the patient) in the treatment area, such as wearing appropriate eyewear.
- Displaying appropriate signage.
- Setting the laser wattage and exposure appropriately and monitoring activation of the laser and observation of team members for breaks in safety.
- Completing a safety checklist and optional laser log.

All healthcare personnel in the vicinity of the nominal hazard zone should be trained in implementation of all laser safety precautions to avoid inadvertent exposure to laser hazards. All personnel, including the patient, within the NHZ should use appropriate personal protective equipment (PPE).

## 14.7 Maintenance and Service

Preventative maintenance should be done every 6 months. Only properly educated, trained, and approved technicians should be allowed to work on the laser or handle the electrical components [5].

## 14.8 Protective Equipment

### 14.8.1 Eye Protection

The eye is the organ that is most susceptible to laser injury. The optics of the eye can concentrate and focus laser light, at wavelengths ranging from 400 to 1400 nm, on the retina which increases the potential ocular hazard. Ultraviolet and far-infrared wavelength regions (outside 400–1400 nm) principally produce corneal effects. Also, laser radiation at certain wavelengths may cause damage to the lens of the eye [6]. Appropriate laser safety eyewear filters out the hazardous wavelength of laser radiation. In addition to direct exposure from misdirected and damaged fibers, scattered, diffused, and reflected laser beams can cause eye injuries. Laser protective eyewear may include goggles, face shields, prescription glasses with special filters or coatings and corneal shields.

The patient's eyes and eyelids should be protected from the laser beam by appropriate methods when the eyes are in the NHZ. Protective methods may include wet eye-pads, laser protective eyewear, or laser-specific eye shields. Corneal eye shields may be necessary when goggles or glasses interfere with the laser treatment.

All personnel in the nominal hazard zone should wear protective eyewear that is labeled with the appropriate optical density and wavelength while the laser is in use [1]. Ocular hazards may transpire during operational pre-testing of the laser to confirm beam alignment and calibration. Potential for ocular hazards is also present during fiber-optic procedures as a result of the fiber becoming disconnected or breaking. Both instances also require protective eyewear to be utilized to prevent exposure of the eye. Protective eyewear should be available outside the room near the posted warning signs designating the specific type of laser in use. For optimal protection, inspect eyewear for pitting, cracking, discoloration, coating damage, frame condition, and light leaks [1]. If any of these are present, the eyewear is considered inadequate for eye protection and should be discarded.

### 14.8.2 Skin Protection

Whenever there is a potential hazard of thermal burns from high-powered lasers, all persons in the laser treatment area should be protected from the laser beam exposures to their skin and other non-targeted tissues. Overexposure to ultraviolet radiation can lead to skin sensitivities or even burns from direct or reflected laser energy [1]. Surgical gloves, tightly woven fabrics, and flame-retardant material, depending on the laser being utilized, may provide skin protection. Protection of exposed tissues around the operative site may be accomplished by covering the areas with saline-saturated or water-saturated, fire/flame-retardant materials (e.g., towels, sponges, drapes, fabrics). These materials must remain moist to absorb or disperse the energy of the laser beam. Polypropylene or plastic drapes can melt if a laser beam strikes them and woven or non-woven fabrics can be ignited. Laser handpiece or fibertip should be covered with a moist towel or sponge to minimize the potential for a fire (2).

## 14.9 Laser Safety and Training Programs

A laser safety program establishes and maintains policies and procedures to ensure control of laser hazards. Laser safety programs policies and procedures should include, but are not limited to, the following:

- LSO guidelines defining the authority and responsibility for evaluation and control of laser hazards. A laser committee may need to be developed when increased laser usage necessitates maintaining enforcement of SOPs.
- Criteria and education for procedures for all personnel working in a nominal hazard zone. All personnel working with lasers should attend laser safety education courses periodically.
- Credentialing and clinical practice privileges of the medical staff are the facility's responsibilities. Credentialing should be for specific laser procedures with specific laser types.
- Implementation of laser hazard control measures.
- A continuous quality improvement program to include appropriate use and maintenance of equipment, management and reporting of accidents as well as prevention.

A laser program should be established specific for the laser wavelength and specialty, for a facilities specific laser(s) and for specific to the procedures being performed in the facility, must be implemented. The program must comply with applicable standards and regulations covering all procedures necessary to provide a safe environment. Personnel should demonstrate and complete competency skills periodically.

## 14.10 Medical Surveillance

Medical Surveillance referes to the baseline eye exams on all personel prior to entering the NHZ. Baseline eye exams are no longer required and are referenced in ANSI 136.1 (1). If an occurrence is thought to occur, an immediate evaluation to determine the extent of exposure should be completed. Surveillance is specific to the personnel category and the known risks associated with the particular laser operated. Personnel categories are broken into laser personnel who routinely work in the NHZ and incidental personnel who are unlikely to be exposed to laser energy (e.g., custodial, supervisory, clerical). Surveillance may be required to assess a level of visual performance to assist in the evaluation of laser damage in the case of inadvertent exposure to the eye. Surveillance can also identify those individuals that may be at risk from ultraviolet hazards, specifically to the skin. Laser accidents must be documented to define the need for further evaluation of the injured person.

## 14.11 Non-beam Hazards

Hazards other than directly related to exposure to the laser (e.g., eye, skin, and other tissues) are known as non-beam hazards. Potential hazards related to non-beam hazards are diverse and the LSO must determine the appropriate control methods to be implemented. Evaluations of the hazards may necessitate the need to enlist the assistance of safety and/or industrial hygiene personnel from OSHA.

### 14.11.1 Electrical Hazards

Lasers contain high-voltage electrical circuits that may lead to shock, electrocution, or fire. Injuries from these types of hazards are some of the leading causes of laser-related accidents and deaths. Potential electrical hazards from damaged electrical cords, faulty grounding, lack of compliance with training programs, and inadequate or inappropriate use of Lockout/Tagout procedures can be prevented by adherence to SOPs of the facility. Visual inspection of the laser including electrical, plumbing, accessory equipment, delivery systems, gas supply, and sterile draping prior to use may prevent injuries from occurring. Observance of general electrical safety (e.g., no fluids placed on or near lasers, extension cords not used to power lasers) will also support the maintenance of safety.

### 14.11.2 Smoke Plume

Vaporization of tissues may release toxic substances (e.g., acetone, isopropanol, toluene, formaldehyde, metal fumes, and cyanide), including carcinogens and viruses, from the cells. This laser plume contains water, carbonized particles, mutated deoxyribonucleic acid (DNA), and intact cells (1). At certain concentrations, ocular, upper respiratory tract irritation and unpleasant odors may transpire. These substances should not be inhaled, thereby initiating the need for some type of smoke evacuation system to be utilized to prevent personnel and the patient from inhaling plume. Removal of plume will also enhance the visualization of the surgical/treatment site and may prevent the laser beam from potentially be reflected.

Smoke plume inhalation should be reduced to a minimum by utilizing multiple controls. These controls may include the use of high-filtration masks, wall suction units with in-line filters, and smoke evacuators. High-filtration masks should be used in conjunction with other controls and not as a sole means for protection. Masks should fit securely and filter to a .1 micron filtration. Masks are not the first line of defense with the creation of laser smoke and engineering controls should be implemented (3). Wall suction systems may be used when the generation of a minimal amount of plume is expected, such as laparoscopic cases. Wall suctions generate low suction rates and are designed for fluids, and thus an in-line filter should be used to collect particulate matter. A mechanical smoke evacuator or suction with a high-efficiency filter should be used when a large amount of laser plume is expected. These systems should be turned on simultaneously with the activation of the laser energy and placed as close as possible to the laser site. Standard precautions (gloves and mask) should be taken when using lasers, as well as when handling contaminated filters due to the amount of potential contaminants generated.

### 14.11.3 Fire and Explosion Hazards

Lasers are an ignition source and the protection is not limited to the patient but the staff, physicians and anesthesia (6). Fire is a potential hazard that can have devastating consequences. Laser energy can ignite flammable liquids, solids, and gases. Fire occurring with these types of materials most often occurs outside the patient, but fires can occur inside of the patient. Becoming aware of the safeguards and adherence to them can protect the patient as well as healthcare personnel.

Personnel should be aware of the items that have a potential for causing fire, burns, or explosions. These may include surgical drapes, endotracheal tubes, paper or gauze materials, gases (e.g., oxygen, methane, anesthetic gases), and flammable liquids or ointments (e.g., skin prep solutions, oil-based lubricants) (4). Water or saline and fire extinguishers should be readily available where lasers are used.

Methane gas from the anus or large bowel should be prevented from entering the area where laser energy is dispersed by covering the area with wet towels or packing the anus with wet gauze or packing. Prep solutions should be non-flammable [1]. Any compound or solution containing alcohol (e.g., Hibiclens, chlorhexidine, tape removers, degreasers, benzoin, tinctures) can ignite from contact with laser energy. Alcohol vapors should not be allowed to accumulate under drapes. Overheating of iodoforms, which are to pool on or around the skin, or aerosolized povidone-iodine can lead to flash fires when laser energy is utilized.

Oxygen concentration in the room should be kept to a minimum. The anesthesia provider should be aware of the hazards of oxygen leaking from around a patient's face mask. They should be prepared to turn off the free flow of oxygen.

## 14.12 Specialty Procedures

### 14.12.1 Endoscopy

#### 14.12.1.1 Fiber Optic Delivery

When a fiber is used to deliver laser energy, whether through a flexible or rigid endoscope, the fiber should extend beyond the end of the endoscope. This will prevent laser beam exposure with the sheath. Endoscope lenses can be easily damaged resulting in lens pitting or even shattering. The endoscope sheath may become overheated if the laser energy is activated while still within the sheath, resulting in thermal damage not only to the scope but also potentially to the adjacent or surrounding tissues.

#### 14.12.1.2 Coupling Arm

There are automatic shut-off features incorporated into laser equipment. There is no protection from inadvertent beam delivery if the arm becomes unattached; therefore the laser operator must make certain the coupled attachment is secured.

### 14.12.2 Bronchoscopic Couplers

Couplers used with the $CO_2$ laser in adjunct with bronchoscopy must have an optical system that allows the visible aiming beam to pass co-axially with the invisible $CO_2$ laser beam. Burns to the patient's trachea, larynx, pharynx, and oral cavity have occurred as a direct result of the misaligned beam.

#### 14.12.2.1 Airway

Guidelines to minimize the risks associated with lasers and other energy modalities should be incorporated into the OR team's practices. There are various types of laser-dedicated tubes. The type of laser wavelength utilized dictates the brand of endotracheal tube used. Some tubes have FDA clearances for specific wavelengths of lasers. *The red Rusch™ reusable tube wrapped in the 3 m foil tape is **not** approved for laser usage.* The Rusch™ tube is an evolved practice for which there are articles published in the medical literature stating this is an acceptable tube in the beginning of laser ENT airway applications, but with the advent of new FDA approved laser tubes for specific wavelengths, this wrapped tube should *not* be used. The PVC endotracheal tube is contraindicated with laser airway procedures when the tube is in direct contact with the laser beam. PVC material is very flammable and the by-products are hydrochloric gas and in the presence of fluid, hydrochloric acid. There are no laser-resistant tubes presently on the market. All tubes under pressure are explosive.

The cuff of the endotracheal tube should be instilled with normal saline or water and methylene blue dye is optional. The saline or water will serve as an extinguisher and the methylene blue dye as an indicator that the cuff has been breached. The endotracheal tube cuff is hit 2% of the time even when lasers are utilized by the best technicians.

Water-soluble lubricant is indicated if a laser is used. Petroleum-based lubricant is flammable, and therefore contraindicated.

#### 14.12.2.2 Anesthetic Choice

Considerations should be taken when choosing the appropriate anesthetic agent. No one anesthetic technique is used to the exclusion of others. Helium and compressed air are acceptable gases to use on airway laser procedures. Helium gas is less dense and has the ability to flow through compromised airways easier than compressed air. Helium will also retard burning, but the risks of delivering hypoxic levels can be a problem. Pulse oximetry should always be utilized with helium gas delivery. Nitrous oxide is contraindicated in upper airway laser surgery. Nitrous oxide, in the presence of oxygen, will present as if 100% oxygen is being delivered. Other flammable anesthetics need to be considered with laser airway procedures. The $FIO_2$ of the oxygen range should be no higher than 30%. Above the 30% range supports combustion. ASA recomemends the protocol and is dictated by the clinical status of the patient (1).

### 14.12.3 Airway Fire Management

Before any laser airway procedure, staff should familiarize themselves with the procedural steps to managing an airway fire. The steps are outlined in Table 14.2.

During head and neck surgeries, the patient is mechanically ventilated in the majority of the procedures. If precautionary protocols are not followed and instantaneous action not taken if an airway fire occurs, hot gases can be forced deep into the lungs, causing extensive injuries. Seconds of indecision or confusion can cause irreparable damage or death to the patient. The avoidance, recognition, and management of airway procedures, as well as the collaborative communication between the operating team, are essential in increased patient safety and improved care.

## 14.13 Lasers Used in Radiology

Lasers are extensively utilized in many surgical and medical specialties, and in only the last 15 years there has been an increase in laser applications with radiologic services. The more commonly used lasers are diode lasers in the spectrum of 800–1100 nm. Endovenous laser therapy is a treatment of varicose veins and the diode laser is the predominate laser used. The laser is delivered via a fiber optic with depth gauges located on the fiber. This allows the physicians to advance the fiber to the location needed to treat the varicose vein.

Another wavelength of laser used for interventional approaches is the Holmium Yag laser (Ho:YAG) at 2100–2140 nm. The laser has a low penetration and is pulsed, so the depth of penetration does not exceed the original pulse. The Holmium Yag laser has specific dosimetry when used for laser discectomy, so overtreatment of the disc space does not occur. Fluoroscopy is delivered with 2 C-Arms to set the trajectory of the protruding disc. The laser fiber is directed through a metal spinal needle and the energy shrinks the disc relieving pressure on the nerve.

The Holmium Yag laser has also been used to break up gall bladder stones in conjunction with endoscopic retrograde cholangiopancreatography (ERCP). The Holmium fiber optic catheter is introduced through a specially designed ECRP scope. The Holmium laser fiber is advanced through the working channel of the SpyScope cathcter™ (Boston Scientific).

Cardiovascular applications, e.g., excimer laser coronary atherectomy (ELCA) and for the treatment of peripheral arterial disease (PAD), have increased over the last decade. Excimer is the short of "excited dimer," which means a compound of two identical species that exist only in excited states. The excimer lasers use the noble gas compounds (argon, krypton, or xenon) with a reactive gas (fluorine or chlorine) for lasing. The excimer commonly used for cardiovascular applications is the 308 nm wavelength. With 308 nm excimer laser

**Table 14.2** Steps to manage an airway fire

1. Stop the gas flow to the tube: disconnection of the breathing circuit is the quickest method of stopping the gas flow
2. Extinguish the fire with water/saline. The operating room staff and anesthesia should have water/saline readily available on the operating room back table and anesthesia cart. Removing the tube without extinguishing the fire will allow the tube to continue to burn on extubation
3. Access of the bronchoscopes and tracheostomy trays should be readily available. The location of the instruments should be established prior to any airway procedure. Failure to remove any pieces of the tube will allow the tube to continue to burn in the patient

**Table 14.3** Related links

www.oshs-slc.gov/sltc/laserhazards/
www.fda.gov/cdrh/radhlth/laser.html

light is delivered to the tissue with a fiber optic catheter, in a liquid environment. Because it is a pulsed laser there is not enough time to compound the heating element as with continuous-on lasers.

## 14.14 Conclusion

It is important to understand that regardless of the clinical setting the presence of laser equipment creates a need for unique control measures and work practice controls to be developed and implemented. Whether your setting is a small clinic, a doctor's office, or a large hospital, laser safety is not the responsibility of one individual, but the obligation and duty of everyone involved in the laser surgery process. All personnel involved in the care of a patient may be in the vicinity of the nominal hazard zone and thus should be educated appropriately to maintain a safe environment for patient care. A well-developed laser safety program that is developed according to the ANSI Z136 series can assure safety when implemented properly. When everyone knows the fundamentals of maintaining a laser-safe environment, risk of accidents, resulting from ignorance or noncompliance with policy, is greatly reduced. Two related links are provided for additional reading (see Table 14.3).

## References

1. ANSI, Z. 136.3 for the safe use of lasers in health care facilities. New York: American National Standards Institute; 2018.
2. Castelluccio D. Implementing AORN recommended practices for laser safety. AORN J. 2012;95(5):612–27.
3. Fencl JL. Guideline implementation: surgical smoke safety. AORN J. 2017;105(5):488–97.
4. Spratt D, Cowles CE, Berguer R, Dennis V, Waters TR, Rodriguez M, Groah L. Workplace safety equals patient safety. AORN J. 2012;96(3):235–44.
5. Takac S, Stojanović S. Characteristics of laser light. Med Pregl. 1999;52(1–2):29–34.
6. AORN Recommended Practices (2017). Perioperative Standards and Recommended Practices. https://doi.org/10.6015/psrp.13.01.0043.

# Minimally Invasive Image-Guided Procedures

# 15

Margaret M. Doherty-Simor

## 15.1 Introduction

The first significant advances that forged minimally invasive image-guided procedures (MIIPs) date back to the early 1950s and 1960s. In 1953, a Swedish-born physician first published a technique he pioneered that is known to this day as the "Seldinger technique" for accessing blood vessels without a surgical cut-down [1–4]. A decade later, Dr. Charles Dotter published his experience using this technique by introducing a series of dilating catheters to treat an atherosclerotic lesion in a femoral artery, a technique which became known as "Dottering" [5, 6]. In contrast to minimally invasive surgery, MIIPs do not use cameras inside the body. Instead, MIIPs utilize medical imaging technologies such as fluoroscopy, computed tomography (CT), magnetic resonance imaging (MRI), and ultrasound (US) to see inside the body from the outside avoiding the need for multiple larger incisions required to place cameras and surgical instruments into the body. Most procedures are performed on an outpatient basis or require a hospital stay that is considerably shorter than that following an open surgical procedure. General anesthesia is not usually required which makes MIIPs safer for patients with multiple comorbidities. In select cases, general anesthesia can be helpful or required, as in very lengthy, complex, or potentially painful procedures. Nurse-administered moderate sedation is usually utilized to keep the patient comfortable while maintaining their ability to respond to commands and protect their airway. MIIPs provide many benefits to patients and to the facilities that provide these services. Procedures may be performed on an outpatient basis using moderate sedation with recovery times that are significantly reduced. MIIPs are less invasive and less painful than open surgery, as they are performed through a very small hole that requires little or no stitches with significantly less scarring. The use of targeted image-guided treatment results in higher levels of safety and efficacy and reduces the risk of infection. By avoiding traditional surgery, reductions to the length of stay after procedures, improved patient outcomes, the ability to resume normal activities, and return to work sooner result in a reduction in costs for both the patient and the hospital. MIIPs contribute to higher patient satisfaction.

## 15.2 Principles

### 15.2.1 Evolution of Interventional Radiology as a Specialty

The practice pattern of interventional radiologists (IR) has evolved over the years since Dr. Charles

M. M. Doherty-Simor, MSN, RN (✉)
The Interventional Initiative, Oakland, CA, USA

Dotter performed the first percutaneous transluminal angioplasty (PTA) successfully dilating a tight stenosis of a superficial femoral artery on January 16, 1964. An 82-year-old female was suffering from painful gangrenous toes and refused to undergo an amputation [5, 6]. After the intervention, her pain subsided and she ultimately walked out of the hospital. Dr. Dotter was the first to lecture that the future of diagnostic angiography would not only provide an exact diagnosis but, in fact, would provide the means by which angiographers would be able to treat patients percutaneously with catheters and guide wires [5]. During the 1970s, the early pioneers applied their techniques to other conditions and expanded the indications for percutaneous procedures resulting in the introduction of coronary PTA, vena cava filters, and the use of the first micro coils and polyvinyl alcohol (PVA) for embolization in treating gastrointestinal bleeding. The early coronary balloon catheters were used to dilate peripheral arteries and an industry was born with multiple medical device companies improving upon the technology facilitating the expansion of MIIPs into other areas of the body. By the late 1980s, bare metal balloon-expandable stents became available for treating benign and malignant strictures in the biliary tree as well as coronary and peripheral vascular lesions. Patients with end-stage liver disease with significant morbidity suffering from esophageal bleeding and intractable ascites were very poor candidates for open surgery. These stents provided the solution to manage these patients as IRs were able to percutaneously create an internal shunt between the portal vein and hepatic vein, thus decompressing the liver preventing further bleeding and eliminating ascites. Catheter techniques learned from the treatment of gastrointestinal bleeding are used today in the treatment of liver cancer to deliver chemotherapy and radioactive spheres. Throughout the course of its history, IR has moved away from a diagnostic specialty to a clinical practice model. Increasingly, patients are being seen in clinic for evaluation and informed consent prior to admission for procedures. Advanced level practitioners often are found in clinics providing evaluation through history and physical exams and ordering pre-procedure testing, educating patients about a procedure and obtaining consents, and performing follow-up for patients. At some facilities radiologists may have admitting privileges should the patient need a 24-h stay or an overnight admission following a procedure. Advanced practice providers often are involved in the follow-up care of admitted patients.

In 2017, IR gained official specialty status from the American Board of Medical Specialties (ABMS). The Society of Interventional Radiology has outlined IR training options [7] (see https://www.sirweb.org/learning-center/ir-residency/). As IR became more clinically oriented and patient acuity increased, more clinical radiology nurses were needed to care for the procedure patients, pre-, intra-, and post-procedure. The need for more radiology advanced practitioners has also increased. The Association for Radiologic and Imaging Nursing (ARIN, www.arinursing.org), which supports radiology nurses via education and networking, has grown in response to the needs of all radiology, especially IR (see Chaps. 1 and 2 for more information about the role of the advanced practice nurse in radiology).

### 15.2.2 The Interventional Initiative

The Interventional Initiative (the II, http://theii.org/miips/procedures) is a 501c3 not-for-profit charitable organization founded in 2015 by physicians, patients, and allied healthcare professionals who recognized a healthcare knowledge gap between the public and the availability of MIIPs.

It has been estimated that in the USA only 12% of adults have proficient health literacy, which means that nearly nine out of 10 adults may not have the skills needed to make informed decisions around their healthcare needs and choices [8]. What is striking is that according to the U.S. Bureau of Labor Statistics 12.2% of the nation's workforce reside in the healthcare industry, so a large percent of those who are deemed proficient likely are healthcare workers such as physicians, nurses, and allied health professionals [9] (https://www.bls.gov/emp/tables/employment-by-major-industry-sector.htm).

A study published by members of the II in 2017 found that 65% of radiology department outpatients in a single hospital setting had no prior knowledge of IR [10]. A survey of the general public found that 72% could not identify an interventional radiologist as a physician. Understanding that internet searches are one of the primary methods used by the public to learn about disease and treatment options, the authors also evaluated the activity of internet searches and IR-related coverage in the media and compared findings to those of medical specialties that also perform MIIPs such as cardiologists, vascular surgeons, and nephrologists and found that they were markedly lower.

Low health literacy coupled with a lack of knowledge of interventional radiology highlights the needs to engage the public about MIIPs providing education about the full breadth of diseases treated and empowering them to take an active role in their healthcare decision-making. Despite the general lack of awareness of IR, Heister and colleagues found that the majority of patients would prefer a MIIP to open surgery, especially if it is recommended by their physician [10]. It is therefore imperative that MIIPs providers make available opportunities to educate their referring physicians about the services they provide.

The II supports the beliefs that patients who are empowered to make informed healthcare decisions will have better outcomes [11]. The II produces informative content at the sixth grade health literacy level delivering it through a variety of platforms including visually engaging infographics, medical animation, and short-format video podcasts titled "Behind the Scrubs" and "Ask an IR." The documentary series "Without a Scalpel" (http://www.theii.org/the-docuseries) provides a glimpse inside MIIPs from both the patient and the interventional radiologist perspectives. The Centers for Disease Control (CDC) offers a variety of online health literacy courses including topics such as writing and speaking with the public [12]. For a list of courses see https://www.cdc.gov/healthliteracy/gettraining.html?CDC_AA_refVal=https%3A%2F%2Fwww.cdc.gov%2Fhealthliteracy%2Fwriting-course%2Findex.html.

## 15.3 Description of Techniques and Indications

### 15.3.1 Percutaneous Access

The Seldinger technique provides the foundation of both percutaneous vascular and nonvascular access [1]. A small gauge needle is used to puncture a blood vessel, organ, or anatomical space. A guide wire is then threaded through the needle, the needle is withdrawn, and a catheter is then threaded over the guide wire. The guide wire is removed and contrast is injected to verify that the catheter is in the correct location. For vascular cases, common femoral artery access is often preferred. However, the transradial approach for both diagnostic and interventional procedures has gained popularity due to resulting shorter procedural recovery times and hospital stays, possible reductions in access-site complications, and improved patient satisfaction due to the ability to ambulate sooner.

### 15.3.2 Imaging Equipment

Improvements in the imaging equipment designed specifically for the angiography suite incorporating C-arm technology and digital subtraction angiography (DSA) and adoption of low and iso-osmolar contrast media to improve visibility have significantly improved the patient experience and procedural success. DSA is a technique used in MIIPs to allow the interventionalist to clearly visualize blood vessels that are in close proximity to bone or within dense soft tissue environments. This is accomplished by digitally subtracting an image that was acquired before contrast came into contact with the area under investigation. DSA decreases the procedure time, radiation dose, and the amount of contrast required. Three-dimensional (3D) technologies include "road mapping" which allows the interventionalist to overlay a DSA-acquired image of the area to be treated or integrate a 3D "reconstructed" image of structures attained during rotational angiography, CT or MRI over live images to help navigate guide wires and catheters

**Table 15.1** Equipment/supplies

Puncture needle
Guide wire(s)
Introducer sheath/peel-away sheath
Syringes
Contrast media
Power injector
Diagnostic catheter(s)
Guiding catheter(s)
Balloon catheter(s)
Stent(s)
Vascular closure device (VCD)

**Table 15.2** List of common vascular interventions

Balloon angioplasty
Central line placement
Dialysis graft or stent maintenance
Foreign body retrieval
Inferior vena cava (IVC) filter placement
IVC filter removal
Mechanical thrombectomy
Stent and stent graft placement
Thrombolysis
Transarterial embolization
Transjugular intrahepatic portosystemic shunt (TIPS)
Transjugular biopsy
Vein ablation
Vein embolization

across complex lesions or vascular structures. See Table 15.1 for a list of equipment and supplies utilized in a typical IR procedure.

### 15.3.3 Vascular Interventions

"Lower extremity PAD is a common cardiovascular disease that is estimated to affect approximately 8.5 million Americans above the age of 40 and is associated with significant morbidity, mortality, and quality of life impairment. It has been estimated that 202 million people worldwide have PAD" [13] (https://www.ahajournals.org/doi/full/10.1161/CIR.0000000000000470). Vascular intervention is not limited to the lower extremities. The same techniques for accessing blood vessels in the lower extremity are used to provide interventions in the brain, chest, and abdomen. See Table 15.2 for a list of common vascular intervention procedures.

#### 15.3.3.1 Balloon Angioplasty

Percutaneous balloon angioplasty is utilized to open a blood vessel and is performed utilizing a catheter with a balloon mounted on the distal end. Once inflated, the balloon will open a blocked or narrowed blood vessel by stretching the walls of the vessel. However, the resulting injury to the vessel may lead to an inflammatory response known as intimal hyperplasia which has been shown to cause narrowing in the vessel or in the stent, called in-stent restenosis [14, 15]. Subsequent endothelial growth may necessitate later interventions such as angioplasty, stenting, or surgical bypass. A number of therapies are available to use in conjunction with or as an alternative to angioplasty in an effort to minimize the incidence of in-stent restenosis including drug-coated balloons, drug-eluting stents, and atherectomy [16, 17].

#### 15.3.3.2 Endovascular Stents

Stents are permanent tubes made of metal mesh. Stents are deployed to open vessels that do not respond sufficiently to angioplasty. Stents can be self-expandable, which have the benefit of exerting high radial force, or balloon-expandable, which have the benefit of precise placement. Stents can be bare metal or covered. Stents covered by material such as polytetrafluoroethylene (PTFE) are called stent grafts. Stent grafts create a barrier to intimal hyperplasia and leaks. They are commonly used to treat aneurysms in the iliac arteries and abdominal aorta. The choice of stent size, deployment, and type depends on the indication and anatomy (Fig. 15.1).

#### 15.3.3.3 Transcatheter Arterial Embolization

Embolization is the intentional closure of a bleeding or diseased blood vessel using any of a variety of materials delivered through a catheter. Embolization techniques were first utilized by interventional radiologists in the early 1970s to treat gastrointestinal bleeding and spinal vascular malformations [2]. Embolic agents include small particles, coils, plugs, and glue. The choice of

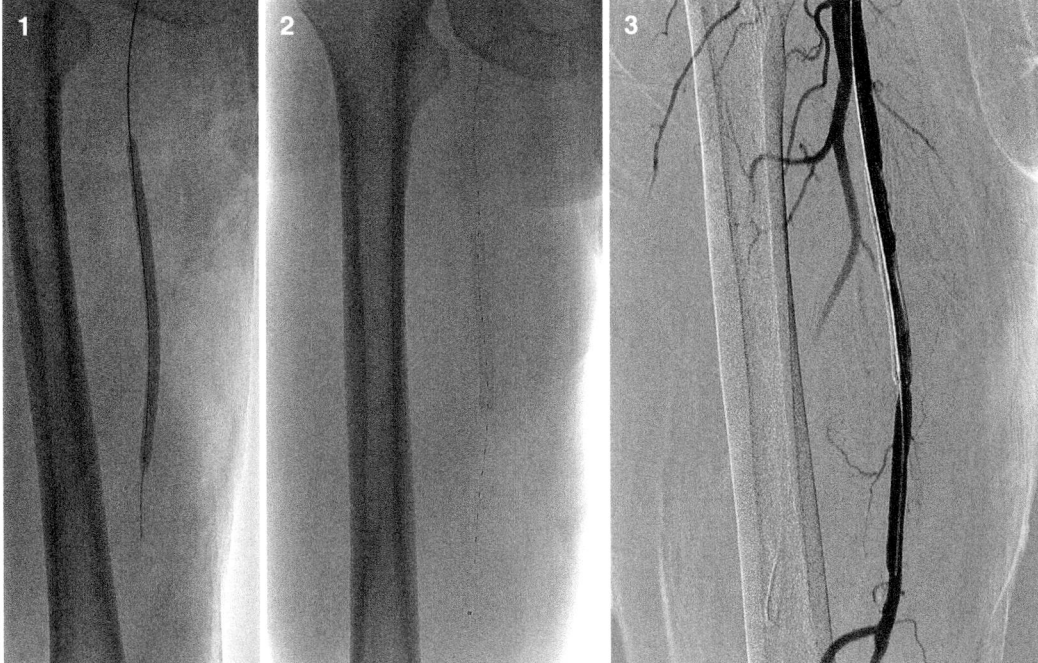

**Fig. 15.1** Seventy-one-year-old male with claudication due to narrowing in the superficial femoral artery (SFA). Image 1 shows percutaneous balloon angioplasty of SFA. Image 2 shows a metal stent with guide wire in SFA. Image 3 with contrast flow through SFA stent

agent depends on several factors: the vascular territory to be treated, the type of abnormality being treated, the possibility of superselective delivery of an occlusive agent, the goal of the procedure, and the permanence of the occlusion [18, 19]. Careful placement of the correct catheter is essential to decrease the risk of complications from embolization of nontarget vessels.

#### 15.3.3.4 Vascular Closure Devices

Manual compression of the vascular entry site can be utilized to achieve hemostasis. A mechanical device can be used to maintain pressure but should be attended by personnel who can verify correct placement without slippage of the device and possible hemorrhage. Compression of arterial access points typically takes 20 min whereas compression of venous access site typically takes less than 5 min. After arterial access, patients are required to stay on bed rest with the affected limb immobilized for a length of time depending on the point of access. All manufacturer recommendations should be followed after deployment of a vascular closure device. Some products include a "sticker" of identification that can be temporarily placed at the puncture site to inform staff of the device used. There has been a shift from the femoral artery access to the radial artery approach (see Chap. 9); however, a percentage of cases will require a crossover to the femoral approach either due to failed radial access or to perform an intervention. The utilization of vascular closure devices provides an alternative to manual compression with the benefit of shorter time to hemostasis and ambulation [20, 21].

### 15.4 Nonvascular Interventions

Nonvascular MIIP treatments have emerged as an alternative to open surgery through the application of techniques that were utilized in the early vascular MIIPs. MIIPs can be performed on essentially any organ or location in the body, depending on the disease process and the patient's clinical presentation including laboratory workup and imaging findings. Under real-time imaging guidance, IRs insert a small gauge needle into the structure of interest, such as dilated biliary ducts, a dilated ureteral system, or a pocket of abnormal fluid. Once placement is confirmed fluid is aspirated. If the fluid is infected or expected to recur, a catheter can be inserted to provide external drainage (Fig. 15.2). In the case of biliary or ureteral obstruction, temporary drainage catheters can be exchanged for chronic or permanent stents to treat benign and malignant strictures. See Table 15.3 for a list of common nonvascular interventions.

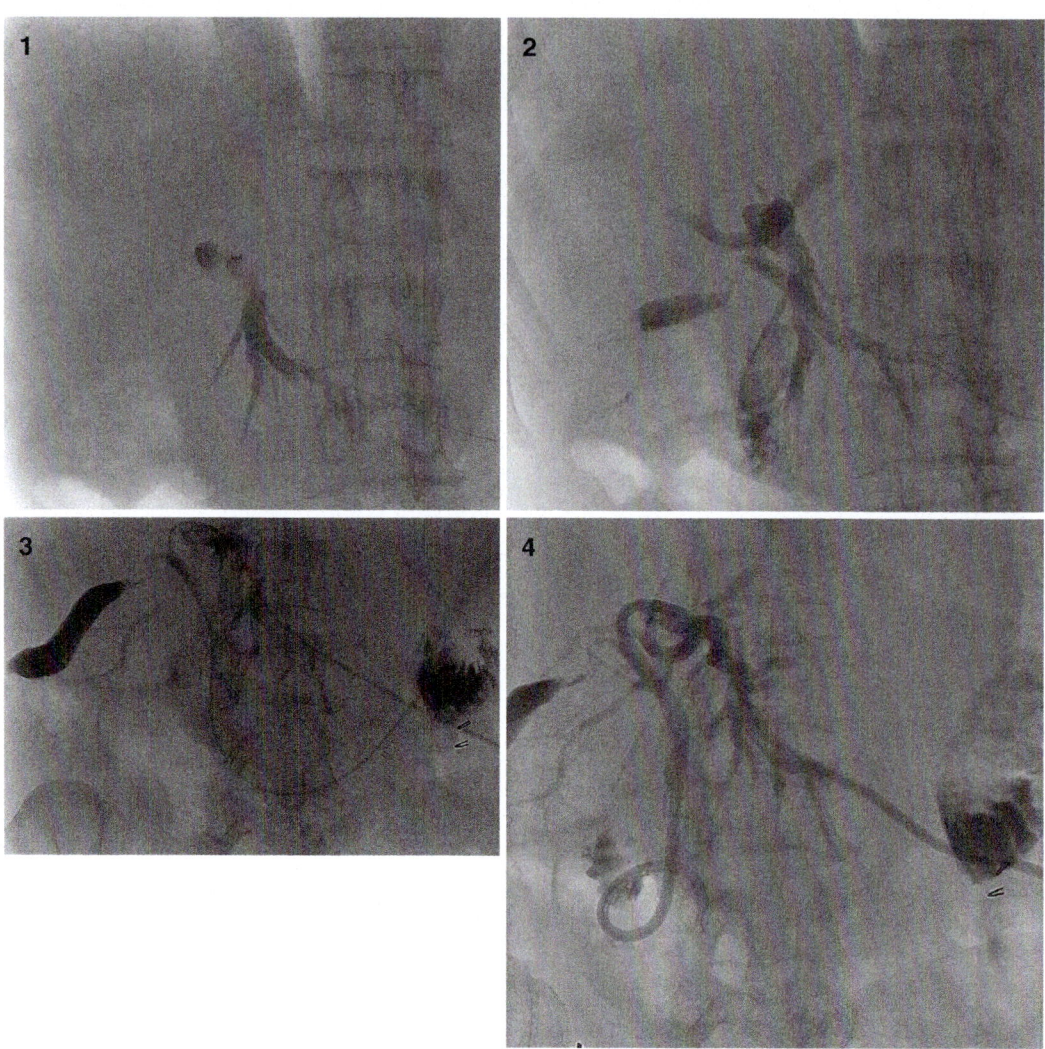

**Fig. 15.2** Sixty-eight-year-old male with pancreatic cancer. Image 1 shows percutaneous transhepatic cholangiogram using a left side or anterior approach with contrast filling of left biliary duct. Image 2 shows further filling of the biliary tree, gall bladder with flow into the duodenum. Image 3 shows guide wire through left biliary duct, common bile duct into duodenum. Image 4 shows an internal/external biliary drainage catheter. The drainage catheter has side holes that allow bile to drain internally to the duodenum and externally to a drainage bag

**Table 15.3** Common nonvascular interventions

| | |
|---|---|
| Percutaneous biopsy | Abdominal |
| | Lung and mediastinum |
| | Neck |
| Percutaneous ablation (alcohol, heat-based [radiofrequency or microwave ablation], Cryoablation) | Liver, lung, kidney, bone |
| Percutaneous abscess and fluid collection/drainage | Throughout the body |
| Biliary duct intervention | Percutaneous transhepatic cholangiography |
| | Biliary drainage for benign and malignant obstructions |
| | Common bile duct stent placement |
| Gallbladder intervention | Percutaneous cholecystostomy |
| | Percutaneous cholecystolithotomy |
| | Gall bladder ablation |
| Percutaneous genitourinary intervention | Percutaneous nephrostomy, nephroureteral stent, or ureteral stent |
| | Percutaneous lithotripsy and nephrolithotomy |
| | Percutaneous stent placement and removal |
| | Ureteral brush biopsy |
| | Ureteral stricture dilatation |
| | Suprapubic cystostomy |
| Musculoskeletal intervention | Biopsy |
| | Facet joint infiltration |
| | Percutaneous epidural/nerve root block |
| | Percutaneous kyphoplasty/vertebroplasty/sacroplasty |
| | Thermal ablation of bone tumors |
| Image-guided breast intervention | Breast biopsy |
| Gastrointestinal tract intervention | Percutaneous gastrostomy |
| | Percutaneous gastrojejunostomy |
| | Percutaneous jejunostomy or cecostomy |
| | Stricture dilatation |

## 15.5 Interventional Oncology

Interventional oncology (IO) is a subspecialty of IR that utilizes image guidance for cancer care across the continuum. This includes diagnosis through biopsy, MIIPs such as ablation and embolization, and the palliation of symptoms such as those which accompany obstructive jaundice with biliary drainage and stenting. Ablation and embolization procedures allow for selective targeted distribution of therapy to cure or control the spread of tumors, relieving symptoms while sparing normal organ tissue, preserving organ function and causing as little collateral damage to nearby structures and minimizing the body's exposure to therapy, as in systemic approaches [22, 23].

### 15.5.1 Tumor Ablation

Ablations are accomplished through the image-guided delivery of energy via a probe inserted directly into the tumor to destroy the tissue in situ through cytotoxic high or low temperatures to either burn or freeze the tumor using US or CT guidance. Success is dependent upon the size of the tumor and the accessibility of the probes. The most common forms of ablation are radiofrequency ablation (RFA), microwave ablation (MWA), cryoablation, and high-intensity focused ultrasound (HIFU).

### 15.5.2 Tumor Embolization

The two most common forms of IO embolization are transarterial chemoembolization (TACE) and transarterial radioembolization (TARE). In both procedures, a small catheter is carefully placed into the artery feeding the tumor and small particles are delivered. In TACE, the small particles are either mixed with or conjugated to chemotherapy agents. Iodinated poppy seed oil, which treats liver cancer and is also visible on fluoroscopy and CT, may or may not be included in TACE. Real-time fluoroscopic imaging is used to determine when the procedure has successfully disrupted blood flow to the tumor(s). In TARE, the microspheres are about ten times smaller than those in TACE. The TARE microspheres are loaded with a beta-emitting form of radioactivity.

## 15.6 Patient Considerations

It is important to determine that the planned procedure is the most appropriate one for the patient. The American College of Radiology (ACR) has established appropriateness criteria to assist clinicians in determining the right procedure for the patient. "The ACR Appropriateness Criteria are evidence-based guidelines funded solely by the American College of Radiology to assist referring physicians and other providers in making the most appropriate imaging or treatment decision for the specific clinical condition. By employing these guidelines, providers enhance quality of care and contribute to the most efficacious use of radiology" [24] (https://www.acr.org/Clinical-Resources/ACR-Appropriateness-Criteria/About-the-ACR-AC). The Society of Interventional Radiology (SIR) has published a number of evidence-based clinical practice guidelines with the goal of safeguarding patient safety and the delivery of patient care [25]. See the following for a list of practice guidelines by topic of interest https://www.sirweb.org/practice-resources/guidelines-by-document-type/guidelines-by-service-line/.

### 15.6.1 The American Medical Association (AMA) Implementation and Clinical Decision Support

"Overuse and inappropriate use of many imaging tests may cause harm by unnecessarily exposing patients to excess radiation; they can also impact patient outcomes when incidental findings are present and can increase healthcare costs" [26] (https://edhub.ama-assn.org/steps-forward/module/2702161). Beginning January 1, 2020, in the USA, the Protecting Access to Medicare Act (PAMA) requires referring providers to consult appropriate use criteria (AUC) prior to ordering advanced diagnostic imaging services (ADIS) including CT, MRI, Nuclear Medicine, and positron emission tomography (PET) for Medicare patients. MIIPs providers will be required to include evidence that AUC were used at the time of billing otherwise Medicare will not reimburse for the services rendered [27]. See the ACR clinical decision support page for further information (https://www.acr.org/Clinical-Resources/Clinical-Decision-Support). Appropriate pre-procedure consults should be done to ensure patient safety.

## 15.7 Complications

MIIP procedures provide less risk than open surgical procedures. However, there is still a potential for complications that can range from access site pain to life-threatening bleeding or respiratory complications. Careful planning including a review of the patient history and laboratory results as well as screening for appropriateness of moderate sedation is essential for the prevention or mitigation of complications. Table 15.4 includes a list of potential complications arising from MIIPs.

Table 15.4 Complications of MIIPs

| | |
|---|---|
| Vascular | Bleeding |
| | Dissection |
| | Hematoma |
| | Perforation |
| | Pseudoaneurysm |
| | Reocclusion/intimal hyperplasia |
| | Thrombosis |
| | Vasospasm |
| | Off-target embolization |
| Contrast media | Allergic response/anaphylaxis |
| | Renal impairment/failure |
| Infection/sepsis | Iatrogenic |
| | Spread of infection from abscess or infected viscus |
| Over-sedation | Respiratory depression |
| | Need for reversal agents |
| Stroke | Embolic |
| | Hemorrhagic |
| Death | |

## 15.8 Personnel

Radiology nurses are an integral part of the MIIPs team which includes the radiologist (or other provider), technologists, and, when needed, anesthesia personnel. In the case of hybrid procedures, other medical specialists may also be involved in the procedure. From the advanced practice nurse to the clinical nurse, their involvement facilitates the planning, performance, patient recovery, and follow-up for the procedures.

## 15.9 Conclusion

MIIPs have emerged through a rich history of innovation and disruptive technology that has created the opportunity to cure diseases virtually through a pinhole. The continued proliferation and adaptation of technology to new indications, especially to critically ill patients, will provide new challenges to nursing to keep step and provide informed care to patients across the MIIPs continuum.

**Acknowledgments** In appreciation for the images provided by Christopher J. Friend, MD, MBA.

## References

1. Seldinger SI. Catheter replacement of the needle in percutaneous arteriography: a new technique. Acta Radiol. 1953;39(5):368–76. https://doi.org/10.3109/00016925309136722.
2. Murphy TP, Soares GM. The evolution of interventional radiology. Semin Intervent Radiol. 2005;22(1):6–9.
3. Lakhan SE, Kaplan A, Laird C, Leitor Y. The interventionalism of medicine: interventional radiology, cardiology, and neuroradiology. Int Arch Med. 2009;2:27.
4. Maingard J, Kok HK, Ranatunga D, Brooks DM, Chandra RV, Lee MJ, et al. The future of interventional and neurointerventional radiology: learning lessons from the past. Br J Radiol. 2017;90:20170473.
5. Rosch J, Keller FS, Kaufman JA. The birth, early years, and future of interventional radiology. J Vasc Interv Radiol. 2003;14:841–53. https://doi.org/10.1097/01.RVI.0000083840.97061.5b.
6. Payne MM. Charles Theodore Dotter: the father of intervention. Tex Heart Inst J. 2001;28:28–38.
7. The Society of Interventional Radiology. Becoming and interventional radiologist. https://www.sirweb.org/learning-center/ir-residency/. Accessed 20 Apr 2019.
8. Kutner M, Greenberg E, Jin Y, Paulsen C. The health literacy of America's adults: results from the 2003 national assessment of adult literacy. US Department of Education. 2003. https://eric.ed.gov/?id=ED493284. Accessed 28 April 2019.
9. Bureau of Labor Statistics. Employment projections by major industry sector. 2017. United States Department of Labor. https://www.bls.gov/emp/tables/employment-by-major-industry-sector.htm. Accessed April 28, 2019.
10. Heister D, Jackson S, Doherty-Simor M, Newton I. An evaluation of trends in patient and public awareness of IR. J Vasc Interv Radiol. 2018;29(5):661–8. https://doi.org/10.1016/j.jvir.2017.11.023.
11. Berkman ND, Sheridan SL, Donahue KE, Halpern DJ, Crotty K. Low health literacy and health outcomes: an updated systematic review. Ann Intern Med. 2011;155:97–107. https://doi.org/10.7326/0003-4819-155-2-201107190-00005.
12. Centers for Disease Control and Prevention. Health Literacy. U.S. Department of Health and Human Services. 2019. https://www.cdc.gov/healthliteracy/gettraining.html?CDC_AA_refVal=https%3A%2F%2Fwww.cdc.gov%2Fhealthliteracy%2Fwriting-course%2Findex.html. Accessed 28 Apr 2019.
13. Gerhard-Herman MD, Gornik JL, Barrett C, Barshes NR, Corriere MA, Drachman DE, et al. 2016 AHA/ACC guideline on the management of patients with lower extremity peripheral artery disease: executive summary: a report of the American College of Cardiology/American Heart Association task force on clinical practice guidelines. Circulation. 2017; https://doi.org/10.1161/CIR.0000000000000470. Accessed 1 May 2019
14. Lo RC, Darling J, Bensley RP, Giles KA, Dahlberg SE, Hamdan AD, Wyers M, et al. Outcomes following infrapopliteal angioplasty for critical limb ischemia. J Vasc Surg. 2013;57:1455–64. https://doi.org/10.1016/j.jvs.2012.10.109.
15. Rockley M, Jetty P, Wells G, Rockley K, Fergusson D. Prolonged versus brief balloon inflation during arterial angioplasty for de novo atherosclerotic disease: protocol for a systematic review. Syst Rev. 2019; https://doi.org/10.0086/s13643-019-0955-2.
16. Krankenberg H, Tubler T, Ingwersen M, Schluter M, Scheinert D, Blessing E, et al. Drug-coated balloon versus standard balloon for superficial femoral artery in-stent restenosis: the randomized femoral artery in-stent restenosis (FAIR) trial. Circulation. 2015;132(23):2230–6. https://doi.org/10.1161/CIRCULATIONAHA.115.017364.
17. Ho KJ, Owens CD. Diagnosis, classification, and treatment of femoropopliteal artery in-stent restenosis. J Vasc Surg. 2017;65(2):545–57. https://doi.org/10.1016/j.jvs.2016.09.031.
18. Robertson I. Basic principles of embolization. In: Kessel DO, Ray CE, editors. Transcatheter embo-

lization and therapy. London: Springer; 2010. p. 3–13.
19. Bauer JR, Ray CE. Transcatheter arterial embolization in the trauma patient: a review. Semin Intervent Radiol. 2004;21(1):11–22.
20. Mankerious N, Mayer K, Gewalt SM, Helde SM, Ibrahim T, Bott-Flugel L, et al. Comparison of the femoseal vascular closure device with manual compression after femoral artery puncture – post-hoc analysis of a large-scale, randomized clinical trial. J Invasive Cardiol. 2018;30(7):235–9.
21. Mohanty S, Trivedi C, Beheiry S, Al-Ahmad A, Horton R, Della Rocca DG, et al. Venous access-site closure with vascular closure device vs. manual compression in patients undergoing catheter ablation or left atrial appendage occlusion under uninterrupted anticoagulation: a multicenter experience on efficacy and complications [abstract]. Europace. 2019:euz004. https://doi.org/10.1092/europace/euz004.
22. Erinjeri JP, Fine GC, Adema GJ, Ahmed M, Chapiro J, den Brok M, et al. Immunotherapy and interventional oncologist: challenges and opportunities – a society of interventional radiology white paper. Radiology. 2019:1–10. https://doi.org/10.1148/radiol.2019182326.
23. Solomon SB, Silverman SG. Imaging in interventional oncology. Radiology. 2010;257:624–40. https://doi.org/10.1148/radiol.10081490.
24. American College of Radiology. About the ACR appropriateness criteria. https://www.acr.org/Clinical-Resources/ACR-Appropriateness-Criteria/About-the-ACR-AC. Accessed 18 April 2019.
25. The Society of Interventional Radiology. Standards of practice: clinical guidelines by topic. 2019. https://www.sirweb.org/practice-resources/guidelines-by-document-type/guidelines-by-service-line/. Accessed April 18, 2019.
26. Hames GR, Sowers LR. Clinical decision support and diagnostic imaging. AMA steps forward. 2016. https://edhub.ama-assn.org/steps-forward/module/2702161. Accessed April 18, 2019.
27. American College of Radiology. Clinical decision support. https://www.acr.org/Clinical-Resources/Clinical-Decision-Support. Accessed 18 Apr 2019.

# MR Safety Essentials for Nurses

**16**

Maureen N. Hood

## 16.1 Introduction and Background

Magnetic resonance imaging (MRI, often just termed MR) has been used clinically since the early 1980s. MRI is now ubiquitous in our clinical world with nursing requiring more interaction and thus more education on MR safety and the unique needs of caring for the patient in MRI. To understand MR safety, a brief overview of key aspects of how an MRI scanner works is necessary. If one understands where danger may occur, one will be better prepared to prevent adverse events. This chapter will integrate the physics of MRI with the dangers that relate to safety and how to prevent problems.

### 16.1.1 What Is MRI?

Although most nurses know MRI as a common imaging modality, few actually know what MRI actually is, how it works, or why MR safety is so complicated. Magnetic resonance imaging is actually nuclear magnetic resonance imaging as it focuses on the nucleus of the atom. The word nuclear was dropped when application for medical use was being developed as the general public associated the word nuclear with radiation and being radioactive, a scary entity in the early 1980s due to the Three Mile Island nuclear power plant accident. MR works by exploiting the magnetic properties of the nucleus of certain types of atoms using magnetic fields and radiofrequency energy to create images and other information.

### 16.1.2 Background Physics and Terminology

MR uses a static (main) magnetic field (B0), a switching, gradient magnetic field ($dB/dt$) (the audible time-varying field), and a radiofrequency time-varying magnetic field (B1), simply referred to here as radiofrequency (RF). All of these components relate to the risks unique to MR safety. This section briefly covers these main concepts and additional terms commonly used in MR safety.

To begin our understanding in the physics behind the MR scanners, let's start with the main magnetic field itself. The main magnetic field in MRI is most commonly created according to Ampere's law by sending electric current through loops of wires. The magnetic field strength is typically measured in units of Tesla (T) after Nikola Tesla who explored the rotating magnetic field and is credited with the beginnings

---

M. N. Hood, PhD, RN, RT (R)(MR),
FSMRT, FAHA (✉)
Department of Radiology & Radiological Sciences,
Uniformed Services University of the Health
Sciences, Edward Hébert School of Medicine,
Bethesda, MD, USA

© Springer Nature Switzerland AG 2020
K. A. Gross (ed.), *Advanced Practice and Leadership in Radiology Nursing*,
https://doi.org/10.1007/978-3-030-32679-1_16

of alternating current [1]. The unit of 1 T equals 10,000 gauss, another magnetic field unit used below. Currently, FDA-approved clinical scanners range from approximately 0.02 to 7 T [2].

The magnetic field of the MR scanner has a large uniform region in the middle of the magnet which drops off with distance from the magnet (Fig. 16.1). This is important to know for any MR Conditional equipment taken into the scanner room. The lines you may see on the floor of your MR scanner room are simply the gauss lines demonstrating general levels of magnetic field strength to help staff identify the safe limits for their MR Conditional equipment. Additionally, the rate at which the magnetic field drops off over distance or "Spatial Field Gradient" (SFG) is important information for various MR Conditional devices.

The material properties of any item coming into the scanner room is a point of significant concern, particularly ferrous objects. The term ferrous refers to an object containing iron. However, the related term, ferromagnetic, refers to any metal or metal alloy that contains iron, nickel, and/or cobalt that can become magnetized when exposed to a magnetic field and remain magnetized even when removed from the magnetic source. Thus, ferromagnetic objects taken close to the magnetic field of the MR scanner will experience a displacement force that will attract them towards the strong magnet field. This is commonly referred to as the *"missile" effect*.

Ferromagnetic objects in a magnetic field may also experience a rotational force that can cause long ferromagnetic items to align with the magnetic field.

The time-varying gradient magnetic fields ($dB/dt$) create spatially varying magnetic fields in the orthogonal planes $X$, $Y$, $Z$. The gradients are used to localize position, and thus help define field of view, resolution, and slice position and help with acquiring certain types of image contrast. We can hear the gradients because the frequency of operation is in the audible range. The term $dB/dt$ is defined as the ratio between the change in amplitude of the magnetic field ($dB$) and the time it takes to make that change ($dt$) [3]. This factor is a key determinant for peripheral nerve stimulation considerations.

The last major section of terminology to review before digging into the main safety discussions is a short introduction to the electromagnetic spectrum (Fig. 16.2). MR utilizes radiofrequency (RF) pulses, which are a form of electromagnetic energy. These pulses typically excite the nucleus of hydrogen atoms. The electromagnetic spectrum (Fig. 16.2) shows the relationship between frequency, wavelength, and the energy conveyed in the waves. Furthermore, Faraday's law of induction tells us that time-varying magnetic fields generate an electrical current in any conductive material such as the human body and cause appreciable patient heating. The short RF pulses can induce a current

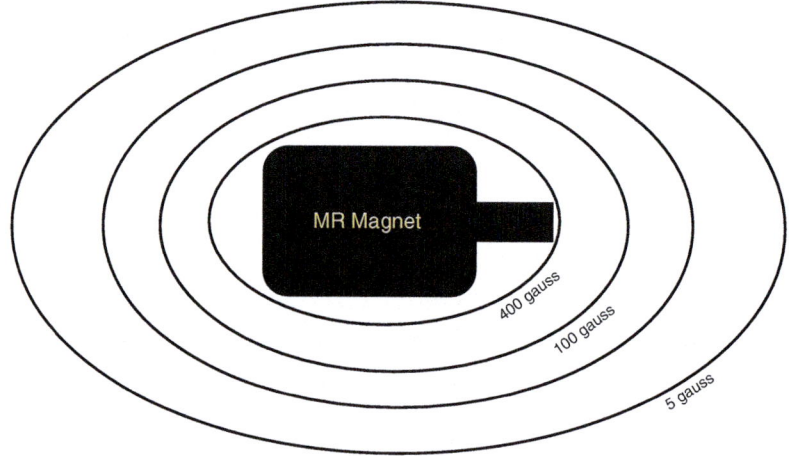

**Fig. 16.1** Simplified depiction of the measured gauss lines. The static magnetic field becomes stronger as you get closer to the magnet. The actual gradation of the field lines vary from scanner to scanner and are not this elliptical nor are the gauss values necessarily found at locations marked. The magnetic field increases rapidly as the distance to the magnet decreases

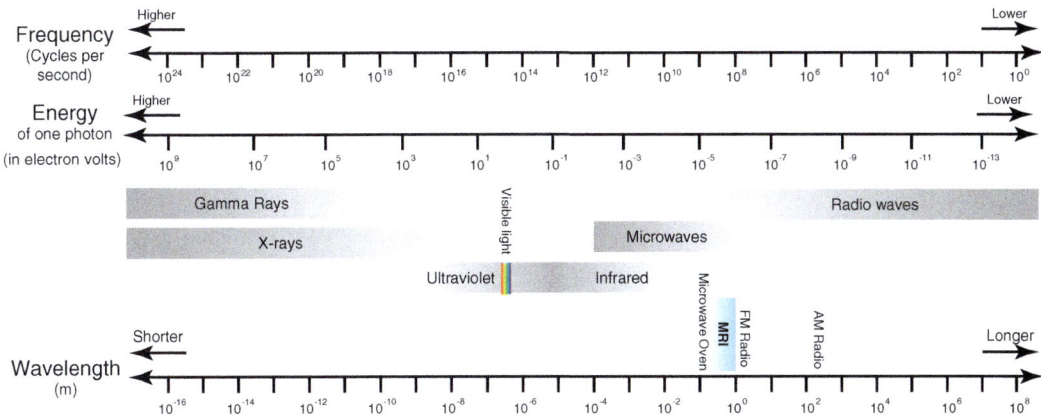

**Fig. 16.2** The electromagnetic spectrum as measured in a vacuum. Note that MRI falls in the overlap range of microwaves and radio waves, but is far from the ionizing energies of gamma rays and X-rays

in any conducting object such as the leads and cables leaving the patient to connect to monitoring equipment and under the wrong conditions can cause severe heating. The time-varying gradients can also induce heating, but is usually not a concern. Thus, it is important to keep all cables together exiting out the center of the bore where possible [4]. Do *not* let the cables touch the bore of the scanner. Remember to only use MR-approved supplies and equipment.

## 16.2 Main Safety Concerns

This section will investigate three concerns, namely, safety concerns of the main magnetic field, safety concerns of the time-varying (switching) gradient fields, and safety concerns of the radiofrequency field.

### 16.2.1 Safety Concerns of the Main Magnet Field—B0

A multitude of people and vendors have advocated for tools to help prevent "missile" accidents from ferromagnetic objects entering the MRI environment. Truth be told, no single method or tool will catch everything. If the clinic owns ferromagnetic detectors, wands, or any type of "stop and check" equipment, it should be utilized prior to the patient entering the MRI scanner room.

Training staff to be aware of the dangers of MR, to screen patients carefully, and to look for hidden objects under garments or blankets is the best protection for working around an MR scanner. Using a tool such as a ferromagnetic detector as an additional layer of checking for MR unsafe items can be helpful. Be mindful that these tools are only sensitive to ferrous metals. Other conducting materials that can cause grievous injury are not ferrous, or necessarily even metallic (e.g., carbon) which is why screening is so critical for safety. Objects being taken into the MRI scanner room must be cleared by MRI staff prior to being taken into the scanner room. Having a handheld magnet or ferromagnetic wand can be used to check certain items. Equipment in the MRI suite should be labeled according to ASTM International (Formerly American Society for Testing and Materials) standards (Table 16.1), which relates to MR safety in general and not just the main magnetic. The labels come in color as well as black-and-white versions. The colors follow the internationally accepted colors of green for safe, yellow for caution, and red for danger.

### 16.2.2 Safety Concerns of the Time-Varying (Switching) Gradient Fields—(dB/dt)

Acoustic noise is a phenomenon caused by Lorentz forces arising from the switching

**Table 16.1** Internationally accepted labeling system for MR safety

| Term | Definition | Label appearance |
|---|---|---|
| MR Safe | An item that poses no known hazards in all MRI environments. | |
| MR Conditional | An item that has been demonstrated to pose no known hazards in a specified MRI environment with specified conditions of use. Additional conditions, including specific configurations of the item, may be required. | |
| MR Unsafe | An item that is known to pose hazards in all MRI environments. MR unsafe items include magnetic items such as a pair of ferromagnetic scissors. | |

Reprinted with permission from ASTM F2503–13 Standard Practice for Marking Medical Devices and Other Items for Safety in the Magnetic Resonance Environment, copyright ASTM International, 100 Barr Harbor Drive, West Conshohocken, PA 19428. A copy of the complete standard may be obtained from ASTM International, www.astm.org

gradients interacting with the main magnetic field of the scanner [5, 6]. As higher field strength scanners tend to use higher-performance gradient systems, the Lorentz forces are higher as well; thus, the combination of higher field strength (B0) and stronger gradients can lead to louder scanners. This is why 1.5 and 3 T MRI scanners are generally louder than low field MRI scanners.

The safe working exposure limit for an 8 h period is 85 dB [7], so it is reasonable to assume that shorter exposures of an hour or two at up to 85 dB should be fine for most people. The cases reported in the U.S. Food and Drug Administration (FDA) Maude Database about hearing loss note inadequate or inadequately placed earplugs [8]. Proper instruction on earplug use followed by visual inspection and a whisper test is essential to help reduce hearing loss. The Noise Reduction Rating (NRR) of earplugs is generally 29–33 dB NRR and most MR hear muff headsets around 24–29 dB NRR. The MRI scanner safety manual will state the minimum NRR required for the particular scanner. Offering both earplugs and headsets is recommended whenever it is possible and/or reasonable to do so. Neonates and young children have more sensitive hearing, which makes the need for hearing protection even more critical. Standard adult earplugs are too big for children and the small yellow ear covers only attenuate about 7 dB and the more expensive headphones for babies only attenuate 22 dB, so extra padding around the sides of the head is recommended. The standard adult earplugs may also be too large for some adults. Therefore having a variety of sizes of earplugs would benefit adults and children.

The hearing risk to the fetus when scanning of pregnant women has been debated for years despite the study performed in 1995 [9]. The fetal environment was simulated by placing an acoustic probe in a stomach full of water, which estimated that the gravid uterus should attenuate more than 30 dB of noise. In a recent study of 751 neonates exposed to MRI during pregnancy, there was no difference in hearing found as compared to neonates that were not exposed to MRI [10].

The time-varying gradient fields also have a potential effect on MR unsafe electrically active devices including implanted cardiac pacemakers, defibrillators, neurostimulators, medication pumps, etc. The time-varying or switching gradient fields can induce currents that can interfere with electrically active devices. In addition, heat and vibration induced by the switching gradients may cause the device to malfunction or cease operating at all [11]. What this means is that the manufacturers guidelines should be followed for implanted active devices.

### 16.2.3 Safety Concerns of the Radiofrequency (RF or B1) Field

The best way to avoid burns is not only to use MR-approved equipment, but also to be aware of all lines, cables, and any other conductive materials. When preparing the patient for scanning, check for any watches, jewelry, metallic patches, etc. as patients often forget to take these items off. For patients with tattoos, they should be counseled to squeeze the alarm ball if they feel any heat or discomfort. If they are an inpatient, be especially mindful to look for ECG electrodes, pulse oximetry components, and anything else that can be hiding under a sheet or blanket. If the patient is a neonate or child, be especially careful to check clothing for snaps, pins, and a pulse oximetry probe on a toe. It is further recommended that the patient change into MRI-provided gowns or scrubs for the exam. Regular clothing can have metallic threads or coatings that can put the patient at risk for harm. For example, copper and silver are now commonly used in many types of clothing. These metallic fabrics have resulted in several patient burns [12]. Also be on the lookout for patients wearing health and exercise sensors. Clothing, including underwear, is now being designed with biosensors [13]. These sensors cannot go into the MR scanner.

If the patient needs to be monitored in the scanner, use only MR-approved equipment and supplies. Keep track of any lines, cables, or other long leads exiting the scanner, keep the cables together away from the bore wall, and preferably running out the center of the bore. For the Wi-Fi monitoring attachments, secure the sensors so that they do not touch the bore of the scanner. Poorly managed cables have resulted in focal burns and fires [14, 15]. MRI scanners also have special pads to use to aid in patient comfort. Using pads between the legs, arms, or other touching body parts help to break the skin/skin electrical contact. Do not let patients clasp their hands together even if they are outside the bore as skin/skin contact has resulted in burns [16]. Always make sure there is a pad between the patient's skin and the bore of the MRI scanner wall to give extra distance from the transmit coil that is located just behind the tunnel wall. Sheets and blankets are not to be considered as padding.

## 16.3 Training

MR safety training is recommend for all persons working routinely in the MRI suite (Table 16.2). According to The Joint Commission (TJC) MR technologists and radiologists are now required to have annual advanced or Level II training every year [17]. Non-MR staff (radiology administrators, schedulers, nurses, housekeeping, first responders, etc.) who work near or sometimes in the MRI scanner room are recommended to have basic, or Level I, training annually. Staff members entering the MRI scanning area must either have annual MRI safety training at Level I or Level II, or be screened by Level II personnel prior to entering the MR scanner room. For staff who do get annual training but do not work regularly in the MRI suite, a quick screen by Level II staff is recommended. It is also important to remind staff to empty their pockets of all non-MRI approved items prior to walking into the scanner room as *the magnet is always on, even when it is quiet*.

**Table 16.2** MR safety training recommendations

| Training level | Type of persons | Responsibilities/expectations |
|---|---|---|
| Level I –Basic | *Must be supervised 100% of time in Zone III and IV* | |
| | Nurses | Work safely in magnet room and manage monitoring equipment |
| | Anesthesiology providers | Work safely in magnet room and manage monitoring equipment |
| | Support staff | Be safe near MR or in magnet room |
| | MR research support staff | Be safe near MR, initial screen of subjects |
| | MR schedulers | Be safe near MR, initial screen of scheduled patients, answer basic questions |
| | Radiology administrators | Be safe near MR |
| | Housekeeping | Be safe near MR or in magnet room |
| | Hospital biomedical engineering | Work safely in near or in magnet room |
| | Hospital facilities/maintenance | Work safely in near or in magnet room |
| *Level I—Basic—Special for first responders*[a] | | |
| | Fire fighters, emergency responders | Work safely in near or in magnet room, be prepared for a fire in magnet room, know who and how to contact should magnetic field need to be ramped down (if possible), know how to turn off power to systems. Know the difference between power off and ramp down magnet and where to find those buttons |
| *Level II—Advanced* | | |
| | MR technologists | Responsible for every non-MR person in Zones III and IV, screening and documenting patient for safety, responsible for all MR exam-related duties and patient care, know when to call radiologist or nurses for assistance, be prepared for emergencies. |
| | Radiologists | Risk benefit decision. Ultimate authority over MR patient care. |
| | MR nurses | Work safely in MR scanner room, know monitoring for MR patients including implanted electronic device patents, assist with screening and patient care, be prepared for emergencies |
| | Other MR providers | Work safely in MR scanner room |
| | MR researcher staff | Work safely in MR scanner room |

[a]First responders should have a written standard operating procedure in the event of a fire involving MRI scanners. Fire departments recommended to communicate with MR department for special safety considerations

It is also important to remind staff that items such as stethoscopes, hairpins, paperclips, and pens can become projectiles. Simply wearing a surgical cap or closing a pocket is not sufficient and will not protect an item from the force of the magnet.

## 16.4 Screening

A multifaceted standard operating procedure with a variety of checks or processes will help reduce the chance of a projectile accident, the wrong equipment, or a patient with an unsafe implant entering the MR scanner room. Every MR clinic or hospital should develop a *multi-layered screening process*. Screening by the MRI clinic should start when the patient makes the appointment. Screening at the time of appointment by trained staff helps to find implanted items in the patient that require additional consideration (Table 16.3). Certain implanted items in a person's body in addition to certain medical conditions may require additional follow-up or special handling such as active medical devices, a history of metal fragments to the eye, allergies (including contrast media), renal impairment, claustrophobia, or a complicated or unstable medical condition. It is also important to get height and weight to make sure the patient will fit for the exam. A patient

**Table 16.3** Implanted medical devices

| Category of implant | Type | Advanced screening required[a] | Advanced monitoring required[b] | Programming required[b] | Post MRI assessment needed |
|---|---|---|---|---|---|
| *Passive* | | | | | |
| | Orthopedic screws, plates, pins | No | No | No | No |
| | Orthopedic rods | Yes | No | No | No |
| | Surgical staples | No | No | No | No |
| | Joint replacements | Maybe | Maybe | No | No |
| | Filters | Yes | No | No | No |
| | External fixation device | Yes | Yes | No | Maybe |
| | Stents—coronary | Maybe | No | No | No |
| | Stents—other than coronary | Yes | Yes | No | No |
| | PDA/VSD closure devices | Yes | No | No | No |
| | Aneurysm clip | Yes | No | No | No |
| | Artificial heart valve | No | No | No | No |
| | Dental devices (nonremovable) | No | No | No | No |
| *Passive, but adjustable by a magnet or other device* | | | | | |
| | Spinal rods | Yes | Yes | Maybe | Maybe |
| | Breast tissue expanders | Yes | Yes | Maybe | Maybe |
| | External fixation device | Yes | Yes | Maybe | Maybe |
| *Electronically active* | | | | | |
| | Cardiac pacemaker | Yes | Yes | Maybe | Yes |
| | Cardiac defibrillator | Yes | Yes | Maybe | Yes |
| | Neurostimulator | Yes | Yes | Yes | Maybe |
| | Cochlear implant | Yes | Yes | Yes | Yes |
| | Implanted medication delivery | Yes | Yes | Maybe | Yes |
| | Cardiac loop recorder | Yes | No | No | Maybe |
| | Programmable shunt | Yes | Maybe | Maybe | Yes |

A short table of examples of the categories of devices. This is **not** a complete list. Manufacturer's guidelines must be followed carefully. Not all devices in a certain category are the same. Some devices may have additional recommended or required processes
[a]Documentation of implanted medical devices is the best practice for safety
[b]Not all implanted medical devices have been tested to be safe for MRI

weight is needed for proper MR system operation. When the patient arrives in the MRI clinic, some sort of written or electronic documentation must be completed by the patient or legal representative able to provide medical information about the patient. The MR technologist/radiographer who is to perform the exam should do an interview with the patient. The patient should change into MR-approved clothing. The clothing should be supplied by the MR clinic as street clothes can be problematic and screening for some items per above is nearly impossible. For patients with prosthetics, the prosthetic cover needs to be either removed or checked as silver is now being used in the material of some covers. In addition, prior to the patient entering the MRI scanner room, a last verbal check by the MR team members taking care of the patient, often referred to as a "Time-Out," should occur to check for inadvertently missed items and to remind staff to do a self-check.

## 16.5 Implanted Medical Devices

Medical implants come in a variety of types, sizes, shapes, composition, and function. When speaking in terms of MR safety, implanted medical devices are generally categorized as active or passive. Active devices are defined as those devices that are acted upon by an energy source that does not come from the human tissue such as a pacemaker, neurostimulator, programmable shunt, or adjustable spinal rods [18]. Passive implants are not operated by a power source but may have movable parts that can be manipulated through the use of a power source or some other mechanisms. Passive implants (Table 16.4) are items such as stents, joint replacements, dental fillings, and orthopedic screws [19].

Scanning active implanted medical devices is becoming routine in major medical centers, but they are also a major struggle to handle in a timely manner. The FDA and other international regulatory bodies have been working with industry manufacturers for proper testing and labeling of implanted medical devices, with the electrically active devices being the most complicated. Each implanted active device will have its own labeling and special requirements that have been approved by the FDA based on testing. It is in the best interest of nurses proving care in MRI to learn about the monitoring requirements specified by the manufacturers as they may be different than in other areas of the hospital or clinic. In addition, your facility should have written guidelines on how patients with these devices are to be handled.

MR Conditional devices come with labeling documentation that needs to be followed for the patient to be safely scanned in MRI. The label may contain certain technical terms that define the MR conditional requirements. The details of these terms are beyond the scope of this chapter; however, the main terms are Specific Absorption Rate (SAR) and B1+rms [20]. B1+rms is a more recent term, but it is preferred for active implanted devices, but support for this term may not exist on all MRI scanners.

Many pacemakers and implanted cardiac defibrillators (ICDs) are now MRI approved at 1.5 and 3 T. Nurses are frequently called upon to support the scanning of patients with cardiac pacemakers and defibrillators. The manufacturer's guidelines must be followed for each make and model. Checklists are available from some companies that make it easy to meet the monitoring requirements and steps. For example: A patient calls to schedule an MRI. The patient says yes to having a pacemaker. If the patient has the pacemaker information or card, it's your lucky day and a simple check of the patient's records can confirm make, model and leads. If not, the desig-

Table 16.4 Center for Medicare and Medicaid Services (CMS) Guidelines for the safe scanning of cardiac devices not labeled for MR use. Extras precautions, training and staff are required to support off-label devices safely. These guidelines are available at: https://www.cms.gov/Outreach-and-Education/Medicare-Learning-Network-MLN/MLNMattersArticles/downloads/MM10877.pdf

| Cardiac-implanted devices | Expand coverage for implanted Pacemaker (PM), implanted cardioverter defibrillator (ICD), cardiac resynchronization therapy pacemaker (CRT-P), or cardiac resynchronization therapy defibrillator (CRT-D) device that does not have FDA MR labeling |
|---|---|
| 1.5 Tesla using normal operating mode | |
| No fractured, epicardial, or abandoned leads | |
| The facility has a checklist which includes the following: | |
| | Patient assessment |
| | Informed consent |
| | Prior to MRI, device interrogated and programmed into appropriate MRI scanning mode |
| | *A qualified physician, nurse practitioner, or physician assistant with expertise with PMs, ICDs, CRT-Ps, or CRT-Ds must directly supervise the MRI scan (i.e., immediately available)* |
| | Patients observed in MRI scanner via visual and voice contact, and monitored with equipment to assess vital signs and cardiac rhythm |
| | *An ACLS provider must be present for the duration of the MRI scan* |
| | A discharge plan that includes re-interrogated immediately after the MRI scan to detect and correct any abnormalities |

nated safety person will hunt through the patient records and/or call the pacemaker manufacturer to confirm. The patient may need to be scanned on a day when a properly trained pacemaker programmer can be available as most pacemakers and defibrillators must go through a series of checks and programming to MRI mode before the MRI. The patient must be monitored by qualified medical personnel (determined by your institution's practice guidelines), and then the patient's pacemaker will go through a series of checks and programming after the MRI exam to confirm the patient is fine before being released. There is currently a company that has designed cardiac devices to auto-detect being in the presence of a magnetic field and it will automatically program itself into MRI-mode [21]. Patients with auto MR detection devices must still be monitored while in MRI. For those devices, pulse oximetry is generally recommended as the preferred monitoring according to manufacturer's guidelines, but ECG may be placed on the patient as well for general assessment.

The nursing staff may also be called upon to assist with implanted medication devices. The manufacture's guidelines should be followed carefully as over- and under-infusion, unintended boluses, and device malfunctions have been reported [22]. A careful check of the device should occur before the patient is scanned. Some MR Conditional medication pump models recommend the patient have the device checked following the MR procedure as pump problems such as a stalled pump have been reported. There are actually many active devices such as neurostimulators and programmable shunts that call for the patient to contact their provider for a safety check after the MRI.

## 16.6 Off-Label Devices

### 16.6.1 Electrically Active

It is estimated that over 75% of all persons with a cardiac device will need an MR at some point; thus, the need to scan patients with MR unsafe cardiac devices is great [23]. The Centers for Medicare and Medicaid Services (CMS)[24] has expanded coverage for beneficiaries with certain cardiac devices that do not have FDA labeling specific for an MRI, but under certain conditions (Section 220.2(B)(3)) (Table 16.4). However, scanning patients off-label increases the risk to the patient, so extra precautions must be taken to monitor and care for the patient should something go wrong. For those patients, a serious risk-benefit decision should be made by the referring and imaging physicians. The good news is that because off-label scanning typically occurs in large institutions with careful selection, screening, monitoring, and back up, thousands of patients have been successfully scanned in MRI with off-label devices.

### 16.6.2 Passive

Many passive implants such as pins, screws, and staples are scanned off-label. Some passive devices (stents, closure devices, heart valves, etc.) are tested for the appropriate MR Conditional labeling. Many orthopedic devices such as screws may not have been tested for MRI, but may be made of potentially acceptable materials such as titanium or certain grades of stainless steel. Deciding on how to handle these devices depends on your institution's written MR safety policies. Size, shape, composition, and location all play into the safety of a passive implanted item. Items such as external fixation devices and halos should be tested with a handheld magnet to check for ferromagnetic parts and then the patient must be instructed to squeeze the emergency ball should the patient feel any heat or unusual sensations during the exam. Unfortunately, the configuration of some external fixation devices or halos can heat up during scanning even if the components are non-ferromagnetic, but conductive. Shrapnel is another tough decision as it could be any metal. For potential metal in the eye, X-rays or an available head CT can be used to rule out a foreign object in the eye. For shrapnel in other body parts, most patients can be safely scanned, but they should always be reminded to squeeze the emergency ball if they feel any unusual sensations while being scanned. Each institution should have a written policy specifically for how to handle patients with shrapnel.

## 16.7 Contrast Agents

Most contrast agents being used in MRI are gadolinium-based contrast agents (GBCAs). For a contrast agent to work in the MRI environment, it must have a characteristic that can be exploited by MR imaging, which is why the iodinated contrast agents used in X-ray and computed tomography do not work in MRI. MRI contrast agents must affect the local tissue magnetic environment. Paramagnetic substances can alter the MRI contrast in certain tissues acquired in MRI [25]. GBCAs are primarily extracellular agents, have good stability, exit the body relatively rapidly and are generally nonspecific in their distribution (except they do not cross the blood brain barrier). Iron and manganese agents have also been developed, but are currently not available clinically in the United States for numerous reasons ranging from lack of sales to high adverse reaction rates.

Adverse reactions to GBCA are relatively uncommon (0.07–2.4%) and most are mild such as injection site complaints, nausea, headache, vomiting, and paresthesia [26–29]. Allergic-like reactions can occur (0.004–0.7%) that are similar to allergic-like reactions found with iodinated contrast agents [27, 29]. Severe reactions and death are extremely rare (0.006–0.001%) [26–29].

The main risk associated with the use of contrast agents is nephrogenic systemic fibrosis (NSF). The GBCAs are primarily filtered from the body via the kidneys, and since almost all cases of NSF have occurred in end-stage chronic renal failure or acute renal injury (AKI), renal function laboratory screening used to estimate the glomerular filtration rate (eGFR) is used to help the physician to determine a patient's risk potential. The American College of Radiology (ACR) has updated the classification of GBCAs in 2018 to divide the currently available agents into three classes (Table 16.5) [30]. The main change is that a much more clear distinction has been made regarding the stability of the agents. GBCAs with lower stability have an increased risk of NSF, and thus have more restrictions for screening and use (Table 16.6).

One other aspect of the gadolinium contrast agents that needs to be addressed in this chapter is gadolinium deposition, first discovered in 2013 [31]. It is postulated that the gadolinium contrast in vivo can, in small amounts, dechelate and deposit into our tissues [32]. The MR community is searching for answers as to the clinical significance of this finding. Currently, there are no known clinical symptoms, but that doesn't mean there aren't any since we never knew to look before. Since gadolinium is toxic when not chelated, potential toxicity is a concern [33]. It appears that all gadolinium agents have documented some level of gadolinium deposition, but not all contrast agents are equal. Current research is reporting that the less stable, linear agents appear to have a greater gadolinium deposition, as well as with increased NSF risk [32]. Administration of linear gadolinium che-

**Table 16.5** Classes of gadolinium-based contrast agents

|  | Agent name | Trade name | Company |
|---|---|---|---|
| Class I Agents associated with the greatest number of NSF cases ||||
|  | Gadodiamide | Omniscan® | GE Healthcare |
|  | Gadopentetate dimeglumine | Magnevist® | Bayer HealthCare Pharmaceuticals |
|  | Gadoversetamide | OptiMARK® | Guerbet |
| Class II Agents associated with few, if any, unconfounded cases of NSF ||||
|  | Gadobenate dimeglumine | MultiHance® | Bracco Diagnostics |
|  | Gadobutrol | Gadavist®, Gadovist | Bayer HealthCare Pharmaceuticals |
|  | Gadoterate acid | Dotarem® | Guerbet |
|  | Gadoteridol | ProHance® | Bracco Diagnostics |
| Class III Agents with *limited data* regarding NSF risk, but for which few, if any unconfounded cases of NSF have been reported ||||
|  | Gadoxetate disodium | Eovist®, Primovist | Bayer HealthCare Pharmaceuticals |

*Adapted with permission from:* ACR Committee on Drugs and Contrast Media, ACR Contrast Manual, 2018, V10.3, p81–89, ACR

**Table 16.6** How to manage patient screening according to gadolinium-based contrast agent class

| Class I and III | Must screen for risk factors |
|---|---|
| Complete lab testing and eGFR calculation | |
| Inpatients | Within 48 h |
| Outpatients No prior eGFR at scheduling | No risk factors—No eGFR required With risk factors—Obtain eGFR |
| Most recent eGFR > 45 at scheduling | NO risk factor and eGFR 60 or above, no new eGFR required WITH risk factors and/or eGFR 45–59, no new eGFR if labs within 6 weeks, otherwise obtain a new eGFR |
| Most recent eGFR 45 or below | Obtain eGFR within 2 days of the MRI study |
| | Risk factors* 1. History of renal disease, including: a. Prior dialysis b. Renal transplant c. Single kidney d. Kidney surgery e. Renal cancer 2. Hypertension requiring medical therapy 3. Diabetes mellitus |
| | *Other risk: Recent iodinated contrast—contrast-induced nephropathy (CIN) risk, therefore new labs recommended |
| Class II | *Standard dose or less, assessment of renal function is optional as long as contrast is deemed medically necessary* |
| | Preferred if: On dialysis, severe or end-stage CKD (eGFR < 30 mL/min/1.73 m²), or AKI |

Patients with acute kidney injury (AKI) on dialysis (any type)—eGFR deemed not useful, therefore group II agents strong preferred
Children: Use updated Schwartz equation for eGFR
*Adapted with permission from:* ACR Committee on Drugs and Contrast Media, ACR Contrast Manual, 2018, V10.3, p81–89, ACR

lates, despite normal renal function, leads to long-term deposition of gadolinium in the skin, bone, liver, and a focal, specific distribution in the brain [31–35]. Gadolinium deposition is an active area of research. In the meantime, clinicians should be prudent with their use of gadolinium-based contrast agents, following established best practice clinical guidelines.

## 16.8 Anxiety Issues

Anxiety is a common problem for any radiologic procedure, but MRI tends to increase the anxiety levels in some people. Patient screening and education in advance of the MR exam are critical steps to help decrease the fear factor of "going into the tunnel." Unfortunately, marketing professionals have coined the terms "open" and "closed" to describe scanners. Conventionally open, or lower field scanners (below 1.2 T), tend to have a more open shape whereas the more common, higher field (currently 1.5 T and higher) are a cylindrical, oval, or tunnel shape. The higher field scanners also come in a variety of sizes. It is best to educate patients MR scanners are open at both ends, have lights, communication systems, and air that blows through the tunnel. The patient will be able to talk to the technologist during the scan and they will be given a squeeze ball that works as a secondary way to alert the technologist that the patient needs something. Educating and reassuring the patient that the MR staff is here to help them at any time can aid in reducing patient anxiety.

Some patients know in advance that they do not tolerate the MRI scanner well. Some of these patients just need the widest bore MR scanner the clinic has and extra communication to get through the exam. Some clinics allow a family member to stay in the room with the patient (this person must be screened for MRI as well), unless the patient is being care for by a sedation or anesthesia team (who also need to be screened). A wide variety of antianxiety medications are available. It is important for MR staff to know when a patient has taken any kind of antianxiety medication as they should be monitored while in the scanner. Some patients need more than just a simple oral antianxiety medication. Every MR center needs to have a written policy for handling sedated patients. Large facilities have sedation and anesthesia teams that work with MR regularly and have all of the appropriate MR Conditional equipment to manage sedated and anesthetized patients safely. For children, it is recommended to have a pediatric team that can not only provide the sedation care, but screen and prepare children for the MRI. The use of videos, mock MRI scanner, and even virtual reality techniques have been used to help children get through their MRI exams without the use of medication [36, 37].

## 16.9 Patient Monitoring

Nurses are becoming increasingly involved in monitoring patients in MRI. Sedation and anesthesia cases used to be the main types of cases that nurses were involved in for MRI, but now the active implanted medical devices are becoming more common with nursing being utilized for monitoring and charting care. Nurses need to familiarize themselves with the MR specific equipment. Patient monitoring systems, medication infusion pumps, respirators, anesthesia machines, and other specialty equipment are made specifically for use in MRI scanner rooms [38]. It is critically important the MR Conditional equipment and supplies are used for monitoring while in MRI, including the ECG electrodes.

There is currently only a single vendor providing MR Conditional medication infusion pumps for use in sedation and anesthesia procedures in the United States. This system requires special tubing as well. Do not assume the MR technologists will know how to use the medication pump. Make sure nursing gets training on this infusion pump as it is slightly different from the regular equipment used in the rest of the facility.

One of the hardest things to get used to in MRI is the unreliable ECG signal [39]. ECG in MRI should not be used as the primary method to monitor your patient as the magnetic fields interfere with the ECG signal. Pulse oximetry and end-tidal $CO_2$ are more reliable than ECG when the patient is in the scanner. That can make nurses new to MRI very uncomfortable when monitoring patients in the MR environment. End-tidal $CO_2$ is becoming the gold standard for monitoring sedated or anesthetized patients as it is a more robust method for anesthetized patients. When monitoring a patient in MRI, it is a good idea to position yourself to see both the monitors and the patient. Sometimes you can see the patient move before you see changes on the monitoring equipment. Also, sometimes the pulse oximetry signal can be temporarily lost, which can sometimes happen simply because the patient was moving their fingers or hand.

## 16.10 Facility Recommendations

The physical layout of the MRI suite can enhance safety. TJC now recommends the MR safety white papers from the ACR that promotes the four-zone system physical layout and labeling system [40]. Zone I is the public area where people may come and go freely, Zone II is generally the reception and waiting area. The screening process starts here. It is highly recommended that Zone II be the patient changing area as well. Zone III is the MR-controlled zone as it has direct access to the MR scanner room (Zone IV). In Zones III and IV, MR personnel must supervise non-MRI personnel and all patients 100% of the time. All persons in Zone III and IV must also be screened and educated on how to keep safe while in the MRI suite.

## 16.11 Code Procedure

If the patient is having a medical emergency in the MRI, the first thing you need to do is get the patient out of the scanner room as the last thing you need is a projectile accident happening during the code. One member of the MR team should be designated to call the code while others are getting the patient to the designated safe code location, preferably away from the immediate MR scan room. Although extremely rare, the MR staff must be familiar with how to call a code and how to direct the care team to the safe area to care for the patient. The crash cart should be located near the designated safe location or be easily and quickly moved to the safe location where the patient is being worked on. Crash carts should *never* be taken into an MR scanner room as the cart itself, things in and on the cart maybe ferromagnetic, plus the defibrillator will not work properly in a magnetic field. The MR technologists must ensure that the MR scanner room is secured so that non-MR personnel cannot accidentally enter the MR scanner room during or after the code.

## 16.12 iMR: Interoperative and Interventional MR

Interventional/interoperative MR (iMR) in a formal surgical suite has been around since 1994, but is still only in major medical or research institutions [41, 42]. iMR is expanding in use and in the variety of techniques being performed. Since MR provides three-dimensional anatomical detail quickly, plus can provide flow information as well as monitor thermal changes, blood oxygenation, perfusion, and diffusion, MR makes for a desirable interactive tool for certain procedures and without the risk of ionizing radiation.

With the increase in growth of iMR and its associated specialized equipment, the need for MR safety knowledge and vigilance also grows. The iMR team is made up of a wide variety of medical professionals, many of whom are not MR specialists; therefore, MR safety protocols and education are particularly critical. The iMR suite should have a written policy on how to handle all equipment within the iMR suite as there will be a variety of equipment in the iMR suite that isn't always MR safe or MR Conditional [43]. The medical director for the iMR should have a written policy for how all items in the iMR suite are to be tested before bringing into the iMR suite. All equipment used in the iMR must be tested by personnel appointed by the iMR medical director and labeled using a system of coding such as the ASTM labeling for MR safety (Table 16.1). The ASTM color-coding system (green = MR safe, yellow = MR conditional, and red = MR unsafe) can be used to mark tools and other items where stickers may be hard to see or are impractical to place a sticker. The ASTM labels can be purchased. Some equipment may be MR unsafe, but needed for parts of the procedures when the patient is kept in an area away from the MR or in an adjacent room. iMR suites should have a system for demarcating the room for those times when the MR scanner will be used. Having your suite designed with visual cues for safety such as colored floors, barrier tapes, lights, and movable partitions can also help. A system of checks and procedures should also be in place to ensure MR unsafe items are removed and secured from the MR area prior to the MR being used during the procedure. Procedures such as time-outs or similar team safety checks at key points in the procedure are highly recommended. It is also prudent to have a well-trained MR technologist acting as the MR safety specialist who is responsible for checking and screening all people (staff and patient) as they enter the MR suite. The MR safety restrictions are the same for iMR as they are for any other MR room, with the addition of hearing protection for staff that remains in the scanner room during scanning.

For combination suites that involve the use of X-ray or CT, assess all safety equipment, including lead shields. Lead aprons should be free of ferrous metal buckles or fasteners, plus movable lead shields must not contain ferromagnetic components. Written plans for multimodality suites must be in place and followed by all staff.

## 16.13 Cryogen Safety

Most MRI scanners that are 0.5 T or higher (or of the tunnel shape) are superconducting scanners. They use liquid helium to maintain the powerful magnetic field. The MR scanner systems have a special venting system to let the helium gas vaporize out through a venting system if the magnetic field needs to be reduced rapidly (in the event of a person pinned by a large ferromagnetic object or a fire in the scanner room), or if the scanner has a rare spontaneous quench. The rapid reduction in the magnetic field is called a fast run down or quench. The helium gas should vent out through the venting safely, but venting malfunctions including explosions have occurred. If the venting system fails, the helium gas may vent into the scanner room. The escaping gas can be heard as a loud hissing sound and the white cloud of helium gas will form near the ceiling, displacing oxygen in the room. The helium cloud is cold (liquid helium is −268.93 Centigrade). Because the helium cloud poses a potential asphyxiation and cold burn hazard, the patient and all personnel must exit the MR suite while keeping lower than the helium cloud, and avoiding any dripping liquids. The MR staff will have a written procedure on how to evacuate all patients and personnel until the area is safe for return.

## 16.14 Fire Safety

Fires can happen anywhere in a hospital or clinic, including MR. In the event of a fire, the patient needs to be removed from the MR suite and standard fire emergency guidelines followed. The MR suite should have MR Conditional fire extinguishers that are checked regularly just as any other fire extinguisher. The local fire department should be educated regarding the MR environment and be familiar with the MR clinic spaces. Fire department training should include how to turn off the power to the MR equipment (the emergency power off button is different from a quench button) and a policy in place should a quench of the magnetic field be required.

## 16.15 Summary

Nurses are being more frequently called upon to work in the MR suite. Understanding the theory of MR safety, knowledge of the support equipment specifically designed for use around an MR, and the safety fundamentals to keep staff and patient safe is essential. MRI has unique safety issues that nurses need to become familiar with in order to provide optimal care to their patients in the MRI environment.

**Acknowledgements** The author acknowledges the MR safety and physics discussions with Michael Steckner, PhD, MBA.

*Disclaimer*: The opinions and assertions expressed herein are those of the author(s) and do not necessarily reflect the official policy or position of the Uniformed Services University or the U.S. Department of Defense.

## References

1. Tesla N. My inventions the autobiography of Nikola Tesla. Seaside, OR: Rough Draft Printing.; Reprinted; 2013. p. 92.
2. U.S. Food and Drug Administration. FDA clears first 7T magnetic resonance imaging device. https://www.fda.gov/news-events/press-announcements/fda-clears-first-7t-magnetic-resonance-imaging-device. Accessed 6 Aug 2019.
3. Mansfield P, Morris PG. NMR imaging in biomedicine. In: Waugh JS, editor. Advances in magnetic resonance, suppl 2. New York: Academic Press; 1982. p. 32–83.
4. Sprawls P, Bronskill MJ, editors. The physics of MRI: 1992 AAPM Summer School Proceedings. Woodbury, NY: Published for the American Association of Physicists in Medicine by the American Institute of Physics; 1993. p. 748.
5. Röschmann P. Human auditory system response to pulsed radiofrequency energy in RF coils for magnetic resonance at 2.4 to 170 MHz. Magn Reson Med. 1991;21(2):197–215.
6. Mansfield P, Glover PM, Beaumont J. Sound generation in gradient coil structures for MRI. Magn Reson Med. 1998;39(4):539–50.
7. U.S. Department of Health and Human Services, Public Health Service Centers for Disease Control and Prevention National Institute for Occupational Safety and Health. Criteria for a Recommended Standard: Occupational Noise Exposure Revised Criteria. Cincinnati, Ohio June 1998. Accessed 6 Aug 2019. https://www.cdc.gov/niosh/docs/98-126/pdfs/98-126.pdf
8. Steckner M. A Review of MRI acoustic noise and its potential impact on patient and worker health. In: Shrivastava, editor. Safety and biological aspects in MRI. Hoboken, NJ: Wiley. Submitted June 2019.
9. Glover P, Hykin J, Gowland P, Wright J, Johnson I, Mansfield P. An assessment of the intrauterine sound intensity level during obstetric echo-planar magnetic resonance imaging. Br J Radiol. 1995;68(814):1090–4.
10. Strizek B, Jani JC, Mucyo E, De Keyzer F, Pauwels I, Ziane S, Mansbach AL, Deltenre P, Cos T, Cannie MM. Safety of MR imaging at 1.5 T in Fetuses: aretrospective case-control study of birth weights and the effects of acoustic noise. Radiology. 2015;275(2):530–7.
11. G. Schaefers, W. Goertz, Y. Noureddine, C. Koch and M. J. Pawlenka, "Magnetic resonance (MR) safety testing of implants using numerical simulation for worst-case determination," *2011XXXth URSI General Assembly and Scientific Symposium*, Istanbul, 2011, pp. 1–4.
12. Pietryga JA, Fonder MA, Rogg JM, North DL, Bercovitch LG. Invisible metallic microfiber in clothing presents unrecognized MRI risk for cutaneous burn. AJNR Am J Neuroradiol. 2013;34(5):E47–50.
13. Bryson D, McCann J, editors. Smart clothes and wearable technology. 1st ed. Sawston, Cambridge: Woodhead Publishing; 2009. p. 484.
14. Friedstat JS, Moore ME, Goverman J, Fagan SP. An unusual burn during routine magnetic resonance imaging. J Burn Care Res. 2013;34(2):e110–1.
15. Knopp MV, Essig M, Debus J, Zabel HJ, van Kaick G. Unusual burns of the lower extremities caused by a closed conducting loop in a patient at MR imaging. Radiology. 1996;200(2):572–5.
16. Takahashi T, Fujimoto N, Hamada Y, Tezuka N, Tanaka T. MRI-related thermal injury due to skin-to-skin contact. Eur J Dermatol. 2016;26(3):296–8.

17. The Joint Commission. Diagnostic imaging requirements. 2015. https://www.jointcommission.org/assets/1/18/AHC_DiagImagingRpt_MK_20150806.pdf. Accessed 6 Aug 2019.
18. EUR-Lex. Council Directive 90/385/EEC of 20 June 1990 on the approximation of the laws of the Member States relating to active implantable medical devices. 1990. https://eur-lex.europa.eu/legal-content/EN/TXT/?uri=CELEX:31990L0385. Accessed 6 Aug 2019.
19. ASTM F2182-11a, Standard Test Method for Measurement of Radio Frequency Induced Heating On or Near Passive Implants During Magnetic Resonance Imaging, ASTM International, West Conshohocken, PA, 2011., www.astm.org
20. Woods TO. Standards for medical devices in MRI: present and future. J Magn Reson Imaging. 2007;26(5):1186–9.
21. Biotronik, BIOTRONIK Pacemakers that Automatically Adapt to MRI Environments Get CE Approval. Berlin, Germany 2016. https://www.biotronik.com/en-ca/newsroom/press-releases/press-release-e-series-ce-mark-july01-en/. Accessed 6 Aug 2019
22. U.S. Food and Drug Administration. Safety Concerns with Implantable Infusion Pumps in the Magnetic Resonance (MR) Environment: FDA Safety Communication. 2017. https://www.fda.gov/medical-devices/safety-communications/safety-concerns-implantable-infusion-pumps-magnetic-resonance-mr-environment-fda-safety. Accessed 6 August 2019
23. Indik JH, Gimbel JR, Abe H, Alkmim-Teixeira R, Birgersdotter-Green U, Clarke GD, Dickfeld TL, Froelich JW, Grant J, Hayes DL, Heidbuchel H, Idriss SF, Kanal E, Lampert R, Machado CE, Mandrola JM, Nazarian S, Patton KK, Rozner MA, Russo RJ, Shen WK, Shinbane JS, Teo WS, Uribe W, Verma A, Wilkoff BL, Woodard PK. 2017 HRS expert consensus statement on magnetic resonance imaging and radiation exposure in patients with cardiovascular implantable electronic devices. Heart Rhythm. 2017;14(7):e97–e153.
24. The Centers for Medicare and Medicaid Services Decision Memo for Magnetic Resonance Imaging (MRI) (CAG00399R4). 2018. https://www.cms.gov/medicare-coverage-database/details/nca-decision-memo.aspx?NCAId=289&bc=AAAAAAAACAA&. Accessed 6 Aug 2019.
25. Hao D, Ai T, Goerner F, Hu X, Runge VM, Tweedle M. MRI contrast agents: basic chemistry and safety. J Magn Reson Imaging. 2012;36(5):1060–71.
26. Behzadi AH, Zhao Y, Farooq Z, Prince MR. Immediate allergic reactions to gadolinium-based contrast agents: asystematic review and meta-analysis. Radiology. 2018;286(2):471–82.
27. Hunt CH, Hartman RP, Hersley GK. Frequency and severity of adverse effects of iodinated and gadolinium contrast materials: retrospective review of 456,930 doses. AJR Am J Roentgenol. 2009;193:1124–7.
28. Costello JR, Kalb B, Martin DR. Incidence and risk factors for gadolinium-based contrast agent immediate reactions. Top Magn Reson Imaging. 2016;25(6):257–63.
29. Tasker F, Fleming H, Mcneill G, Creamer D, Walsh S. Contrast media and cutaneous reactions. Part 1. Immediate hypersensitivity reactions to contrast media and gadolinium deposition. Clin Exp Dermatol. 2019; https://doi.org/10.1111/ced.13990.
30. American College of Radiology. Manual on Contrast Media, V 10.3, 2018. https://www.acr.org/-/media/ACR/Files/Clinical-Resources/Contrast_Media.pdf. Accessed 6 Aug 2019.
31. Kanda T, Ishii K, Kawaguchi H, Kitajima K, Takenaka D. High signal intensity in the dentate nucleus and globus pallidus on unenhanced T1-weighted MR images: relationship with increasing cumulative dose of a gadolinium-based contrast material. Radiology. 2014;270(3):834–41.
32. Runge VM. Dechelation (Transmetalation): consequences and safety concerns with the linear gadolinium-based contrast agents, in view of recent health care rulings by the EMA (Europe), FDA (United States), and PMDA (Japan). Investig Radiol. 2018;53(10):571–8.
33. Arsenault TM, King BF, Marsh JW Jr, Goodman JA, Weaver AL, Wood CP, Ehman RL. Systemic gadolinium toxicity in patients with renal insufficiency and renal failure: retrospective analysis of an initial experience. Mayo Clin Proc. 1996;71(12):1150–4.
34. Ramalho J, Ramalho M. Gadolinium deposition and chronic toxicity. Magn Reson Imaging Clin N Am. 2017;25(4):765–78.
35. Kanda T, Fukusato T, Matsuda M, Toyoda K, Oba H, Kotoku J, Haruyama T, Kitajima K, Furui S. Gadolinium-based contrast agent accumulates in the brain even in subjects without severe renal dysfunction: evaluation of autopsy brain specimens with inductively coupled plasma mass spectroscopy. Radiology. 2015;276(1):228–32.
36. Jaimes C, Gee MS. Strategies to minimize sedation in pediatric body magnetic resonance imaging. Pediatr Radiol. 2016;46(6):916–27.
37. Barkovich MJ, Xu D, Desikan RS, Williams C, Barkovich AJ. Pediatric neuro MRI: tricks to minimize sedation. Pediatr Radiol. 2018;48(1):50–5.
38. Deen J, Vandevivere Y, Van de Putte P. Challenges in the anesthetic management of ambulatory patients in the MRI suites. Curr Opin Anaesthesiol. 2017;30(6):670–5.
39. Jekic M, Ding Y, Dzwonczyk R, Burns P, Raman SV, Simonetti OP. Magnetic field threshold for accurate electrocardiography in the MRI environment. Magn Reson Med. 2010;64(6):1586–91.
40. Expert Panel on MR Safety, Kanal E, Barkovich AJ, Bell C, Borgstede JP, Bradley WG Jr, Froelich JW, Gimbel JR, Gosbee JW, Kuhni-Kaminski E, Larson PA, Lester JW Jr, Nyenhuis J, Schaefer DJ, Sebek EA, Weinreb J, Wilkoff BL, Woods TO,

Lucey L, Hernandez D. ACR guidance document on MR safe practices: 2013. J Magn Reson Imaging. 2013;37(3):501–30.
41. Jolesz FA, Blumenfeld SM. Interventional use of magnetic resonance imaging. MagnReson Q. 1994;10(2):85–96.
42. Tempany CM, Jayender J, Kapur T, Bueno R, Golby A, Agar N, Jolesz FA. Multimodal imaging for improved diagnosis and treatment of cancers. Cancer. 2015;121(6):817–27.
43. White MJ, Thornton JS, Hawkes DJ, Hill DL, Kitchen N, Mancini L, McEvoy AW, Razavi R, Wilson S, Yousry T, Keevil SF. Design, operation, and safety of single-room interventional MRI suites: practical experience from two centers. J Magn Reson Imaging. 2015;41:34–43.

# Alarm Fatigue

Stacey Trotman

## 17.1 Introduction

Alarm fatigue is described as the reactionary effect that occurs when clinical staff or healthcare providers unavoidably experience an increased amount of alarms. Alarm fatigue can further be described as a causative response which arises due to sequential alarms of clinical equipment in the healthcare setting. Alarm fatigue occurs when clinical staff or healthcare providers become desensitized as a result of the overwhelming amount of alarms, real or false.

Clinical alarms are installed in most medical equipment utilized in the healthcare setting today. Common medical equipment includes cardiorespiratory monitors, pulse oximetry, capnography, ventilators, fall alarms, patient warming equipment, hypothermia equipment, and infusion pumps including intravenous and feeding pumps. In providing care to patients, multiple pieces of medical equipment are utilized increasing the risk of alarm fatigue and creating confusion in determining the device alarming [1]. Clinical staff may not prioritize alarm responsiveness appropriately due to the confusion created by multiple alarms.

S. Trotman, DNP, RN, CMSRN, RN-BC, NE-BC (✉)
Department of Nursing and Critical Care Unit,
Mercy Medical Center,
Baltimore, MD, USA

## 17.2 Purpose of Alarms

Clinical monitors are utilized in healthcare settings to provide care and continuous monitoring of a patient. Clinical monitors are designed to provide constant oversight to the patient's physiological state. Clinical alarms in medical devices are designed to alert clinical staff and healthcare providers by means of cognitive distress to physiological changes in the patient's medical state or systems errors within the clinical monitor. Clinical staff and healthcare providers experience both audio and visual cognitive recognition to clinical alarms. The alarms are meant to alert clinical staff or healthcare providers to address any changes identified by the alarm based on alarm settings.

## 17.3 Alarm Settings

Clinical alarms are preliminarily programmed by device manufacturers based on medical algorithms. Algorithms utilize a conservative approach to alarms in order to decrease risk and liability related to patient harm from a missed physiological change or system error [2]. Alarm algorithms are driven and developed by multifaceted events including human, organization, and technical factors. Standards for alarms are set by national governing bodies including the International Electrotechnical Commission (IEC, available at https://www.iec.ch) and the American National Standards Institute (ANSI, available at https://www.ansi.org) [3].

Levels of alarms vary based on predetermined factory settings or parameters. The most common alarm levels include crisis, warning, advisory, message, and system warning [4]. The predetermined levels alert clinical staff and healthcare providers based on the severity of the alarm identified by the medical device. Predetermined levels utilized include medical device manufacturer settings, organizational settings, unit-based settings, or individualized patient settings. Alarm tones vary based on equipment type, manufacturer, and organization settings. For the focus of alarm fatigue, clinical alarms can be further separated into non-actionable or nuisance alarms and actionable alarms [5].

## 17.4 Scope of Problem

Clinical staff and healthcare providers may experience between 350 and over 900 alarms per day [2, 3]. Components of alarm fatigue are alarm desensitization related to overload and delayed responsiveness and alarm apathy directly driven by a lack of trust in alarms [6]. The ECRI Institute has cited alarm hazards in their Top 10 Hospital Health Technology Hazards for 2019 which includes "Improper Customization of Physiologic Monitor Alarm Settings May Result in Missed Alarms" [7].

### 17.4.1 Non-actionable Alarms

Alarm fatigue typically occurs when the amount of non-actionable or nuisance alarms are prevalent causing clinical staff or healthcare providers to have decreased reactivity [8]. Studies have shown between 72% and 99.4% of alarms are non-actionable or nuisance alarms [4, 8, 9]. High percentages of non-actionable alarms increase the probability of clinical staff and healthcare providers delaying response or failing to respond to clinical alarms. Non-actionable or nuisance alarms are designed to create an awareness not requiring clinical staff or healthcare provider action or represent an invalid alarm. Alarm fatigue is a direct result of non-actionable or nuisance alarms.

### 17.4.2 Actionable Alarms

Actionable alarms are small in comparison to non-actionable or nuisance alarms. Approximately 10% of alarms occurring are actionable [4, 8, 9]. Actionable alarms require clinical staff or healthcare providers to intervene, address, and treat based on alarms occurring. Actionable alarms may be patient dependent and can be categorized in levels from crisis to message [4].

## 17.5 Response to Alarms

Clinical staff and healthcare providers respond to alarm fatigue utilizing measures directly impacting patient safety. Examples include failure to respond to alarms, silencing alarms, decreasing alarm volumes, setting inappropriate alarm parameters, or turning alarm parameters off [3]. Patients and clinical staff suffer when a failure to address actionable alarms occur as a result of alarm fatigue. The first sentinel event published by the ECRI Institute occurred in 1974 and was related to a hypothermia machine alarm resulting in patient burns [9]. Since 1974 The Joint Commission (TJC) has released sentinel events related to alarm fatigue. The most recent release spanned 3 years and included 98 events with 80 of those events leading to patient death [10]. In January 2019 TJC Hospital National Patient Safety Goals included *Goal 6: Reduce the harm associated with clinical alarm systems* [10]. Nursing personnel are overwhelmed with multiple healthcare noises including pagers, phones, healthcare personnel calling for assistance, patient call bells, and overhead paging. In addition to healthcare noises, nurses face additional challenges of interruptions by other healthcare personnel which may cause further overload and a delay in response to alarms. The culture set within the organization can directly impact alarm fatigue—addressing interruptions should be set within the organizations culture.

## 17.6 Impact of Alarm Fatigue

Alarm fatigue has a direct impact on the patient and the clinical staff or healthcare provider. Research has shown negative impacts on care provided and satisfaction related to alarm fatigue. The occurrence of negative outcomes and a poor provision of care can be directly correlated to alarm fatigue in the setting of increased non-actionable or nuisance alarms. Cardiorespiratory monitoring equipment and intravenous infusion pumps are the most common equipment utilizing alarms that play a role in the prevalence of alarm fatigue.

Alarm fatigue has been studied on multiple levels focusing on clinical staff and healthcare providers. Alarm fatigue causes increased cognitive distress related to anxiety, burnout, and negative clinical outcomes due to the response, or lack thereof [1].

The patient also experiences negative impacts and outcomes related to the occurrence of alarm fatigue. Patient impacts may range from poor patient satisfaction to, in some cases, death related to missed clinical events [11]. Alarm fatigue impacts patients by causing cognitive distress, difficulty sleeping, and may lead to an increased length of stay [12]. Further, patients may experience delirium from increased alarms, physiologic distress, and weakened immune systems [3, 13, 14]. Patients suffer the consequences of alarm fatigue related to cardiac arrest, respiratory arrest, and death.

The Joint Commission released information on examples of patient impact related to alarm fatigue. Examples include the death of a 60-year-old man related to the lack of responsiveness to an apnea alarm and the cardiac arrest of a patient due to a lack of response to a cardiac alarm for over 75 min [15]. Additional data on alarm consequences related mechanical ventilation alarms showed out of 23 events 19 deaths occurred, 65% were related to alarms [16].

## 17.7 Occurrence of Clinical Alarms

Clinical alarms occur for a multitude of reasons. They are preset by the equipment manufacturer and further individualized based on the healthcare setting or patient. Specifically, clinical alarms driven by physiologic changes have the greatest variance in audio alarm settings. The most significant and actionable alarm is a *crisis alarm*. Crisis alarms are commonly programmed for arrhythmias including asystole, ventricular tachycardia, ventricular fibrillation, and ventricular bradycardia. *Warning alarms* are commonly set for tachycardia, bradycardia, and ventricular tachycardia non-sustained for greater than two beats. *Advisory alarms* are commonly set for pulse oximetry outside of normal limits and premature ventricular contractions. *Message alarms* are commonly set for couplets—regular or irregular. *System warnings* are commonly set for lead failures or arrhythmia suspend [4].

### 17.7.1 Etiology of Clinical Alarms

Common causes of clinical alarms related to the patient's physiologic state include poor lead placement or connection, dried electrocardiogram (ECG) electrodes, physiologic alarm parameters set with a small window of variance, and pulse oximetry monitors placed incorrectly [10]. Common causes of mechanical ventilation alarms include high pressure, low pressure, or disconnection alarms; this requires patient assessment to ensure the alarm is not patient condition related [17]. Common causes of infusion pump alarms can be divided into mechanical alarms or dosing alarms. Mechanical alarms are related to air in the line, occlusions, or low battery; dosing alarms are related to exceeding or not meeting standard dosing alarm limits [18].

## 17.8 Reducing the Prevalence of Alarm Fatigue

Alarm fatigue is the responsibility of the organizations leadership with a strict focus on the utilization of proper equipment alarms, development and implementation of policies, and staff education [19].

Reducing the prevalence of alarm fatigue remains a significant patient safety initiative. Clinical staff and healthcare providers are tasked with addressing the safety concerns related to alarm fatigue and implementing practices to reduce the occurrence of alarms in the healthcare setting. Healthcare professionals should work closely with device manufactures to individualize alarm systems for clinical equipment.

Throughout the literature, healthcare professionals have shown positive impacts in patient safety initiatives related to alarm fatigue. The following is a review of practices related to clinical alarms shown to have successful outcomes in reducing the number of alarms which occur.

Utilizing an evidence-based approach to addressing alarm fatigue is imperative for patient and staff safety. Throughout the literature, evidence-based practice is being utilized to combat alarm fatigue. Recent literature identifies multiple approaches including daily electrode changes, proper skin preparation, eliminating non-actionable alarms, patient alarm customization, and alarm volume individualization [6, 20].

Smart alarms utilize variability in the patient's state to learn physiologic variances individualized to the monitored patient. This can be described when the patient-specific variances are identified by the equipment which then limits the occurrence of nuisance alarms while maintaining normal parameters for the patient [21]. Setting individualized, specific parameters which are patient based are imperative in reducing the prevalence of alarm fatigue. Alarm threshold settings should be customized based on the patient's condition, known normal, and prioritization of arrhythmias. Patient-specific conditions can set preliminary alarms which can be further individualized for each patient. Patient monitoring should be utilized in patients with specific indications [8].

Alarms should be set based on urgency and actionable response. Utilizing proper lead placement, proper probe placement, and increased amplitude in physiologic monitors can reduce the number of clinical alarms [8]. *Non-crisis* alarms may be programmed with a 6 s delay to allow for false readings to re-correct before alarming.

## 17.9 Staff Education on Alarms

Clinical staff and healthcare providers require education on the types of alarms, alarm reduction and prioritization, and equipment use impacting alarms. Organizations must work closely with equipment manufactures to ensure staff are properly trained on the types, levels, and acuity of alarms utilized in specific pieces of equipment. Staff should be educated on safe practices in alarm response, established protocols or practices for response, and documentation of alarm parameters [3] (Fig. 17.1). A recent study on nursing staff and alarm fatigue provided insight, validating most nursing staff are not aware of the scope of the problem or the level of alarm fatigue suffered [19].

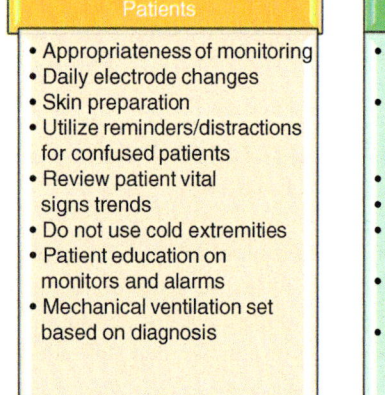
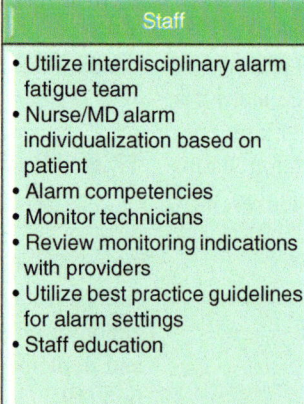
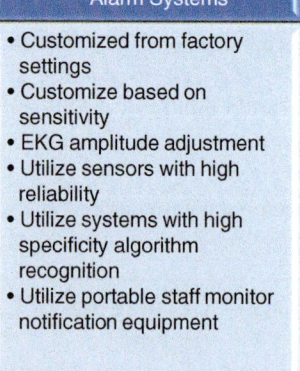

**Fig. 17.1** Alarm reduction education. Additional information for staff education can be found at the Association for Advancement of Medical Instrumentation (AAMI, available at www.aami.org/htsi/alarms) [22]

## 17.10 Conclusion

In conclusion, clinical alarms are developed and implemented for patient safety, clinical staff safety, and a prevention method to life-threatening outcomes. Due to the potential life-threatening impacts, addressing and implementing initiatives to combat alarm fatigue is essential.

Utilizing a multimodal approach to addressing alarm fatigue can be the most effective and have significant positive impacts on outcomes. Alarm fatigue must be a top priority in patient safety and organizational outcomes.

## References

1. Ruppel H, Funk M, Clark T, Gieras I, David Y, Bauld TJ, et al. Attitudes and practices related to clinical alarms: a follow-up survey. Am J Crit Care. 2018;27(2):114–23.
2. Mikta M. Joint commission warns of alarm fatigue: multitude of alarms from monitoring devices problematic. JAMA. 2013;309(22):2315–6.
3. Bach TA, Berglund LM, Turk E. Managing alarm systems for quality and safety in the hospital setting. BMJ Open. 2018;7(3) https://doi.org/10.1136/bmjoq-2017-000202.
4. Graham KC, Cvach M. Monitor alarm fatigue: standardizing use of physiological monitors and decreasing nuisance alarms. Am J Crit Care. 2010;19(1):28–37.
5. Casey S, Avalos G, Dowling M. Critical care nurses' knowledge of alarm fatigue and practices towards alarms? A multicenter study. Intensive Crit Care Nurs. 2018;48:36–41.
6. Turmell JW, Coke L, Catinella R, Hosford T, Majeski A. Alarm fatigue: use of an evidenced-based alarm management strategy. J Nurs Care Qual. 2017;32(1):47–54.
7. ECRI Institute Top 10 Hospital Technology Hazards for 2019 Available at. https://www.ecri.org/top-ten-tech-hazards/. .
8. Hravnak M, Pellathy T, Chen L, Dubrawski A, Wertz A, Clermont G, et al. A call to alarms: current state and future directions in the battle against alarm fatigue. J Electrocardiol. 2018;51(6):s44–8.
9. Sendelbach S, Funk M. Alarm fatigue: a patient safety concern. AACN AdvCrit Care. 2013;24(4):378–86.
10. The Joint Commission. [Internet] Hospital National Patient Safety Goals. Available at https://www.jointcommission.org/assets/1/6/NPSG_Chapter_HAP_Jan2019.pdf. .
11. American Association of Critical-Care Nurses [Internet]. Practice alert outlines alarm management strategies. 2018 May 24. Available from https://www.aacn.org/newsroom/practice-alert-outlines-alarm-management-strategies.
12. Winters BD, Cvach MM, Bonafide CP, Hu X, Konkani A, O'connor MF, et al. Technological distractions (part 2): a summary of approaches to manage clinical alarms with intent to reduce alarm fatigue. J Crit Care Med. 2018;46(1):130–7.
13. Drew BJ, Harris P, Zègre-Hemsey JK, et al. Insights into the problem of alarm fatigue with physiologic monitor devices: a comprehensive observational study of consecutive intensive care unit patients. PLoS One. 2014;9 https://doi.org/10.1371/journal.pone.011027.
14. Xie H, Kang J, Mills GH. Clinical review: the impact of noise on patients' sleep and the effectiveness of noise reduction strategies in intensive care units. Crit Care. 2009;13(2) https://doi.org/10.1186/cc7154.
15. Zhang JJ, Weathers N. Electrocardiographic alarms in the acute care setting. J NursHealthc Chronic Illn. 2017;5(1) https://doi.org/10.5176/2345-718X_5.1.187.
16. Larson, A. Clinical alarms management in the Intermediate cardiology and cardiovascular intensive care units at the University of Iowa Hospital and clinics. Iowa Research Online Honors Theses at the University of Iowa. 2018 Spring.
17. Caple, C. & Heering, H. Mechanical Ventilation: Troubleshooting. Cinahl Information Systems. 2016. Retrieved from https://www.ebscohost.com/assets-sample-content/Mechanical_Ventilation_Troubleshooting_-_NSP.pdf.
18. Shah P, Irizarry J, O'Neill S. Strategies for managing smart pump alarm and alert fatigue: a narrative review. Pharmacotherapy. 2018;38(8):842–50. https://doi.org/10.1002/phar.2153.
19. Hannah C, Little B. Nurses' perception and practices related to alarm management: a quality improvement initiative. J Contin Educ Nurs. 2018;49(5):207–15. https://doi.org/10.3928/00220124-20180417-05.
20. Sowan AK, Reed CC. A complex phenomenon in complex adaptive health care systems – alarm fatigue. JAMA Pediatr. 2017;171(6):515–6. https://doi.org/10.1001/jamapediatrics.2016.5137.
21. Srinivasa E, Mankoo J, Kerr C. An evidence-based approach to reducing cardiac telemetry alarm fatigue. Worldviews Evid Based Nurs. 2017;14(4):265–73.
22. Association for Advancement of Medical Instrumentation (AAMI, Available at www.aami.org/htsi/alarms).

# Patient Falls in Radiology

**18**

Greg Laukhuf

## 18.1 Introduction

The Agency for Healthcare Research and Quality (AHRQ) estimates 700,000 to 1000,000 people suffer a fall yearly in the United States [1–3].

The Joint Commission (TJC) under Provision of Care, Treatment, and Services (PC) PC.01.02.08 states: "The hospital assesses and manages the patient's risk for falls." Additional statements contained in this section include EP 1: "The hospital assesses the patient's risk for falls based on the patient population and setting" and EP 2: "The hospital implements interventions to reduce falls based on the patient's assessed risk." The National Patient Safety Goal NPSG.09.02.01 states "Reduce the risk of falls," with additional falls emphasis in subsections EP1–EP5 [4]. The Safe Practices of the National Quality Forum states, "Take actions to prevent patient falls and to reduce fall-related injuries by implementing evidence-based intervention practices" [5].

Falls are an upsetting occurrence that can happen when providing medical care. In good circumstances, these events may result in a near miss. In lesser circumstances, these events result in fractures, lacerations, or internal bleeding. Falls impact healthcare and add cost for consumers, families, and providers [6, 7].

Radiology is a high volume, ever-changing, dynamic workspace filled with many obstacles including Mayo stands and procedure tables, anesthesia equipment, portable ultrasound machines, oxygen tanks, and electrical or other cables that can lend to patient falls. The fact that the patient maybe weak from a nothing by mouth (NPO) status, the present illness, and/or the effect of sedative/anxiety and other medications increases the falls risk. The potential for liquids (contrast or other) on the floor after a procedure and dim lights in radiology areas also make navigating a room hazardous. Multiple personnel may be milling about as they prepare the procedure room and the patient if elderly may possess sensory deficits that can contribute to the risk of falling [8].

Fall prevention involves many facets of the patient's care, including managing a patient's risk factors for falls and the department's physical structure [3, 8]. As hospitals and ambulatory care sites continue to strengthen falls programs while decreasing falls risk, ancillary areas such as radiology offer additional opportunity.

## 18.2 Background

Most of the research regarding falls has occurred in hospitalized patient populations [9] and in elderly populations located in community or long-term care facilities [10–13]. Data regarding

G. Laukhuf, ND, CRN, RN-BC, NE-BC (✉)
Department of Radiology, University Hospitals Cleveland Medical Center, Cleveland, OH, USA

falls in a supplemented service, such as radiology-nursing, is limited. A ten-year literature review of review of the *Journal of Radiology Nursing* (www.sciencedirect.com/journal/journal-of-radiology-nursing) [14] revealed no articles dedicated to patient falls. The *Core Curriculum for Radiologic and Imaging Nursing, third edition* (https://www.arinursing.org/resources/publications/) [15] does mention a paragraph regarding falls prevention for patients in radiology, so clearly there is a need for more research into this problem in radiology.

### 18.2.1 Fall Rates

Research studies have found falls occur at a rate of 3–5 per thousand hospital bed days [2]. From 30 percent to 35 percent of these patients sustain an injury as a result of the fall, and approximately 11,000 falls are fatal [2, 3]. Falls injuries result in increasing length of stay 6.3 hospital days with the average cost for a serious fall at $14,056 per patient [3]. The Pennsylvania Safety Authority cites 620 radiological falls in 2009 resulting in 5% serious safety event (SSE) [8].

### 18.2.2 Etiology and Consequences

Table 18.1 outlines a general issues patient falls map. Death or serious injury resulting from a fall at a healthcare facility is considered a never event [2, 3]. The Centers for Medicare and Medicaid Services (CMS) do not reimburse hospitals for additional costs associated with patient falls [2, 6, 16]. As noted in a 2018 PSNet publication, even "no harm falls" are stressful to patients, family members, and healthcare staff [2]. "A patient fall can start the beginning of a negative cycle that can lead older patients to restrict activities leading to loss of strength and independence" [2].

## 18.3 Fall Risk Assessment

Falls prevention has been the subject of extensive research and articles in the quality literature. Prevention efforts begin with assessing the individual patient's risk of falls [2]. There are many tools for identifying patients at risk for falls, success is dependent on the patients predisposing issue [2]. Most falls occur in elderly patients who are experiencing delirium, are prescribed psychoactive medication, or have baseline difficulties with strength, mobility, or balance [17, 18]. Non-elderly patients who are acutely ill also have a higher falls risk [2, 19]. Table 18.2 presents a current list of commonly used patient screening tools to determine falls risk.

## 18.4 Preventing Patient Falls

As with all successful programs, it is important for patients and their families to feel empowered, educated, and involved in their treatment plan [24]. There are two major considerations when considering a fall prevention program. First, the prevention measures must be individualized to the client [24]. There is no single method to prevent falls. The most impactful programs include a combination of environmental interventions such as bed alarms, slippers, and ensuring patients are within the nurse's line of sight coupled with clinical intervention such as minimizing medications that may predispose patients to falls and implementing a falls tool [25]. The use of a standardized risk assessment tool and cultural interventions are executed as well [25, 26]. Emphasizing falls prevention is a multidisciplinary responsibility [2, 17].

**Table 18.1** General falls issues

| Falls Issue |
|---|
| Fall risk assessment issues, e.g., physical surroundings, patient mobility |
| Handoff communication issues |
| Toileting issues |
| Call light issues |
| Organizational cultural and educational issues |
| Patient medication issues |

Source: Adapted from *Health Research & Educational Trust* [3]

**Table 18.2** Falls assessment tools

| Scale | Development | Rating system | Principle constructs |
|---|---|---|---|
| Morse fall scale | Developed by Janice Morse in 1985 | Elements rated either "yes" or "no," and assigned a point value. Score used to determine risk | • History of falling<br>• Use of ambulatory aid<br>• Intravenous therapy<br>• Gait<br>• Mental status |
| STRATIFY scale | Developed in 1997 by D. Oliver | Score used to determine risk | • Falls history<br>• Patient agitation<br>• Frequent toileting<br>• Transfer and mobility (number score of how much aid patient requires) |
| Hendrich II fall risk model | Developed by Ann Hendrich in 2003 | Score used to determine risk | • Confusion, disorientation, impulsivity<br>• Symptomatic depression<br>• Altered elimination<br>• Vertigo<br>• Male patients<br>• Administration of antiepileptics (or dosage changes)<br>• Benzodiazepine administration<br>• Poor performance in rising from a seated position test |
| Johns Hopkins fall risk assessment tool | Developed by Johns Hopkins Medicine in 2005 | Score used to determine risk | • Patient age<br>• Fall history<br>• Elimination<br>• Medications<br>• Use of patient care equipment<br>• Mobility<br>• Cognition |
| STEADI (stopping elderly accidents, deaths and injuries) | Developed in 2013 by the CDC | Score used to determine risk | • Toolkit contains educational materials geared toward patients and their families |

Source: Adapted from Wong C, Recktenwald A, Jones M, Waterman B, Bollini M, Dunagen W [20].; Centers for Disease Control and Prevention, [21]; Poe SS, Dawson Patricia B, Cvach M, Burnett M, Kumble S, Lewis M, et al. [22]; Han J, Xu L, Zhou C, Wang J, Li J, Hao X, et al. [23]

### 18.4.1 Multifactorial Approach to Fall Reduction

Literature has suggested that focusing interventions on specific components of falls and fall risks has been unsuccessful in reducing falls [3]. Patient falls can result from many factors. Prevention programs that utilize synchronized strategies such as improving the fall risk assessment process, using visual cues or systems to alert staff to patients at risk, improving communication among staff regarding fall risk status, ensuring safe patient transfers while toileting [25, 27], using equipment such as low beds with mats, and improving staff and patient education are instrumental in successfully reducing patient falls [3, 25, 27].

### 18.4.2 Successful Fall Prevention Interventions

Innovative falls programs must confront a common fallacy held by many healthcare providers; falls are inevitable, not necessarily preventable [2]. Measures to improve overall safety in a unit may be helpful. A 2018 PSNet perspective discusses the specific components used in successful fall prevention intervention [2]. Table 18.3 summarizes these interventions as reported in

**Table 18.3** Successful components in fall prevention strategy

| Hospital | Interventions | Results | Lessons learned |
|---|---|---|---|
| Bassett Medical Center, Cooperstown, New York | • Call don't fall campaign targeted at patient toileting issues<br>• Post-fall huddles to identify contributing factors and root causes | • 43% falls reduction | • Staff concerned with patients' privacy to assist with toileting<br>• Reluctance of patients to ask for help |
| Baylor Scott & White Medical Center—Garland, Texas | • Revised patient educational materials<br>• Revised patient workflows for toileting and falls risk communication | • Unspecified falls reduction | • Post-fall assessments to identify contributing factors and root causes |
| Kaiser Permanente Zion Medical Center, San Diego, California | • Educating patients and families about the danger of falls<br>• Staff work with resistant patients to determine the cause and address their concerns<br>• Continual assessment of each patient's risk level based on medical condition, medications and ambulation | • Unspecified falls reduction | • Interdisciplinary falls committee created<br>• Unit huddles at the beginning of each shift and 2 h later reviewing patient changes and observations |
| Memorial Hermann Memorial City Hospital, Houston, Texas | • Current falls allowed for increased subjectivity, inconsistent ratings and assessment<br>• Post fall huddle started<br>• Bed alarms not standardized or functional | • Falls in cardiology decreased 50.5% in the study and falls with injuries decreased 49.2%<br>• Success credited to robust process improvement, safety culture and leadership commitment | • Video of best practices produced including a checklist of critical steps to ensure patient safety<br>• Preventing falls with injury is a continuous effort due to patients and family member variability |
| Wake Forest Baptist Medical Center, Winston-Salem, North Carolina | • Impaired mobility and impaired cognitive function confirmed as key risk factors for falls<br>• Diuretics administered close to bedtime identified as risk factor | • Unspecified falls impact | • Unit-based huddles pass on critical information to staff<br>• Falls added to daily system check-in, for quality and safety issues |

Source: Adapted from Health Research and Educational Trust [3]

The Joint Commission Center for Transforming Healthcare Project [3].

## 18.5 Robust Process Improvement® (RPI)

Preventing patient falls is a complex issue that requires analysis to determine contributory factors and analyze the data trends. As part of The Joint Commission Center for Transforming Healthcare: Preventing Falls with Injury project, seven U.S. hospitals used Robust Process Improvement®, which integrates tools from Lean Six Sigma and change management procedures, to decrease falls with injury on targeted units. The seven participants followed the Six Sigma DMAIC (Define, Measure, Analyze, Improve, and Control) framework to discover the causative factors and root causes for falls and falls with injury in the test areas [3, 24]. The seven study sites identified 30 root causes and developed 21 specific solutions to address those root causes [3, 24].

The study participants set an initial collective goal to reduce the rate of falls with injury by 50% and to decrease the overall falls rate by 25%. The participating institutions began with a collective baseline falls with injury rate of 1.31 (falls with injury per 1000 patient days) and a combined baseline falls rate of 4.00 (falls per 1000 patient days) [3, 24].

### 18.5.1 Targeted Solutions Tool

Recognizing that every organization has its own unique combination of contributing factors, the Center for Transforming Healthcare developed an online application called the Targeted Solutions Tool® (TST®) to guide organizations through a method for fall prevention. Embedded within the software application is a data collection tool that helps an organization in measuring and analyzing the contributory factors for falls. When the data is entered in the TST®, the software tool provides analysis and listing of the organization's falls and falls with injury deficiencies. After reviewing the provided analysis, the TST® provides solutions targeting the top contributing factors for falls and falls with injury in the unit examined [3]. The Preventing Falls TST® is available to all Joint Commission-accredited organizations. Further information on TST® is available at: (https://www.centerfortransforminghealthcare.org/what-we-offer/targeted-solutions-tool).

### 18.5.2 Success

Examination of the project outcomes had surprising results. Leadership support was critical to the project success, confirming that those involved had the time to perform data collection for measurement with subsequent analysis and providing institutional knowledge for project navigation. This leadership support was vital during the solution implementation phase [3].

The first key for falls prevention success was to effectively measure and analyze the contributory factors. A misperception discovered among the participants was the belief that specific contributing factors had already been addressed at their organization. Examples included tasks such as having a fall risk assessment consistently used or proactive toileting and educating patients. The healthcare organizations that measured and analyzed their specific contributing factors were able to identify the most impactful factors for their areas and focus their time and resources on solution implementations targeting their needs [3].

Sustainable success was achieved by the careful measurement and analysis of the specific causative factors at each participating institution. For example, an organization may employ a fall risk assessment but through data-driven analysis the organization was able to discover whether or not staff consistently scored the fall risk assessment (interrater reliability), whether or not the assessment captured those patients at the greatest risk for falls, and whether or not the patients' falls assessment was updated with changes in medical condition. This process led to learning and several "aha" moments for the teams involved [3].

The second key for a successful fall prevention initiative was to address culture change. It is imperative to have project support from leadership and staff, including senior management, medical staff, and patient advisory council. Having this support will help ensure a robust fall prevention culture and will help raise expectations for fall prevention. The healthcare organizations with the most success were those that developed a philosophy of "zero falls" among all staff, from the chief executive officer to the maintenance crews. Successful falls prevention organizations developed a culture of pride and ownership over "zero falls." Preventing falls became a mission that reverberated throughout the entire hospital. Successful cultures effectively used change management tools and approaches to support the culture changes. In addition, they engaged and partnered with patients and families to adopt an organization-wide commitment to improving safety and preventing falls [3, 24].

The Joint Commission Center for Transforming Healthcare: Preventing Falls with Injury project was successful. Participating organizations tallied a 62 percent reduction in the falls with injury rate and a 35 percent reduction in the falls rate. A 200-bed hospital utilizing this approach to reduce patient falls with injury could see 72 fewer injuries and net $1 million in costs avoidance. A 400-bed hospital would experience 134 fewer injuries and realize a $1.9 million savings in costs [3].

## 18.6 Radiology

Radiology is not immune from the risks outlined. In a 2011 American Journal of Radiology article, a fall rate of 0.46 per 10,000 imaging examinations performed in the radiology department was identified [28]. The ratio of falls among outpatients and inpatients was proportionate to the volume of imaging examinations performed in similar categories [28]. A 2016 Chinese study by Lee et al. listed falls as a concern in the radiology department as well [29]. This elevates falls in radiology to a level of global concern.

The rate of falls is one piece of information all radiology nurse managers needs to know. Fall rates and prevention practices should be tracked as an element of your unit's quality improvement program [9]. With tracking, you can determine if care is improving, staying the same, or worsening in response to efforts to change. Monitoring allows you to track your progress and identify areas for further interventions. It allows you to compare falls rates with like units such as in NDNQI benchmarks. It also allows a tangible means to celebrate successes with staff and build sustainable success.

There are several crucial strategies for the implementation of a fall reduction program. They include first, assessing and reassessing patient risk factors for falls with medical and/or environmental causes in the department. Second, identifying patients at risk of falling should be done. Third, communicating patient's fall risk status to staff is important. Fourth, educating patients, families, and staff about how to prevent falls, and finally conducting analysis when a fall occurs should be done. The analysis can be conducted by using a root cause analysis (RCA) [30], conducting a structured, systematic technique for failure analysis to identify risks and hazards such as a radiology failure mode and effect analysis (RFMEA)

[31], or maintaining improvements and revisiting the subject with programs such as the Deming cycle of Plan-Do-Check-Act (Adjust) (P-D-C-A) [32]. Implementing some of those strategies has succeeded in reducing the number of falls among hospitalized patients and may be applicable to radiology areas [9, 33, 34].

The research literature in preventing falls has shown intercessions to be effective in reducing the rate and risk of falling [35]. Due to the unique patient population in ambulatory care including radiology, modifications in the methods used to identify those at risk of falling may be required. The Joint Commission recommends in radiological settings, consideration of gait, balance, cognition, and environmental factors that may contribute to falls. These patient attributes maybe more important for considerations than the patient's medication use [36].

The environment of care should be evaluated for safety issues that could predicate a fall. Periodic assessments of individual patients and the service environment play an important role in preventing falls and limiting the harm they cause. Ward et al. [37] developed a fall reduction program for their transitional care unit at an acute care facility that resulted in a 57% reduction in fall rates after 1.5 years of implementation. They emphasized the use of a unit-specific program to identify patients at high risk and to design interventions to protect at-risk patients who may differ in different units of care.

To develop a fall reduction program in a radiology department, specific aspects may need to be considered. Patient education in the prevention of hospital falls is an important facet of falls reduction. Simple interventions such as consistent assistance by staff, avoidance of walking in socks, careful observation of surroundings, slow and steady mobilization, use of eyeglasses, and use of extra caution if taking certain medications should be a part of the educational program [2, 9].

Even with the best intentions, a fall can occur. If an unfortunate fall does occur, it is important to report the event and follow institutional policies and procedures when caring for the injured patient or staff. Filling out the appropriate paperwork for your quality committee or risk management department allows for a review of the case and implementation of safety practices if indicated. This may help prevent others from suffering a similar fate.

## 18.7 Conclusion

It is not just patients but also the radiology staff who are at risk for falls in the department, so all environmental hazards need to be taken seriously. Preventing falls is a complicated process made more complicated by the diverse patient population, rapid patient turnover, and technological nature of radiology. While the solutions appear logical on the surface and many are thought already to be in practice, organizations have found that common practices were not implemented consistently. By targeting solutions to their own specific circumstances, radiology departments can be confident that they are addressing the right problems within all the imaging modalities and using scarce time and resources for the greatest impact in the department and organization. Taking a close examination of issues within each individual modality gives radiology departments the opportunity to implement targeted solutions that lead to impactful, sustained reduction in falls and falls injuries.

## References

1. Currie L. Fall and injury prevention. In: Hughes RG, editor. Patient safety and quality: an evidence-based handbook for nurses. (AHRQ publication no. 08–0043). Rockville, MD: Agency for Healthcare Research and Quality; 2008. p. 195–250.
2. AHRQ Patient Safety Network. Patient Safety Primer Falls. [Internet] 2018. [updated 2018 August; cited 2019 Apr 30]. Available from: https://psnet.ahrq.gov/primers/primer/40/falls
3. Health Research & Educational Trust. Preventing patient falls: asystemic approach from the joint Commission Center for Transforming Healthcare project. Chicago IL: Health Research & Educational Trust. [Internet]. [2018 Oct; cited 2019 Apr 30]. Available from: www.hpoe.org/preventingfalls
4. The Joint Commission. Sentinel Event Alert #55: Preventing Falls and Fall-related Injuries in Health Care Facilities: Joint Commission Requirements Relevant to Falls [Internet]. [cited 2019 Apr 30]. Available from: https://www.jointcommission.org/sea_issue_55/
5. National Quality Forum (NQF). Safe practices for better healthcare–2009 update: aconsensus report. Washington, DC: NQF.; [Internet] 2009. Safe Practice 33: Falls Prevention [cited 2019 Apr 30]. Available from: http://www.qualityforum.org/Publications/2009/03/Safe_Practices_for_Better_Healthcare–2009_Update.aspx
6. FieldsJ, AlturkistaniT, KumarN, KanuriA, SalemDN. MunnS. Prevalence and cost of imaging in inpatient falls: the rising cost of falling. [Internet]. Dovepress; 3 June 2015 Volume 2015: 7 [cited 2019 Apr 30]. P 281—6. Available from: https://www.dovepress.com/prevalence-and-cost-of-imaging-in-inpatient-falls-the-rising-cost-of-f-peer-reviewed-fulltext-article-CEOR
7. Dykes PC, Carroll DL, Hurley A, Lipsitz S, Benoit A, Chang F. Fall prevention in acute care hospitals. JAMA. 2010;304(17):1912–8.
8. Pennsylvania Safety Authority. Falls in Radiology: Establishing a Unit-Specific Prevention Program. Pa Patient Saf Advis. 2011;8(1):12–7. [Internet]. [cited 2019 Apr 30]. Available from: http://patientsafety.pa.gov/ADVISORIES/Pages/201103_12.aspx
9. Fischer ID, Krauss MJ, Dunagan WC, Birge S, Hitcho E. Patterns and predictors of inpatient falls and fall-related injuries in a large academic hospital. Infect Control Hosp Epidemiol. 2005;26:822–7.
10. Vassallo M, Sharma JC. Incidence and prognostic implications of falls associated with acute medical illness: a medical inpatient study. Int J ClinPract. 1998;52:233–5.
11. Parker R. Assessing the risk of falls among older inpatients. Prof Nurse. 2000;15:511–4.
12. Tinetti ME, Williams CS. Falls, injuries due to falls, and the risk of admission to a nursing home. N Engl J Med. 1997;337:1279–84.
13. Carroll NV, Slattum PW, Cox FM. The cost of falls among the community-dwelling elderly. J Manag Care Pharm. 2005;11:307–16.
14. *Journal of Radiology Nursing*. Available from: www.sciencedirect.com/journal/journal-of-radiology nursing.
15. Gross, K., ed. *Core curriculum for radiologic and imaging nursing, 3rd edition*. Association for Radiologic and Imaging Nursing, 2014. Available from: https://www.arinursing.org/resources/publications/
16. Growdon ME, Shorr RI, Inouye SK. The tension between promoting mobility and preventing falls in the hospital. JAMA Intern Med. 2017;177:759–60. [Intranet] [cited 2019 Apr 30]; Available from: https://www.psnet.ahrq.gov/resources/resource/31064/the-tension-between-promoting-mobility-and-preventing-falls-in-the-hospital. https://doi.org/10.1001/jamainternmed.2017.0840.
17. Ganz DA, Huang C, Saliba D, Berlowitz D, VanDeusen Lukas C, Pelczarski K, et al. Preventing falls in hospitals: a toolkit for improving quality of care. (Prepared by RAND Corporation, Boston University School of Public Health, and ECRI Institute under Contract No. HHSA290201000017I TO #1.) AHRQ Publication No. 13-0015-EF. Available from: https://www.ahrq.

gov/sites/default/files/publications/files/fallpxtoolkit.pdf [Intranet]. Rockville, MD: Agency for Healthcare Research and Quality; 2013.
18. Schwendimann R, Buhler H, De Geest S, Milisen K. Falls and consequent injuries in hospitalized patients: effects of an interdisciplinary falls' prevention program. BMC Health Serv Res. 2006. [Intranet]. [cited 2019 Apr 30] Available from: https://www.ncbi.nlm.nih.gov/pmc/articles/PMC1534028/;6(69):669–7. https://doi.org/10.1186/1472-6963-6-69.
19. Fischer ID, Krauss MJ, Dunagan WC, Birge S, Hitcho E, Johnson S. Patterns and predictors of inpatient falls and fall-related injuries in a large academic hospital. Infect Control Hosp Epidemiol. 2005. [Intranet]. [cited 2019 Apr 30] Available from: https://digitalcommons.wustl.edu/open_access_pubs/909;26(10):822–7. https://doi.org/10.1086/502500.
20. Wong C, Recktenwald A, Jones M, Waterman B, Bollini M, Dunagen W. The cost of serious fall-related injuries at three Midwestern hospitals. Jt Comm J Qual Patient Saf. 2011. [Intranet]. [cited 2019 Apr 30] Available from: https://www.jointcommissionjournal.com/article/S1553–7250(11)37010–9/fulltext;37(2) https://doi.org/10.1016/S1553-7250(11)37010-9.
21. Centers for Disease Control and Prevention. Algorithm for fall risk screening, assessment, and intervention [Internet]. 2017 [cited 2019 Apr 30]. Available from: https://www.cdc.gov/steadi/pdf/STEADI-Algorithm-508.pdf
22. Poe SS, Dawson Patricia B, Cvach M, Burnett M, Kumble S, Lewis M, et al. The Johns Hopkins fall risk assessment tool: a study of reliability and validity. J Nurs Care Qual. 2018. [Internet]. [cited 2019 Apr 30] Available from: https://jhu.pure.elsevier.com/en/publications/the-johns-hopkins-fall-risk-assessment-tool-a-study-of-reliabilit;33(1):10–9. https://doi.org/10.1097/NCQ.0000000000000301.
23. HanJ, XuL, ZhouC, WangJ, LiJ, HaoX, et al. Stratify, Hendrich II fall risk model and Morse fall scale used in predicting the risk of falling for elderly inpatients Safety. Special Issue Article - Biomedical Research (2017) Health Science and Bio Convergence Technology: Edition-II [Intranet]. 2017 January 31 [cited 2019 May 15]. Available from: http://www.alliedacademies.org/articles/stratify-hendrich-ii-fall-risk-model-and-morse-fall-scale-used-in-predicting-the-risk-of-falling-for-elderly-inpatients.html
24. DuPree E, Fritz-Campiz A, Musbeno DA. New approach to preventing falls with injury. J Nurs Care Qual. 2014;29(2):99–102. https://doi.org/10.1097/NCQ.0000000000000050.
25. Quigley P. Taking appropriate precautions against falls: learn about key fall precautions for patients in acute or long-term settings. Am Nurse Today. 2015. [Intranet]. [cited 2019 Apr 30] Available from: https://americannursetoday.com/wp-content/uploads/2015/07/ant7-Falls-630_FULL.pdf;10(7):32–3.
26. Haines T, Hill A, Hill K, Brauer S, Hoffmann T, Etherton-Beer C, et al. Cost effectiveness of patient education for the prevention of fall in hospital: economic evaluation from a randomized controlled trial. BMC Med. 2013. [Internet]. [cited 30 Apr 2019] Available from: https://bmcmedicine.biomedcentral.com/articles/10.1186/1741-7015-11-135;11(135) https://doi.org/10.1186/1741-7015-11-135.
27. Hitcho E, Krauss M, Birge S, Dunagan W, Fischer I, Johnson S, Nast P, Costantinou E, Fraser V. Characteristics and circumstances of falls in a hospital setting. J Gen Intern Med. 2004;19(7):732–9. https://doi.org/10.1111/j.1525-1497.2004.30387.x.
28. Abujudeh H, Kaewlai R, Shah B, Thrall J. Characteristics of falls in a large academic radiology department: occurrence, associated factors, outcomes, and quality strategies. AJR. 2011;197(1):154–9.
29. Lee Y, Chen C, Lee S, Chen C, Wan Y, Guo W, et al. Patient safety during radiological examinations: a nationwide survey of residency training hospitals in Taiwan. BMJ Open. 2016. [Intranet]. [cited 2019 Apr 30]. Available from: https://www.ncbi.nlm.nih.gov/pmc/articles/PMC5051322/;6:e010756. https://doi.org/10.1136/bmjopen-2015-010756.
30. Kruskal JB, Siewert B, Anderson SW, Eisenberg RL, Sosna J. Managing an acute adverse event in a radiology department. Radiographics. 2008;28:1237–50.
31. Abujudeh H, Kaewlai R. Radiology failure mode and effect analysis: what is it? Radiology. 2009. [Intranet]. [cited 2019 Apr 30] Available from: https://pubs.rsna.org/doi/10.1148/radiol.2522081954;252(2) https://doi.org/10.1148/radiol.2522081954.
32. Adams HG, Arora S. Introduction to total quality management. In: Adams HG, Arora S, editors. Total quality in radiology: a guide to implementation. Boca Raton, FL: CRC Press; 1993. p. 3–16.
33. Fonda D, Cook J, Sandler V, Bailey M. Sustained reduction in serious fall-related injuries in older people in hospital. Med J Aust. 2006;184:379–2.
34. Oliver D, Connelly JB, Victor CR, Shaw F, Whitehead A, Genc Y, et al. Strategies to prevent falls and fractures in hospitals and care homes and effect of cognitive impairment: systematic review and meta-analyses. BMJ. 2007. [Internet] [cited 2019 Apr 30] Available from: https://www.bmj.com/content/334/7584/82;334:82. https://doi.org/10.1136/bmj.39049.706493.55.
35. Chang JT, Morton SC, Rubenstein LZ, Mojica W, Maglione M, Suttorp M, et al. Interventions for the prevention of falls in older adults: systematic review and meta-analysis of randomized clinical trials. BMJ. 2004. [Intranet]. [cited 2019 Apr 30] Available from: https://www.bmj.com/content/328/7441/680;328:680. https://doi.org/10.1136/bmj.328.7441.680.
36. The Joint Commission. NPSG.09.02.01 Fall reduction program [Internet]. [Updated December 9, 2008. February 19, 2010; cited 2019 Apr 30]. Available from: www.jointcommission.org/AccreditationPrograms/LongTermCare/Standards/09_FAQs/NPSG/Patient_falls/NPSG.09.02.01/Fall+reduction+program.htm.
37. Ward A, Candela L, Mahoney J. Developing a unit-specific falls reduction program. J Healthc Qual. 2004. [Intranet]. [cited 2019 Apr 30]. Available from: http://www.hcpro.com/content.cfm?dp=NRS&content_id=51244;26:36–40.

# Adverse Events

**19**

Shawna M. Butler

## 19.1 Introduction

Falls were discussed in the previous chapter. There may be times in radiology or other areas in healthcare organizations that falls (or some of the earlier discussed events from Sect. 19.3) become an adverse event and/or medical error. In this chapter, adverse events and patient safety will be discussed.

When discussing patient harm, many terms may be used by clinicians, facilities, regulatory agencies, or even the legal system. Healthcare is purportedly one of the most heavily regulated industries in existence. Regulatory oversight covers providers, practices, and hospitals. State and local agencies, private associations, and specialty societies are some of the regulatory agencies. Examples in the United States (US) include The Joint Commission (TJC), state boards of medicine and state departments of public health. As a foundation, it is important to understand what these terms used by these different areas of healthcare mean.

The Agency for Healthcare Research and Quality (AHRQ) considers an **adverse event** "to be harm from medical care as opposed to underlying disease" [1]. **Medical errors** are described as either an act of commission or omission leading to either an undesirable outcome or potential for that [1]. You may see adverse event and medical error used interchangeably at times in the literature. *For purposes of healthcare quality and safety and regulatory purposes, adverse event is typically the more accurate language to use*. Medical error is a broader term. When reviewing an adverse event, it is necessary to determine if the event was *preventable as opposed to unpreventable*. When reporting some events to external regulatory agencies, they will require in-depth information regarding whether it would be deemed preventable or unpreventable. If deemed preventable, the third-party payers may not be obligated to pay for the patient's expenses related to the event. There is more to come on this later in this chapter.

There are unique challenges in radiology that may lead to the risk for adverse events. Many patient interactions in radiology may be shorter in comparison to clinicians who interact with their patients for an entire shift on a medical unit for example. This leaves detailed information regarding the patient lacking at times. A patient who is at risk for falls may not be well known to those caring for them and therefore a thorough assessment is necessary to prevent serious harm from a fall. Clinicians in the radiology setting may be meeting patients for the first time briefly before an emergent procedure or testing. Retrieving a thorough history may be challenging at this time. It may lead to missing an allergy

S. M. Butler, DNP, JD, RN, CPHRM (✉)
Massachusetts General Hospital, Boston, MA, USA

University of Massachusetts, Boston, MA, USA

for example. A language barrier may also present a potential risk since waiting for an interpreter may not be possible in emergent situations. Being aware of the potential risks related to radiology patients and having systems in place to attempt to account for that are necessary for prevention of radiology adverse events.

## 19.2 Near Miss, Never Event, and Serious Reportable Events

An event that does not rise to the level of being an adverse event may be a **near miss**. The World Health Organization (WHO) defines a **near miss** as "an error that has the potential to cause an adverse event (patient harm) but fails to do so because of chance or because it is intercepted" [2]. Understanding **near misses** are important even though the event was intercepted and/or caused no harm to the patient. The root causes of near misses and adverse events are similar. They both should be reported and reviewed internally (possible external reporting to a regulatory agency may be required for some adverse events as mentioned above) for areas of improvement and to prevent in the future.

A **never event** is a term that may not be heard as much anymore but is still vital to understanding the background of patient safety. The term was initially endorsed by the National Quality Forum (NQF) in 2002 as events that were particularly egregious and therefore should never happen. An example of a never event is wrong site surgery. "Never events" are rare. Healthcare facilities that experience these types of events would risk consequences from the regulatory agencies who oversee them. An example of a consequence might be revoking their eligibility for reimbursement from Medicare or Medicaid.

Since the initial term "never event" was introduced, it has evolved, and these types of events are now commonly referred to as **serious reportable events (SREs)**. SREs have evolved over time as events are better understood and as the complexity of the healthcare system progresses. The NQF frequently updates the list of official SREs on their website. The NQF considers this list "a compilation of serious, largely preventable, and harmful clinical events, designed to help the healthcare field assess, measure, and report performance in providing safe care" [3]. The purpose of the list is to hold the facilities accountable to the public and to assure robust patient safety systems are in place to prevent them from occurring again to any other patients in the future. As of May 2019, there are 29 event types under 7 different categories and these can be found here: http://www.qualityforum.org/Topics/SREs/List_of_SREs.aspx [4]. The Centers for Medicare and Medicaid (CMS) have also primarily adopted most of the SRE definitions and therefore can withhold reimbursement as a penalty to institutions where these events occur. Most states also require licensed healthcare facilities to report SREs to the appropriate external regulatory agency. Where to report the SREs varies from state to state. It may be the Department of Public Health, the quality division of the State Board of Medicine, the Joint Commission, or a combination of agencies.

## 19.3 The Joint Commission and Sentinel Event Alerts

The Joint Commission (TJC) is an independent, nonprofit organization that accredits and certifies healthcare organizations. As part of TJC's work, they identify and notify healthcare facilities and the public about **sentinel events**. **Sentinel events** relate to adverse events. TJC considers a **sentinel event** to be a patient safety event that involves one of the following: death, permanent harm, or severe temporary harm and intervention required to sustain life [5].

TJC adopted a sentinel event policy in 1996 to assist hospitals that experience adverse events improve safety and learn from those events [5]. They are considered "sentinel" because "they signal the need for immediate investigation and response" [5]. TJC also publishes **sentinel events alerts** for all to learn from. These alerts (see https://www.jointcommission.org/sentinel_event.aspx) include the incident details, the determined root cause, and recommendations for prevention. They are adopted from a pool of events reported to TJC. Reporting to TJC (by healthcare facilities) is voluntary in most circumstances (this is different from the required reporting to the external regulatory agencies noted earlier in this chapter) so the list may not be comprehensive, but the items are still important to the study of patient safety.

## 19.4 Malpractice

Everything addressed up to this point has focused on either internal policies or external regulatory reporting agencies. In addition to understanding the terms related to patient safety and regulatory reporting, adverse events may also be an unfortunate pathway into the judicial civil system for clinicians and/or healthcare facilities. An adverse event may end up as a nursing or medical **malpractice** case.

**Malpractice** is defined by any act or omission by a clinician during a treatment of a patient that deviates from accepted norms of practice and causes injury to a patient. It is the failure to exercise proper care in healthcare. **Malpractice** (professional negligence) requires the following elements:

- **Duty**—the healthcare provider must conduct oneself according to a certain standard, so as to avoid unreasonable risk to their patients
- **Breach**—a failure to conform one's conduct to the reasonable professional in that situation standard (often thought of as carelessness)
- **Causation**—healthcare provider's failure to act with reasonable care was the "cause in fact" of the injury to the patient
- **Damages**—a physical injury to the patient for which there is a monetary remedy [6]

If an adverse event occurs but there is no harm, this cannot be deemed malpractice. All elements must be present for there to be malpractice. As you can see above under "Damages," there must be an actual injury. An error without injury is not malpractice. Malpractice or professional negligence falls under civil law, not criminal.

## 19.5 Clinician Accountability Beyond Malpractice

It is necessary to understand that because no harm results from an error that there are still potential consequences to you as the clinician. Most clinicians learn in their educational/training programs that there is a risk of malpractice in the profession. However, they may not realize the other potential measures for accountability of clinicians. Being exposed to an investigation by the external regulatory agencies noted earlier in this chapter are possible. Clinicians are also subject to the consequences that their professional licensing board may apply as well. The boards are public advocacy boards. If a patient or facility reports a nurse, physician, or other clinician to their professional licensure board, an investigation will be conducted. A hearing may occur, and findings will be determined. It is important to note the distinction between a malpractice case and a board complaint. Harm is not required in a board complaint. The state nursing board, for example, may find the nurse still violated their state nursing practice act or acted out of their scope of practice and may penalize the nurse with a censure, suspension, revocation, etc. There are similar licensing board ramifications for physicians and other licensed healthcare clinicians as well. According to Nurses Service Organization (NSO), there are 10 to 30 times more licensing complaints than malpractice claims filed against healthcare professionals (NSO) [7]. This means clinicians should be more concerned with a licensure complaint than malpractice.

In addition to malpractice cases, external regulatory agency investigations and board complaints, a clinician may find themselves as a defendant party to the criminal system. This is much rarer than being in a civil malpractice case, but it is still possible. If the state prosecutor determines that the act (the adverse event) rises to the level that it should be criminal, they may choose to charge the clinician criminally. If a patient dies due to an adverse event, they may deem this worthy of charging the clinician defendant with manslaughter, wrongful death or even homicide under certain circumstances. They only typically rise to this level when particularly egregious and/or include malicious intent. However, there are examples where an ambitious prosecutor has criminally charged nurses without apparent intent, but instead they focus on the recklessness or negligence aspect of the event.

In February 2019 a nurse in Tennessee was charged with reckless homicide after administering the wrong medication to a patient, which led to criminal charges. This was somewhat controversial because many disagree with the idea of criminalizing malpractice. It is necessary to understand why criminalizing malpractice affects patient safety. While many may consider the fatal error so serious that it warrants serious consequences, many dispute that criminalizing these inadvertent errors is the appropriate path. When systems contribute to the occurrence and even help lead to adverse events, should the nurse hold sole liability and suffer criminal consequences? Instead, the systems issues should be investigated and resolved so that no future patient suffers the same harm. Penalizing the nurse does not solve the problem if the system set the nurse up for failure in the transaction.

## 19.6 Reporting and Managing Patient Safety Events Internally

Harvard physician and professor, Lucien Leape, M.D. (deemed to be the "father of the modern patient safety movement") considers punishing errors as the single greatest impediment to error prevention in the medical industry (for more information see http://www.hcpro.com/NRS-252640-975/Tips-from-BESD-Its-time-to-stop-punishing-people-for-making-medical-errors.html).

If errors are punished, then the likelihood of clinicians coming forward and revealing their errors is minimal. Instead, the clinicians should be involved in the event review and are encouraged to be part of the investigation follow-up so that the true underlying issues are identified. Allowing those involved in the event helps to illuminate why the transaction did not go as intended. If not, the mistakes will be "pushed under the rug" like the old days before reporting events were encouraged. In healthcare patient safety departments all over the USA, an increase in reports is now viewed positively as opposed to negatively because it means that clinicians feel comfortable coming forward and reporting. This exhibits an open, transparent, and "just culture" (more to come on this later) practicing institution. Reporting structure may vary at different institutions, but all healthcare facilities must have an internal reporting process. They may be referred to as incident reports, occurrence reports, variance reports, or safety reports. Safety report is the preferred language since it is a focus on safety as opposed to an "incident" and removes some of the negative connotation of reporting. Safety reports should not be thought of as clinicians being "written up." Instead they are internal documents that help everybody improve. They are the gateway to initiating the investigation and thorough follow-up to determine root causes and underlying systems issues that contribute to adverse event occurrence.

## 19.7 Current State of Patient Safety in the United States

Now that a foundation of patient safety terms and parts of the system that may be involved (regulatory, judicial; civil and criminal, etc.) have been reviewed, it is necessary to address why it is so important to understand patient safety at this juncture in time in the history of healthcare. As noted earlier, healthcare is considered one of the most heavily regulated industries in existence, but issues continue to persist despite this.

Patients experience medical errors at an alarming rate. This is despite the 1999 landmark report by the Institute of Medicine (IOM) stating that the approximately 98,000 patients were dying each year due to medical error [8]. Twenty years later, preventable medical harm still accounts for more than 100,000 deaths per year. A 2016 study attributed 251,454 deaths to medical error [9]. This makes it now the third leading cause of death in the United States [9]. This is so even with countless programs and extensive funding to improve patient safety along with it being more widely known publicly.

### 19.7.1 Second Victims

Adverse events are traumatic for those closest to the event. Patients and/or their families are the primary victims who suffer the consequences of these events for obvious reasons. However, the involved clinicians may experience trauma as well and this is much less known and much less discussed. The literature refers to this phenomenon as "second victimization." The term second victim was first coined by Albert Wu, M.D., MPH at the Johns Hopkins School of Public Health in 2000 [9]. It is important to acknowledge the significance of identifying this as a known issue that occurs to clinicians daily all over the United States. It is a term that is not received well in some circles. Both patients/families and clinicians alike do not prefer the term "victim" when applied to the clinicians involved in the adverse event. For now, it is the recognized term for this type of harm and will be used for purposes in this chapter.

It is estimated that half of all clinicians will be involved in a serious adverse event during their career [10]. Some degree of emotional distress is likely when a clinician is involved directly or peripherally in an adverse event [10]. "Some clinicians are affected profoundly and with potentially lasting consequences" [10]. Across studies, the clinicians involved in these types of events report shame, anger, failure, depression, loss of confidence, post-traumatic stress, and more [10]. Scott reports that second victims involved in these types of events are also traumatized by the event [11]. "[M]any second victims described a stigma they felt after they sought assistance; they often felt that others saw their efforts to seek help as a sign of professional/personal weakness and vulnerability" [11]. There must be supports in place that assist clinicians with these events. This not only helps the clinician process the event, but it is ultimately better for patients to have healthy and well-supported clinicians caring for them. It is vital to patient safety and better patient outcomes. Studies show there is an unmet need to provide support to this group of healthcare clinicians after adverse events [12].

Some may disregard the study of second victims and say it is all part of the profession. They may suggest that the clinician develop "thicker skin" and learn how to get beyond it. However, this is dismissive of the long-term consequences of what can occur to not only to the clinician themselves, but also to their loved ones, their workplace, patients, and the healthcare system as a whole. One real-life example of the consequences of adverse events on clinicians is that of the story of Kim Hiatt in 2010. She was long time critical care nurse at Seattle Children's Hospital. She had been a nurse for over 20 years with a good record and had a long expert history of caring for the pediatric population (all at that same hospital). She was involved in a medication error involving an 8-month-old baby. She had inadvertently administered more than 10 times the intended amount of the medication and the child ultimately died 5 days later. It is impossible to definitively determine whether the overdose explicitly caused the death since the baby died days later and had been very sick prior to the event. The event led to an investigation, a board complaint and termination of employment. The investigation that ensued revealed it was the only serious mistake she had ever made in her career. She ultimately died by suicide on April 3, 2011. Reports revealed how this devastated her life and how she was punishing herself more than any system could have. The local author of the article detailing Kim Hiatt's death and the story that led to this referred to it as the "twin tragedies" of medical errors [13]. This is one example of how clinicians become second victims. Systems must be in place to protect patient safety and our hardworking clinicians.

### 19.7.2 Just Culture

Some strategies to prevent adverse events and the subsequent external regulatory or legal actions include facilities practicing the just culture model. The just culture and the systems thinking concepts apply to the study of second victimization. As noted above, having systems in place that support our hardworking clinicians is necessary. This is part of the just culture model. Within the just culture model, staff are also not terminated for simple human error. It may also be referred to as the "no blame" approach.

The American Nurses Association (ANA) Position Statement (2010) on just culture states that "a just culture recognizes that individual practitioners should not be held accountable for system failings over which they have no control" [14]. The just culture recognizes that humans by nature will make errors and that this does not automatically equate to incompetence or being a sloppy clinician. The just culture algorithm can help institutions with accountability and provider error (Fig. 19.1). The algorithm below has been adapted from the original work of David Marx.

Suspending or revoking one's license, criminalizing unintended patient complications, and/or terminating an employee implies that whatever caused an error is habitual and likely to harm another person. This is rarely the case. Often, it is a systems error that can be fixed by the facility by streamlining the process or implementing an institutional policy. Furthermore, a lack of support to clinicians may promote turnover and turnover is expensive to institutions [15].

The just culture does not mean that clinicians are not accountable for their clinical judgment or professional decision-making related to patient care. The just culture movement has promoted systems thinking, but there still needs to be a reasonable balance between the "no blame" approach and the need for accountability. Accountability is necessary in certain circumstances, such as failure to heed reasonable safety standards [16]. An example of this may be violating a policy without good reason. Accountability and just culture are not mutually exclusive concepts. Even if the just culture is practiced and no blame is placed, counseling for the staff involved may still be needed. There may even be times where an employee needs to be terminated, but this should not be the first line of defense. Use of the just culture algorithm (see Fig. 19.1) can help serve as a guide.

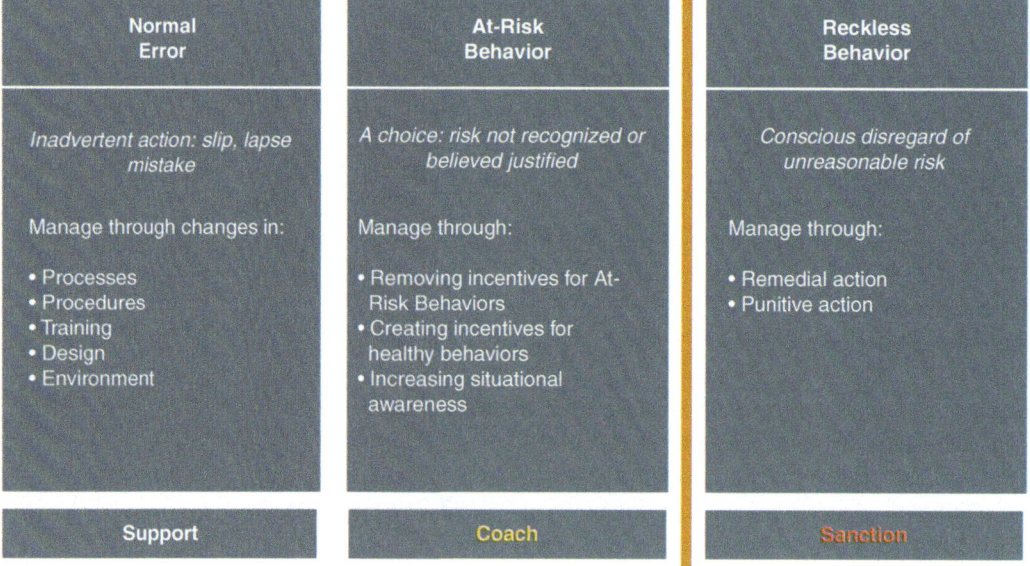

**Fig. 19.1** Just culture. In http://2.bp.blogspot.com/-31n-YIIgdHQ/UXCCCkdME1I/AAAAAAAABdI/CaHzsvDmft0/s640/justculture.gif, adapted from https://www.outcome-eng.com/david-marx-introduces-just-culture/

Promoting the just culture in combination with encouraging a sense of professional accountability is necessary to a healthy organization.

### 19.7.3 Person v. Systems Approach

James Reason, a psychologist who studied human factors, compared the person v. systems approach in his seminal work [17]. The "person-centered approach" focuses on the individual who makes the error. This individual may receive education, training, or possibly discipline if the error was serious. The person-centered approach is doomed to fail, however, because errors have been shown to continue when you replace the people. The "system centered approach" is focused on three principles:

- Error is unavoidable
- Processes can be designed to reduce the possibility of error
- Processes can be designed so that errors are detected and corrected before harm occurs [17]

The systems-centered approach aligns with the just culture because it promotes learning from errors. It promotes systems fixes and including things like forcing functions or hard stops when dispensing or administering medications. The intention of the non-punitive/just culture concept is to perpetuate the safe environment where providers can openly discuss errors. The goal is to avoid the shame and blame of errors and to include those involved in the event to promote learning and prevent future errors.

### 19.8 The Overall Safety Culture of an Organization

Attribution of accidents as human failures does not provide a full picture of all that was involved and contributed to the occurrence of an event. The leadership of the organization must take responsibility for the decisions that impact safe functioning of the organization in its entirety [18]. The term "Safety Culture" was first introduced after the Chernobyl disaster in 1986 [18]. An organization either exhibits a safety culture that is positive or negative. It is ultimately the product of the individual and groups that determine the proficiency of an organization's health and safety processes and protocols [18]. A positive safety culture is one in which shared perceptions of the importance of safety and confidence in preventative measures are experienced by all levels of an organization [18]. Factors that create this positive safety culture include:

- Leadership and the commitment of the chief executive
- A good line management system for managing safety
- The involvement of all employees
- Effective communication and understood/agreed goals
- Good organizational learning/responsiveness to change
- Manifest attention to workplace safety and health
- A questioning attitude and rigorous and prudent approach by all individuals [18]

### 19.9 Investigation and Follow-Up of Adverse Events

When investigating events, there are many formats, strategies, and templates that patient safety experts and organizations have published for use. A root cause analysis (RCA) is necessary to getting to the true underlying cause of the event. The RCA is a structured method used to analyze serious adverse events [19]. Initially developed to analyze industrial accidents, RCA is now widely utilized as an error analysis tool in healthcare [19]. Since 1997 the Joint Commission has mandated use of RCA to analyze serious patient safety events (such as wrong-site surgery) [19].

A "perfect storm" often leads to an adverse event. The systems in place do not set the transaction up for success. The Swiss cheese model by James Reason displays how the error falls through the cracks. When the hole perfectly aligns then the error slips through (Fig.19.2).

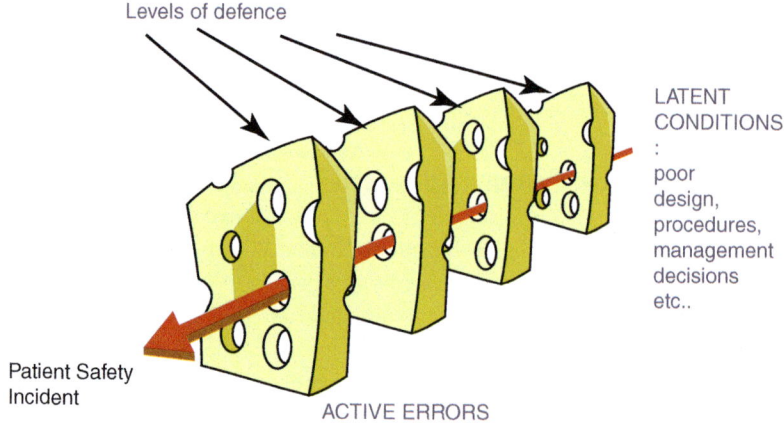

**Fig. 19.2** Reason's Swiss Cheese Model. Source: https://www.researchgate.net/publication/265177684_Understanding_Safety_in_Healthcare_The_System_Evolution_Erosion_and_Enhancement_Model/figures?lo=1) [20]

One example is when a provider intends to order a mild sedative prior to an interventional radiology procedure but orders the wrong drug. The pharmacy then dispenses the wrong drug and the nurse administers the wrong drug. The system allowed this error to fall through the cracks and not get caught at least three different points of contact (ordering by provider, dispensing by pharmacy, and administering by nursing).

When human error is determined to be the cause, safety analyst experts presume the analysis was not in-depth enough. Instead, it is important to uncover the systems issues that led to the ease of ability for the human to make the errors. In addition to the Swiss cheese model, some other methods to assist in conducting an RCA may include the five Why's and the fishbone diagram.

The five Why's is a simple process of asking why up to five times. The intention is that doing so "will lead to better understanding, to possible solutions, and to easier implementation of the solution through staff involvement" [21]. The Institute for Healthcare Improvement (IHI) encourages you to not stop asking why until you get to the true final root cause [22]. This may take more than five times. The initial responses may be things like "because it is my job" or "because we have always done it that way", but the why questions must persist in order to get beyond the superficial layers and get to the underlying rationales as to why a step is truly being done and whether there is waste in the system [22]. If there are unnecessary steps that can be removed from a process than it can be removed as to prevent errors in the future from wasteful steps that interfere with the overall process and contribute to adverse events. Extraneous steps that do not add value risk patient care as well because clinicians learn to do "workarounds" and skip steps as customary part of their practice and sometimes the steps they skip may be the vital steps to maintaining patient safety. Eliminating unnecessary steps may lead to compliance with necessary steps.

The cause and effect diagram also referred to as the "fishbone diagram" or Ishikawa diagram is used to display and review possible causes of a certain outcome (or "effect") [23]. This can be used when causes logically align with certain pre-determined areas: materials, methods, equipment, environment, and people [23]. Samples of fishbone diagrams can be found on the web (for example: https://www.conceptdraw.com/samples/fishbone-diagram, see sample 2 for a template that is applicable to healthcare).

A cause and effect diagram has a variety of benefits:

- It helps teams understand that there are many causes that contribute to an effect.
- It graphically displays the relationship of the causes to the effect and to each other.
- It helps to identify areas for improvement [23].

The above represent a few examples of strategies and tools used in healthcare systems to help not only conduct RCAs, but also to develop improvement processes that prevent adverse events.

## 19.10 Conclusion

The study of patient safety and adverse events is not without its challenges. Healthcare is becoming increasing complex as technology advances lifesaving techniques and as it continues to be more multilayered. The fact that humans carrying out activities will always include a certain amount of inherent errors means that patient safety will be an important area to understand for those in all healthcare specialties. Since errors and adverse events still impact human life significantly (one of the leading causes of death in the United States), regulatory agencies will continue to enhance their oversight. A careful review of why errors truly occur is necessary to get to the true root cause. Without honest and open review of events, it is impossible to uncover the root causes and prevent them from happening to future patients.

## References

1. AHRQ:Adverse events, near misses and errors. Retrieved from https://psnet.ahrq.gov/primers/primer/34/adverse-events-near-misses-and-errors, 2019.
2. World Alliance for Patient Safety. WHO draft guidelines for adverse event reporting and learning systems: from information to action. Geneva: World Health Organization; 2005.
3. National Quality Forum.:Retrieved from http://www.qualityforum.org/Topics/SREs/Serious_Reportable_Events.aspx, 2019.
4. National Quality Forum.:Retrieved from http://www.qualityforum.org/Topics/SREs/List_of_SREs.aspx, 2019.
5. The Joint Commission. Retrieved from https://www.jointcommission.org/sentinel_event_policy_and_procedures/, 2017.
6. American Society of Healthcare Risk Managers, 2018. When medical negligence becomes criminal (slides, 5/24/18).
7. NSO: Medical malpractice, 101 (2019).
8. Institute of Medicine: To err is human: building a safer health system, 1999,.
9. BMJ: Medical error—the third leading cause of death in the US, 2016.
10. AHRQ, Patient Safety Primer: Second victims: support for clinicians involved in errors and adverse events. Retrieved from https://psnet.ahrq.gov/primers/primer/30/support-for-clinicians-involved-in-errors-and-adverse-events-second-victims, 2019.
11. Scott, S. The second victim phenomenon: a harsh reality of health care professions. Retrieved from https://psnet.ahrq.gov/perspectives/perspective/102, 2011.
12. Newman L, O'Neill T, Woltman G, et al. Supporting clinicians after adverse events: Development of a clinician peer support program. Retrieved from https://www.researchgate.net/publication/325610752_Supporting_Clinicians_After_Adverse_Events_Development_of_a_Clinician_Peer_Support_Program, 2018.
13. Aleccia, J. Nurse's suicide highlights twin tragedies of medical errors. Retrieved from http://www.nbcnews.com/id/43529641/ns/health-health_care/t/nurses-suicide-highlights-twin-tragedies-medical-errors#.XN3PQ45Kg2w, 2011.
14. American Nurses Association: ANA Position Statement of the Just Culture. Retrieved from https://www.nursingworld.org/practice-policy/nursing-excellence/official-position-statements/id/just-culture/, 2010.
15. McCotter, P. Promoting clinician resilience: ensuring effective support after adverse events. Presentation at the Annual Conference of the American Association of Nurse Attorneys, Las Vegas, NV, October 9–11, 2014.
16. Wachter, RM. Personal accountability in healthcare: searching for the right balance. Retrieved from https://qualitysafety.bmj.com/content/22/2/176.info, 2013.
17. Reason J. Human error: models and management. BMJ. 2000;320(7237):768–70. https://www.bmj.com/content/320/7237/768
18. Manchi, GB, Gowda, S, Hanspal, JS. Study on cognitive approach to human error and its application to reduce accidents at workplace. Retrieved from https://pdfs.semanticscholar.org/94d4/fd47ca2d8c1b1cdac848799e9f6fe985facc.pdf, 2013.
19. AHRQ, Patient Safety Primer. Root cause analysis. Retrieved from https://psnet.ahrq.gov/primers/primer/10/root-cause-analysis, 2019.
20. Carthey, Jane. Understanding Safety in Healthcare: The System Evolution, Erosion and Enhancement Model. Journal of public health research. 2. e25. 10.4081/jphr.2013.e25, 2013.
21. Dahl, O. How the 5 whys can work in healthcare. Retrieved from https://www.physicianspractice.com/operations/how-5-whys-can-work-healthcare, 2017.
22. Institute for Healthcare Improvement: 5 Whys: Finding the root cause. Retrieved from http://www.ihi.org/resources/Pages/Tools/5-Whys-Finding-the-Root-Cause.aspx, 2019.
23. Institute for Healthcare Improvement: Cause and effect diagram. Retrieved from https://www.physicianspractice.com/operations/how-5-whys-can-work-healthcare, 2019.

# Section IV

# The Patient in Radiology

# Legal and Ethical Considerations for Radiology Procedural Consent

## 20

Adrienne N. Dixon and Meghan Stepanek

## 20.1 Introduction

*Patient Jane is referred to you by another physician, Dr. Smith, who suspects that she has a tumor. He would like Jane to get a computed tomography (CT) imaging procedure with contrast to potentially diagnose and locate the tumor in preparation for proceeding with surgical resection. On the day of Jane's CT procedure, you have been assigned as her radiology nurse.*

*You note in Jane's record that Dr. Smith briefly discussed the risks and benefits of undergoing this procedure, however the informed consent form for the procedure has not been completed. It is your understanding the consent form and other documentation must be completed by the radiology team.*

*Dr. Jones, the radiologist has asked for your assistance to obtain the patient's consent and be the witness. You describe to Jane the risks such as pain, swelling, allergic reactions as well as the benefits of the procedure enabling the surgeon to distinguish between normal and abnormal tissues, define function of the organs and if detected, better visualize the tumor. Jane thinks she has signed so many documents and asks you why this consent form is important.*

A. N. Dixon, JD, MS, PA-C (✉)
M. Stepanek, Esq, MPH
Legal Department, The Johns Hopkins Health System Corporation, Baltimore, MD, USA

As we review and discuss the legal and ethical considerations, we will use the Patient Jane vignette to illustrate the issues related to informed consent that can arise in radiology nursing practice.

## 20.2 Medical Ethics

Ethics are the standards that societies, organizations, and professions establish to define expectations for behavior among members of that group[1]. Medical ethics is based on ethical principles that apply to medical practice and patient care [2]. The four basic principles of medical ethics are: (1) beneficence; (2) non-maleficence; (3) respect for autonomy; and (4) justice [3]. The principles of medical ethics are outlined in Table 20.1.

### 20.2.1 Intersection Between Ethics and Law in the Context of Informed Consent

There is a direct correlation between informed consent and patient autonomy. Autonomy is a universal principle within healthcare, which affords the patient the responsibility and the right to make and carryout decisions based on healthcare interventions they will or will not receive [4]. The need to obtain informed consent arises

**Table 20.1** Principles of medical ethics

| | |
|---|---|
| Beneficence | To act in the best interest of the patient |
| Non-maleficence | To do no harm to the patient |
| Respect for autonomy | The ability of a competent patient to make or refuse one's own medical decisions |
| Justice | The distribution of healthcare resources equitably within members of society |

from a physician's ethical obligation to assist patients in making a choice, including addressing therapeutic alternatives, is consistent with good medical practice [1].

Laws, regulations, and policies are used to more clearly define ethical behavior and, when applicable, to impose sanctions for wrongful actions [1]. Regulations and legal requirements vary from state to state and may differ in who can obtain consent, treatments that require consent, and what information should be reflected in written documentation [5].

Legal liability for practitioners who fail to properly obtain consent arose originally through the tort of battery. Battery is a civil cause of action, which is the intentional, wrongful touching of another without his or her consent [1]. There are courts that have held that an informed consent claim may be asserted by a patient in the absence of a battery or affirmative violation of the patient's physical integrity, because it is the duty of a healthcare provider to inform a patient of material information, or information that a practitioner knows or ought to know would be significant to a reasonable person in the patient's position deciding whether or not to submit to particular medical treatment or procedure [6].

## 20.3 Informed Consent

The need to obtain informed consent arises because society believes that legally competent patients have the right of self-determination and to discuss the proposed plan, treatment, or procedure, results, and risks so patients can make decisions based on the information provided to them by their physician [1]. The right to consent is considered a basic patient right that patients or legally authorized decision-makers can make informed decisions related to their medical care [7]. A material risk is defined as "a risk which a physician knows or ought to know would be significant to a reasonable person in the patient's position in deciding whether or not to have the particular medical treatment or procedure" [6]. The informed consent process is a discussion between physician and patient and must include the material aspects of the patient's diagnosis and proposed treatment that would enable a reasonable patient to consider his or her options, including refusing treatment [1]. As was discussed previously, a physician or, by extension, a healthcare provider who is knowledgeable and capable of reviewing the risks, benefits, and alternatives to a procedure or treatment can obtain consent. In addition, this individual may also delegate his or her authority to obtain consent to another member of the patient's healthcare team. The key is the healthcare professional—to which the consent process has been delegated to—must be knowledgeable to explain the risks, benefits, and alternatives to the patient, to ensure they are informed to make a decision.

Ideally, the informed consent process should occur before the date of the procedure to afford patients the opportunity to contemplate their choice to proceed or forego the recommended procedure [8]. However, there may be multiple factors and variables that can impact the ability to consent patients within a certain period of time before the procedure. The physician should build in time within their workflow to ensure adequate consent discussions, including the need for any follow-up with the patient around the date of the procedure.

From a radiological perspective, types of procedures that frequently require informed consent include interventional radiology procedures, computed tomography, magnetic resonance imaging (with special considerations for certain patient populations such as a pregnant patients), use of intravenous contrast administration, and examinations that use ionizing radiation [8]. The material risks to consider, when applicable,

**Table 20.2** Components of informed consent

| |
|---|
| Description of the nature of the proposed treatment or procedure |
| The name of who will perform the treatment or procedure |
| Description of the benefits of the proposed treatment or procedure |
| Description of the material risks associated with the proposed treatment or procedure |
| The alternatives to the particular treatment or procedure |
| The benefits and risks associated with the alternatives to the proposed treatment or procedure |
| Description of the probabilities that the propose therapy will succeed |
| Provider conflicts of interest disclosures |
| The patient's right to refuse a proposed treatment or procedure, or withdraw previous consent |

include potential risks of radiation exposure, adverse reactions to contrast agents, bleeding, infection, perforation, and death [8].

Table 20.2 describes the components of informed consent, which should be considered during the discussion between the competent patient and physician.

### 20.3.1 Emergency Consent

There are exceptions for treatment provided in the absence of consent when a patient lacks capacity and there is no legally authorized decision-maker identified or available. This commonly occurs in the context of emergency care rendered to an unconscious patient and is consistent with the ethical principle of not choosing an irreversible path when faced with uncertainty [9]. In situations presenting substantial risk of death or immediate and serious harm where the patient's life or health would be adversely affected by delaying treatment, and there is no evidence that the treatment is against the patient's wishes, the provision of treatment is ethically and legally permissible. The best practice is for the physician performing the procedure to document the emergent nature of the patient's clinical condition, and once the patient is able to communicate or when applicable, the legally authorized decision-maker is available, the physician should discuss and review the interventions performed.

### 20.3.2 Serial Consent

Serial consent is a mechanism where patients who are undergoing a series of pre-planned procedural interventions can be consented for all of the procedures during one encounter. Examples of multiple procedures where the application of a serial consent could be applicable are—interventional radiology procedures related to removing fluid collections, radiation oncology treatments, chemotherapy administration, and would care debridements. Serial consents should be used for pre-planned procedures that are contemplated in advance, and are not recommended for urgent or acute clinical events. The key when determining whether a serial consent is legally sufficient is understanding whether the patient's clinical condition will remain the same during the series of procedures, to which the material risks, benefits and alternatives do not change. Thus, if the patient's clinical condition changes, the physician must obtain additional consent from the patient before proceeding with the procedure and discuss the enhanced risks, benefits, and alternatives in relation to the patient's current clinical condition.

### 20.3.3 Minors and Consent

In most circumstances, a minor patient's parent, legal guardian, or court-appointed custodian must be provided the risks, benefits, and alternatives related to the proposed procedure. There are certain circumstances where minor patients are considered to have the same capacity as an adult, and can consent to their own procedures or treatment. This may vary at the state level. Examples include: minors who are married, legally emancipated, seeking treatment for sexually transmitted infections, pregnancy, and contraception other than sterilization.

### 20.3.4 Consent Refusal and Withdrawal

A competent patient's right to refuse a recommended treatment is an important principle in the informed consent process [7]. A patient with decision-making capacity can make good or bad decisions. Respect for patient autonomy and self-determination requires that decisions to consent to or refuse treatment originate freely from the patient, and can be freely withdrawn at any time [7]. It is recommended that the conversations regarding informed consent and refusal of the procedure or treatment be documented by the physician in the patient's medical record [10].

*The informed consent process describes material risks, benefits, and alternatives. The informed consent process is the cornerstone of developing a positive relationship between patients and physicians (or their designee) as it demonstrates respect for their rights and interests in making healthcare decisions.*

**Table 20.3** Role of nurses during the informed consent process

| *Role of nurses during the informed consent process* |
| --- |
| Understanding patient rights and autonomy as part of participation in obtaining consent |
| Empowering and advocating for the patient as part of patient education |
| Addressing patient anxiety and apprehension |
| Collecting related documentation or witnessing the informed consent form |
| Identifying the appropriate legally authorized decision-maker when needed |

## 20.4 Nurse's Role During the Informed Consent Process

While it is universally understood that physicians are responsible for informing patients of the risks, benefits, and alternatives of a proposed treatment, nurses play a vital role as patient advocates during the informed consent process [7]. Nurses may advocate to ensure patient autonomy through appropriate participation in the informed consent process [7]. There is an inherent balancing act between witnessing the patient signing a consent form and ensuring that there was adequate discussion between the patient and physician, for the patient to make an informed choice as to whether or not to undergo a specific medical treatment or procedure. While nurses serve in an advocacy role with their patients, it is important to clearly define role and scope with patients and the physician members on the clinical team so as to avoid the appearance of consenting the patient, which could be considered practicing outside his or her scope of practice [7]. Additional consideration as to the nurse's role in the consenting process relates to how the scope of nursing practice is defined within each state's nurse practice act [7].

While the presumption, unless outlined within specific state law, is the nurse does not obtain informed consent on behalf of the physician, there are opportunities where the nurse can play an integral part within the consent process. For instance, as Table 20.3 describes, there are opportunities to advocate for patients, to ensure patients and, when applicable, their legally authorized decision-makers, without directly discussing the material risks, benefits, and alternatives to a procedure or treatment. When appropriate, and pursuant to provisions outlined within the respective state's nurse practice act, nurses with specialized knowledge and judgment can collaborate with physicians during the informed consent process, and, when applicable, obtain consent.

There is a distinction between completion of the consent form—which is often signed and witnessed by the nurse— and the physician's obligation to disclose relevant information to the patient [7]. The form, which is used to obtain the patient, physician proposing to perform a procedure or treatment, and witness signatures, serves as a placeholder within the patient's medical record, to demonstrate compliance with applicable state laws, regulations, standards set forth by accreditation bodies, and hospital policy. The witness, which in most cases is the nurse, when signing the consent form is merely attesting that the patient signed the form—not that the patient understands the risks, benefits, and alternatives related to the procedure or treatment. This is important to understand because while the nurse may serve as a witness, ultimately the physician or appropriate designee remains liable to ensure the consent process was adequate.

While the form can serve as an indication that the patient was adequately informed about the risks, benefits, and alternatives, the form does not replace the discussion between the physician (or appropriate designee) and the patient [11].

*Nurses can perform a collaborative role with the physician to help the patient understand from an advocacy standpoint. Ultimately, it is the responsibility of the physician or other provider who is performing the procedure or treatment, who has knowledge and expertise to describe the material risks, benefits and alternatives to obtain the patient's consent before the procedure. Witnessing an informed consent form does not indicate whether the patient understands the risks, benefits, and alternatives to a procedure.*

## 20.5 Capacity

*Jane's condition deteriorates, and she no longer seems to comprehend her medical status. Her daughter wants to begin making healthcare decisions for Jane. How do you determine whether Jane has capacity to make her own decisions? If she does not, how do you know if it is okay for her daughter to decide?*

All adults are presumed to have capacity to make medical decisions for themselves. If a patient becomes incapacitated, clinicians rely on an individual acting on the patient's behalf to make decisions in the patient's best interest, consistent with the patient's values and preferences. The alternate decision-maker could be a proxy or healthcare agent that the patient identified before they lost capacity or could be a surrogate who is allowed to make decisions for the patient based on their relationship to the patient under operation of law.

Competency is distinguished from capacity in that it is a higher standard referring to a court determination. In general, the four main components of capacity evaluation include a patient's ability to: (1) communicate a choice, (2) understand, (3) appreciate, and (4) rationalize/reason in relation to their healthcare [12]. Under most state laws, capacity determinations are made by any physician involved in the patient's care and familiar with the patient's condition(s) [13]. Some state laws require additional measures for assessing and documenting capacity such as involvement of a second physician, particularly if the patient is conscious and communicative. The capacity to give informed consent does not necessarily require a psychiatrist, and in some instances calling for one can be seen by some patients as an act of hostility, culminating in a risk of mistaken diagnosis [13].

When a patient no longer has decision-making capacity, a patient's advanced directive (also known as a living will) is referred to for decisions regarding care and/or authorization of a proxy decision-maker. The scope of advance directives can vary but typically includes information on the patient's desires for life-saving measures such as cardiopulmonary resuscitation, care transfer, mechanical ventilation, tube feeding, palliative care, and organ/tissue/body donation. Healthcare agency delegation may also be specified in the advance directive such as delegation of a proxy. In the absence of an advance directive or a living will, some states have enacted laws permitting family members, domestic partners, and close friends to serve as a surrogate decision-maker [1]. The priority as to which of the legally authorized decision-makers can consent on behalf of the patient varies across jurisdictions as well as by hospital or healthcare facility policies. If no surrogate is available, the state may need to appoint a public guardian.

In the United States, most states have laws in place that delineate requirements for alternate patient decision-makers and standards for documentation. At the federal level, the Patient Self-Determination Act applies to most providers and plans that participate in Medicare and Medicaid, and reinforces state laws by requiring, for example, written information to be given to patients describing their rights under the applicable state law governing medical care decisions, documentation in the patient's medical record regarding any advanced directives, and protects the patient from discrimination based on the status of an advanced directive [14].

At any point in time, a patient with capacity can decide to override the documented advanced directive. As a patient's clinical condition changes, their capacity may also be effected, so ongoing assessment is necessary to protect the patient's rights to autonomous decision-making.

*Nurses may ask a patient if they have an advance directive in order to collect documenta-*

*tion or if none, to help in identifying and contacting surrogate decision-makers should a patient become incapacitated.*

## 20.6 Communication and Consent

The communication of information is a well-recognized and essential part of the relationship between the physician and patient, and is central to the process of obtaining consent [15]. Informed consent is more than just obtaining the patient's permission to proceed with a procedure or care plan; it is the conversation that addresses in a meaningful way, the proposed plan, including material risks, benefits, and alternatives before proceeding with a mutually agreeable treatment plan or intervention [8]. Informed consent conversations are a key component of radiologic procedures, such as within interventional radiology [8]. The following considerations can assist the physician in advance of procedural consent discussions: (1) preparation through reviewing the patient's history and other needs; (2) encouraging patients to actively participate and ask questions; (3) address material risks, benefits, and alternatives; (4) utilize the "teach back" method to determine patient understanding; and (5) afford the patient the opportunity to contemplate their decision to proceed or forego the procedure [8].

Other communication considerations during the consent process include discussion surrounding patients who have a do-not-resuscitate (DNR) order, and respecting patient autonomy and self-determination while also balancing the patient's treatment goals and personal values [1]. The patient's nurse can be instrumental and can fully participate in end-of-life discussions with patients and families, including discussions surrounding DNR orders [16].

### 20.6.1 Use of Interpreters to Effectively Communicate

The Americans with Disabilities Act of 1990 ("ADA") disallows discrimination in employment, state and local governments, public accommodations and commercial facilities, transportation, and telecommunications. Title II of the ADA covers state and local governments while Title III of the ADA addresses public accommodations and commercial facilities. Both Titles mandate "effective communication" to persons with limited English proficiency (LEP) [17]. The ADA statute requires all public entities to "take appropriate steps to ensure that communications with applicants, participants, members of the public, and companions with disabilities are as effective as communications with others" [18]. Thus, entities which are considered places of public accomodations under Title III of the ADA, are required to "furnish appropriate auxiliary aids and services where necessary to ensure effective communication with individuals (and, to their companion[s]) with disabilities [19]."

Therefore, it is important to ensure for LEP patients that the clinical team is effectively communicating, and, when applicable, appropriate auxiliary aids and services, such as qualified medical interpreters, are provided.

*Communication is a central component to the informed consent process, and it is vital to ensure the communication is effective for all patients.*

## 20.7 Risk Communication in Radiology Practice

*Dr. Smith determines that Jane has capacity to make her own healthcare decisions. Dr. Jones advises Jane that she will also need an interventional radiology procedure. When she begins to explain to Jane the specific risks and hazards, Jane interrupts to say that she does not want to hear any more because it makes her nervous and that she just wants to proceed with the imaging and procedure.*

Patients have a right to agree to or refuse treatment. In order to be informed, the risks and hazards as well as the benefits and advantages must be conveyed in order for patients to weigh the decision to undergo a radiology test or procedures. Researchers Bedetti and Loré describe the different informed consent risk communication strategies as: (1) "don't say a word," assuming that the expert knows best; (2) understatement, reassuring patients; and (3) full disclosure, including a description of risks as variable but also disclosing risk information by the numbers [20].

In diagnostic radiology, there is "…lack of professional consensus on the duty to inform and on a patient's right to consent in diagnostic radiology" [21]. In the past, the predominant approach to informing patients of risk was the "prudent doctor" model, where the doctor weighs the risk-benefit ratio of any patient treatment and omits mentioning rare nonserious complications [22]. The more prevalent modern approach is the "prudent patient" model, which is based on what the average judicious patient would want to know[22].

For the general population and even health professionals, the difficulty in understanding radiology, including radiation biology principles such as the dose-response relationship and acute versus chronic effects is compounded by unfamiliar terminology and units of measure [23]. Some risks of radiation include radiation-induced cancers and teratogenic defects that disturb the growth or development of an embryo or fetus [24]. Risks may differ based on the patient such as in pediatric patients, who are more radiosensitive than adults and have a longer expected lifetime, putting them at higher risk of cancer from the effects of radiation [25]. The complication of communicating risk is also marked by uncertainty as, for example, scientists have noted for radiation cancer risk that "…it is difficult to say that any cancer is solely caused by radiation exposure, as cancer may be caused by a combination of factors" [24]. New research informing exposure guidelines also drives changes such as recent eye radiation exposure limits that were reduced by the U.S. Nuclear Regulatory Commission to an amount four times less [26]. The radiology team is often best suited to inform both the referrer and the patient of radiology risks based on the type of technology and imaging scan protocol used. However, coordination with the referring team is important in order to contextualize the radiology imaging or procedure relative to the patient's underlying conditions, treatment course, and diagnosis so that the consequences of missing imaging or procedures are understood.

To address the complication and uncertainty that patients face when making a healthcare decision, radiology team members can prepare by anticipating information the patient will want to know in dialogue with their providers, and preparing consent forms that convey written information effectively. While individual patients may have a different perceptions of risk and concerns based on factors such as their previous experiences, values, and beliefs, risk communication preparation through message mapping is an effective approach used in public health that can be adapted to the clinical context [27]. Message mapping involves (1) anticipating the questions and concerns of the stakeholders, (2) organizing thoughts and ideas in response to those questions and concerns, and (3) developing key messages and supporting information [27]. In addition to legal and ethical analysis, the development of effective medical disclosure and consent documents (MDCDs) can also be informed by research of patient preferences. For example, in a study by Donovan et al. of patients who received cardiac catheterization, researchers concluded that most effective MDCDs follow the "CLOVE" framework factors of **c**ompleteness (including the range of possible outcomes), **l**anguage (lack of medical jargon), **o**rganization (good layout and categorization), and **v**olume (short and concise) and are the most **e**ffective as to the qualities and structure of the information [28]. Effective disclosure and informed consent depends on providing sufficient amounts of high-quality, usable information [29].

*Nurse dialogue with patients as a means of risk communication helps them better understand their healthcare choices.*

## 20.8 Liability Risks

*Dr. Jones performs an interventional radiology procedure on Jane. As a result, she develops an extremely rare complication and suffers from partial paralysis. After an extended recovery, Jane is still very upset and feels that Dr. Jones did not adequately advise her of the risk of paralysis. How will Jane's case proceed if she decides to initiate a civil lawsuit?*

Jane may initiate a lawsuit by filing a civil complaint against the doctors as defendants based on the cause of action of negligence. Improper consent is rarely a stand-alone civil claim, but when asserted, is typically added to malpractice (medical negligence) cases. In general, the elements of negligence that the plaintiff must prove are that the defendant owed a duty to the plaintiff, the defendant breached that duty, that breach was the proximate cause of the harm suffered by the plaintiff, and that the harm caused damages. Some cases are dismissed if the plaintiff fails to state a claim upon which relief could be granted by the court. Additionally, most jurisdictions have a statute of limitations under state law that sets time limits for when a medical negligence case may be brought before the courts.

If the case proceeds to court, both the plaintiff and defendant would likely call upon expert testimony from medical professionals and/or evidence such as professional medical study publications to support their arguments about whether the standard of care was met by the physician. While the definition of standard of care may vary, generally, it is considered what a reasonable well-qualified physician would do under the same or similar circumstances. Documentation such as consent forms and notes in the medical record is especially important in this type of litigation [30]. In this case, documentation by Dr. Jones of Jane's refusal to hear about risks and consent to proceed would be particularly important.

In some informed consent cases where a patient alleges that a physician failed to inform them of risks, the defendant may assert that the risk was so remote and outweighed by the benefits that they chose not to disclose so as not to alarm the patient [31]. However, this argument of "therapeutic privilege" to support the denial of full disclosure should be invoked "with great caution…for the courts view such physician conduct with suspicion and skepticism" [31]. In malpractice actions alleging failure to warn patients of risks, court decisions have varied based on the jurisdiction. While the "prudent patient" model as previously discussed is the increasingly prevailing approach [22], other court rulings on civil lawsuits alleging negligent informed consent for a radiology procedure have rejected the "reasonable patient standard" because the determination for risk disclosure was seen as a medical judgment [32]. Some jurisdictions have a hybrid standard such as in North Carolina, where patients are barred from recovery based on the consent having been obtained from both a prudent provider and prudent patient standard, or if a reasonable person would have undergone the treatment or procedure had they been informed in accordance with the standard [33].

The following practices could be used to mitigate risks in radiology practice: having written policies on informed consent, directly involving the referring physician to obtain consent, assessing patients for any special risks, confirming a patient's understanding of the risks, properly filling out forms consistently for thorough documentation through use of consent forms (including any specific risks discussed as well as alternatives mentioned), making notations in the patient's record (including any special circumstances), including anesthesia-related issues if not already addressed in a separate form, and being mindful of the scope of the consent when performing tests and procedures. Depending on the jurisdiction, some of these strategies may also be required by law in statute or regulation.

*Nurses play a key role in documentation of the patient's care that is often used to defend against claims of negligence in civil cases.*

## 20.9 Special Issues with Use of Technology

*The hospital where you work has begun using artificial intelligence (AI) technology that draws on patient data and applies predictive analytics to radiological images to inform their decisions. You are concerned about whether existing data sharing consents address use of personally identifiable information of patients as well as cybersecurity risks.*

Emerging technologies such as medical devices and machines have outpaced the development of applicable legal parameters to guide implementation. In some cases, the technology engineers might not even completely understand how data is processed, leading to cybersecurity risks and continuous challenges for regulators [34]. When using a new technology in the clinical context such as AI or telemedicine, existing statutes, regulations, other compliance requirements, policies and contracts need to be reviewed and applied in determining use parameters and modifications to or development of new consent forms, particularly when a significant or material risk exists [35]. For example, many AI technologies rely on algorithm analysis of big data, some of which is medically sensitive personally identifiable information that is subject to federal and state medical confidentiality laws.

*Nurses play a key role in tracking and learning about technological developments in radiology to help facilitate communications with the patient regarding its use.*

## 20.10 Key Points

1. *Ethical considerations:* The right to consent is considered a basic patient right that patients or legally authorized decision-makers can make informed decisions related to their medical care, including the right to refuse treatment.
2. *Informed consent process:* The informed consent process describes the material risks, benefits, and alternatives that is essential information for a patient to receive to make a decisions. The procedural consent form does not replace the conversation between the physician and patient.
3. *Nurse role in consent:* Nurses play a vital role in advocating for patients during the consent process, including engaging physicians in the event the patient may need additional clarification and information to make an informed decision.
4. *Capacity:* If a patient lacks capacity, an alternate decision-maker such as a proxy/healthcare agent or surrogate needs to be identified to make decisions unless an exception exists such as for an unconscious patient in an emergency situation.
5. *Risk communication:* Coordination of risk messaging between the radiology care team and referring care team helps to address patient concerns and provide the information necessary to inform them of the risks and benefits.
6. *Liability risks:* Thorough documentation and patient record notes are key in defending civil cases for negligence that may arise as allegations of failure to provide informed consent.

**Acknowledgement** The authors would like to acknowledge the assistance of J.D. candidates Elodie Jean-Phillipe and Andryse Leukeu.

## References

1. Gerold KB, Dixon AN. In: Barnett SR, editor. Ethical and legal considerations.Manual of geriatric anesthesia. New York: Springer Science + Business Media; 2013.
2. Snyder JE, Gauthier CC. The underlying principles of ethical patient care. In: Evidence-based medical ethics: cases for practice-based learning. New York: Springer; 2008:11–6.
3. Beauchamp TL, Childress JF. Principles of biomedical ethics. 5th ed. Oxford: Oxford University Press; 2001.
4. Universal Declaration on Bioethics and Human Rights, United Nations Educational, Scientific and Cultural Organization:2005. Available from: https://unesdoc.unesco.org/ark:/48223/pf0000142825_eng#page=80
5. Cook W. "Sign here": nursing value and the process of informed consent. Plast Surg Nurs. 2014;34(10):29–33.
6. McQuitty v. Spangler, 410 Md. 1; 976 A.2d 1020 (2009), citing Sard v. Hardy, 281 Md., 432, 444, 379 A.2d 104, 1022 (1977).
7. Menendez JB. Informed consent: essential legal and ethical principles for nurses. JONAS Healthc Law Ethics Regul. 2013;15(4):140–4.
8. Ripley BA, Tiffany D, et al. Improving the informed consent conversation: a standardized checklist that is patient centered, quality driven, and legally sound. J Vasc Inter Radiol. 2015;26:1639–46.
9. Holt GE, Sarmento B, Kett D, Goodman KW. An unconscious patient with a DNR tattoo. N Engl J Med. 2017;377:2192–219.
10. Association for Radiologic and Imaging Nursing Clinical Practice Guideline:Informed Consent for a Radiology Procedure.Board of Directors.2009.

11. American Medical Association:Code of Medical Ethics Opinion 2.1.1. Available from: https://www.ama-assn.org/sites/ama-assn.org/files/corp/media-browser/code-of-medical-ethics-chapter-2.pdf
12. Dastidar J, Odden A. How do I determine if my patient has decision-making capacity? Hospitalist. 2011Aug;2011(8). https://www.the-hospitalist.org/hospitalist/article/124731/how-do-i-determine-if-my-patient-has-decision-making-capacity.
13. Spike J. Informed consent is the essence of capacity assessment. J Law Med Ethics. 2017;45:95–105.
14. 42 U.S.C.§§1395cc(f) and1396a(w), 42 C.F.R. §489.102. 2019.
15. Hodkinson K. The need to know—therapeutic privilege: a way forward. Health Care Anal. 2013;21:105–9.
16. ANA Center for Human Rights and Ethics:Nursing Care and Do Not Resuscitate (DNR) and Allow Natural Death (AND) Decisions. Position Statement. Accessed 12 Mar 2012.
17. 42 U.S.CA. § 12101, 12111, 12132, 12141, 12161, 12181 (West 2015); see e.g. U.S. Department of Justice, ADA requirements: effective communication, Civil Rights Division Accessed 31 Jan 2014.
18. 28 C.F.R. §35.160(a)(1) (West 2015).
19. 42 U.S.C.§1218(7)(F) (West 2015); 28 C.F.R. §36.104(1)(ii)(B)(6) (West 2015) (hospitals run by private entities are considered places of public accommodation).
20. Bedetti G, Loré C. Radiological informed consent in cardiovascular imaging: towards the medico-legal perfect storm? Cardiovasc Ultrasound. 2007;5:35.
21. Doudenkova V, Bélisle Pipon JC. Duty to inform and informed consent in diagnostic radiology: how ethics and law can better guide practice. HEC Forum. 2016;28:75–94.
22. Baheti A, Borges ME. Informed consent in diagnostic radiology practice: where do we stand? Indian J Radiol Imag. 2017;27:517–20.
23. Cardinal J, Gunderman R, Tarver R. Informing patients about risks and benefits of radiology examinations: a review article. J Am Coll Radiol. 2011;8:402–8.
24. Bolus N. Basic review of radiation biology and terminology. J Nucl Med Technol. 2001;29(2):67–73. Available from: http://tech.snmjournals.org/content/29/2/67.full.
25. U.S. Food and Drug Administration: [Internet]. Pediatric X-ray imaging.Accessed22Feb 2019. Available from: http://www.fda.gov/radiation-emittingproducts/radiationemittingproductsandprocedures/medicalimaging/ucm298899.htm
26. Frey D. Radiation cataracts: new data and new recommendations. AJR. 2014 Oct;203:W345–6.
27. World Health Organization: Communicating radiation risks in paediatric imaging. 2016;50–71. Chapter 3.Available from: https://www.who.int/ionizing_radiation/pub_meet/chapter3.pdf
28. Donovan E, Brown L, Crook B. Patient satisfaction with medical disclosure and consent documents for treatment: applying conceptualizations of uncertainty to examine successful attempts at communicating risk. J Commun Healthc. 2015;8(3):220–31.
29. Donovan E, Crook B, Brown L, Pastorek A, Hall C, Mackert M, et al. An experimental test of medical disclosure and consent documentation: assessing patient comprehension, self-efficacy, and uncertainty. Commun Monogr. 2014 June;81(2):239–60.
30. Hill G, Smouse HB. Lessons learned on how to protect an interventional radiologist against malpractice claim. Seminars in Interventional Radiol. 2006;23(4):315–8.
31. Berlin L. Malpractice issues in radiology: informed consent. Radiology Today. 2010;11(4). Available from: https://www.radiologytoday.net/archive/rt0410p20.shtml.
32. Hook v. Rothstein, 281 S.C. 541 (1984).
33. North Carolina General Statutes Annotated, §90–21.13(a)(1).(2018).
34. Pesapane F, Volonté C, Codari M, Sardanelli F. Artificial intelligence as a medical device in radiology: ethical and regulatory issues in Europe and the United States. Insights into Imaging. 2018;9:745–53.
35. Goodwin S, Rozovsky F. Teleradiology: compliance concerns and solutions. Part II J Health Care Compliance. 2007 Mar; 9(2):15–22.

# Telephone Communications

## 21

Mary Elizabeth Greenberg and Carol Rutenberg

## 21.1 Introduction

Patient screening, preparation, post-procedure education, support, triage, follow-up, and referral are often the responsibility of the radiology nurse. Responsibilities will likely also include information intake, update, and care coordination. All these activities require communication with patients, family, providers, and other healthcare team members.

These interventions require effective communication and will occur face-to-face, but it is likely that more often they take place remotely, primarily over the telephone, but also in the patent portal or via other technology. In radiology, patient safety and quality of care depend on effective communication [1]; in fact, communication failure is one of the most common patient safety events in radiology [2]. There is strong evidence linking poor communication and communication errors to patient safety and adverse outcomes; patient willingness to follow care advice or recommendations; patient and healthcare team satisfaction; and malpractice risk [3, 4].

Although this chapter focuses primarily on nurse patient communication over the telephone, radiology nurse communication with providers and other members of the healthcare team must also be recognized as a potential risk factor for patient safety. In fact, errors stemming from hand-off miscommunication have been identified as the leading cause of serious medical errors [5]. These and other communication errors have a high rate of occurrence in radiology settings [6]. Communication errors not only affect patient health outcomes but are also costly in terms of wasted resources and satisfaction for patients, providers, and staff.

It is therefore essential that the nurses involved in telephone or other remote communication with patients and providers remain aware that they *are engaged in nursing practice* and that extra caution is needed due to the inability to see and assess the patient in person. This chapter will address standards of practice for telephone or other remote communication, also known as telehealth nursing, and provide some guidelines for the nurse that, if followed, will ensure safety for the patients.

## 21.2 Telehealth Nursing Practice

Among the sophisticated technology that impacts and defines the role of the radiology nurse, the provision of care utilizing telehealth technology such as the telephone, patient portal, or video

---

M. E. Greenberg, PhD, RN-BC, C-TNP (✉)
School of Nursing, Northern Arizona University, Tucson, AZ, USA

C. Rutenberg, MNSc, RN-BC, C-TNP
Telephone Triage Consulting, Inc.,
Hot Springs, AR, USA

chat is often discounted. However, radiology nurses often utilize the telephone and other technologies to communicate with and provide care to patients both prior to and following many radiologic procedures. Because the telephone doesn't represent sophisticated technology, it is often assumed that provision of care over the telephone doesn't require specialized knowledge or skill. Although often overlooked as a source of risk, the potential for risk associated with this practice is considerable because of the need for the nurse to assess and manage patients who have potentially high-risk problems without the benefit of being able to see or touch their patient. This type of nursing has been identified as "…one of the most sophisticated and potentially high-risk forms of nursing practiced today" [7].

Radiology nurses engaging in telehealth encounters do so with limited sensory input. They must depend on the ability to communicate and their sense of hearing, supported by critical thinking and sound clinical judgment, to provide safe and appropriate care. Thus, provision of care using telehealth technology requires specialized skills and knowledge that are generally not provided in undergraduate nursing education. Although telehealth nursing is potentially risky, some basic principles, if enlisted, will help ensure the provision of safe and effective nursing care in the non-face-to-face setting.

Preparing a patient for a procedure may seem a straightforward interaction, but it is essential that the radiology nurse do an adequate patient assessment to ascertain factors such as health literacy, identify patient concerns, and determine whether previously undiscovered factors exist that might negatively impact the scheduled procedure. However, the greatest challenge and possibly the greatest risks lie in the post-procedure follow-up encounters [8]. This is when the nurse has an opportunity to identify covert complications or other problems and provide the patient with support and collaborative decision-making to address the concern.

For example, patients who have been discharged after a vascular procedure must be carefully assessed for pseudoaneurysm or hemorrhage. Peripheral circulation is always an area of concern in the event of vascular access. Furthermore, embolic phenomena are potential complications associated with virtually any invasive intravascular radiologic procedure. However, alarmingly, a routine follow-up call to a patient might fail to disclose these problems, *if the nurse is not actively looking for them.* In other words, actively inquiring about peripheral circulation (in layman's terms) might be necessary to identify an arterial occlusion. A belief that the patient will bring up the subject unprompted assumes a proactive patient who is either experiencing significant discomfort or has a concern about an unexpected finding.

Because nurse patient interaction primarily occurs over the ubiquitous telephone, regarded as a device that can be used by almost anyone, its use is easily taken for granted. The ability to provide nursing care over the phone is rarely considered a professional competency that requires compliance with the standards of care. Awareness of and adherence to the legal, ethical, and clinical standards of telehealth nursing practice ensures effective and safe communication with the patient.

## 21.3 Standards of Professional Nursing Practice

In the practice of telehealth nursing, just as in any other area of professional nursing practice, the registered nurse (RN) is accountable for compliance with the standards of professional nursing practice. These standards provide important principles to guide the nurse and the organization in provision and evaluation of clinical practice, design of initial and continuing education and training, and policy development that supports safe practice.

Professional standards are promulgated by such organizations as the International Council of Nurses (ICN) and national nurses associations such as the American Nurses Association (ANA) and provide general guidance to nurses. Standards specific to various clinical specialties are developed by specialty organizations such as the Association for Radiologic and Imaging Nursing

(ARIN). The American Academy of Ambulatory Care Nursing (AAACN) [9], an organization with international membership, has developed the *Scope and Standards of Practice for Professional Telehealth Nursing* (2018), which provide guidance and establish minimum standards of care for nurses practicing telehealth nursing in any setting.

Jurisdictional standards provide legal parameters for their country/state/municipality. Because telehealth encounters occur in a remote setting, geographical boundaries don't exist. This raises jurisdictional issues. Depending on jurisdiction, the locus of responsibility may be regarded as being at the location of the patient while in others it might be the location of the nurse. Because the nurse may be providing care in a remote location, the nurse involved in telehealth communication must be aware of the licensure and practice requirements for the jurisdiction in which they are providing care. Scope of practice is an important part of telehealth communication. Nursing care provided over the phone is still nursing care. It is therefore essential for radiology nurses and their colleagues to understand the scope of practice of the registered nurse (RN) in contrast to the more limited scope of practice of licensed practical (LPN) or vocational nurses (LVN).

Organizational standards can significantly impact the quality and safety of care using telehealth technology [7]. Nurses who provide telehealth services must be licensed and adequately trained to assess patients in the potentially ambiguous non-face-to-face setting. Call or message routing can significantly increase risk to the patient if a process doesn't exist to eliminate or reduce a possible delay in care. Lack of policies, procedures, and in some cases decision support tools can further obscure the practice, leaving the nurse without guidance when encountering difficult situations such as a patient who is reluctant to seek care or lacks a reliable source of transportation. The delivery of safe care may also in part be dependent on the presence of established collaborative relationships with radiologists and other members of the healthcare team. Facilitated access to the patient's medical record and other resources is also supportive of the delivery of effective telephonic communications.

## 21.4 Clinical Practice

The clinical skill set required for effective patient communication using technology is similar to the clinical skills necessary for any patient interaction. However, due to the unknown nature of the problem and the potentially ambiguous situation, slight modifications in how information is collected and processed should prove useful.

### 21.4.1 The Interview

Good communication skills and critical thinking are key to a meaningful telehealth encounter. Although messages may present through the patient portal, it is important to keep in mind that it is neither safe nor even possible to conduct an adequate assessment via a portal message or email. The patient interview is a dynamic process in which it is necessary to have a robust, real-time interaction with the patient, listening to *what* they say and *how* they say it. Live, real-time (synchronous) communication permits the nurse to not only listen to the patient's history but to concurrently collect nonverbal information as well, such as breathlessness or confusion. Additionally, *connecting* with the patient on a human level has been shown to facilitate the process [10]. Often, a meaningful outcome will be the provision of collaborative support to the patient, which the human connection helps facilitate [10].

In performing a patient interview over the phone, it is generally best to let the patient tell their story in their own way at their own pace because sometimes important information comes to them as an afterthought. Because most patients are not healthcare professionals, they often don't discern the difference between an inconsequential fact and a critical finding. It is important to *listen* to what the patient is saying (verbally and nonverbally) and avoid common pitfalls discussed later in this chapter. This process yields the *subjective* part of the patient assessment.

## 21.4.2 The Nursing Process

The nursing process is widely regarded as the basic standard of care, providing a blueprint for the practice of professional nursing, including nursing care provided utilizing telehealth technology. In present theory, it exists in six steps. The nurse first performs an adequate assessment to develop a nursing diagnosis regarding the nature and urgency of the patient's problem [11]. Based on that diagnosis, the nurse identifies desired outcomes, which in turn support and inform development of a plan of care. Once the plan is implemented, the RN must evaluate the effectiveness of the encounter [7, 9].

### 21.4.2.1 Assessment

The patient history, or the telling of their story, yields the *subjective* portion of the patient assessment. Because the nurse is most likely seeking specific information, it might be tempting to try to control the pace and direction of the history. However, it is most likely that simply listening is a best practice, interrupting only to seek clarification. It is critical to keep in mind that the patient might be experiencing an unexpected, and thus unknown, problem that might or might not be related to the purpose of the nurse's call and thus what is uppermost on the nurse's mind. For example, although the nurse's reason for the call might be to assess perfusion in an extremity that has been accessed, failure to listen to the patient carefully and with an open mind might result in a missed pulmonary embolus. That is, if the patient is focusing on the temperature, color, and sensation in a distal extremity, the patient might not feel it is related or even appropriate to mention chest pain or shortness of breath. Elements of the patient history that the RN should listen for include the following information at a minimum. The prudent nurse will listen for these elements, asking the specific questions only if the patient fails to volunteer the information on their own. This process allows the nurse to form a caring relationship and *get to know* the patient within the context of the encounter [10].

- *Problem*: What, if anything is concerning the patient? What type of assistance, if any, is the patient seeking? Sometimes the actual problem is not evident until later in the encounter, so it is important for the nurse to keep an open mind until they have actively or passively collected all relevant information.
- *Onset*: When did the symptom begin and was the onset sudden or gradual? What is its temporal proximity to any specific factors such as a recent interventional procedure?
- *Associated symptoms*: What else is the patient experiencing?
- *Medical history*: What procedures or treatments has the patient undergone recently? A review of chronic illnesses and current medications is also in order to identify unexpected complications or events.
- *Influencing factors*: What actions or interventions mitigate or exacerbate the problem? Has the patient taken any medications, altered position, made any other attempts to remedy the situation, and what were the results? Has the patient noticed that anything makes the problem decidedly worse?

As the nurse notes these and other potentially relevant elements of the patient's history, the nurse is thinking ahead, processing the meaning of what the patient is relating, clarifying, verifying, identifying and/or ruling out potential problems. While the identified problem might be as simple as the patient's failure to hold an anticoagulant prior to an invasive procedure, the potential goes beyond the routine screening questions. Really listening to the patient provides an opportunity for the nurse to detect and waylay fear, confusion, or misunderstanding regarding a scheduled procedure. Addressing this type of concern over the telephone will prevent case backlog or waste of resources resulting from a patient's inability or unwillingness to comply due to lack of understanding that they would need to lie very still without movement as a percutaneous tube was placed during the procedure. What may seem to the nurse to be a routine pre-procedure phone call actually provides an opportunity to inform, educate, and support the patient in order to keep things running smoothly and prevent a potentially negative or embarrassing experience for the patient.

As stated before, telephone communication is a dynamic intellectual process involving critical thinking and tapping into the RNs knowledge base born of education and experience. A lot of preliminary decision-making goes on during this process; however, it is critical for the nurse to avoid bias and keep an open mind throughout the data collection phase.

In addition to the *subjective* portion of the patient assessment, it is also possible and usually necessary to identify *objective* findings that might enhance the nurse's thinking. The nurse must assess the patient's respiratory status, identifying findings such as tachypnea or wheezing, which is best done by *listening* to the patient. Likewise, neurological concerns such as confusion and slurred speech might be evident as the nurse talks directly with the patient. Background noises and the patient's affect might also provide clues to the situation. A well-coached patient or caregiver is capable of being the eyes and hands of the nurse, serving as a surrogate to describe physical signs that can provide clarity. For example, the patient or their representative can compare the color and temperature of a potentially compromised distal extremity to the other, unaffected one. For example, the nurse might ask the caller to "look at and touch" the foot, observing color and temperature as compared to the other foot. Likewise, hydration status can be assessed based on information such as condition of mucous membranes and urinary output. Additionally, many patients today have home medical equipment which can provide objective information such as blood pressure, temperature, weight, and blood sugar. Although these instruments may not be accurately calibrated, they nonetheless provide data for day-to-day comparisons.

Finally, the nurse must listen or ask to ascertain what the patient hopes to get out of the encounter. If surmised from the patient history, it is important to directly confirm the patient agenda so that the nurse may meet that request or explain why it is not possible to do so and negotiate an acceptable alternative.

### 21.4.2.2 Diagnosis

The assessment provides the basis of the nursing diagnosis, or a clinical conclusion in a telehealth encounter. Depending on the type of encounter, the assessment might lead to varying types of nursing diagnoses. For example, the nursing diagnosis in a telephone triage call is identification and expression of the *nature* and the *urgency* of the patient's problem. This problem is usually identified through a process of clinical reasoning ideally guided by decision support tools. Because of the complex nature of this process, it often requires extensive knowledge and experience. Likewise, if symptoms or problems are identified in the course of a follow-up call, what was intended to be a quick, routine call must now be recognized as a triage call. Such issues as knowledge deficit or anxiety can also be represented as a nursing diagnosis, thus providing a basis for identification of desired outcomes and eventually informing the plan of care.

### 21.4.2.3 Outcomes

Based on the patient assessment and nursing diagnosis, the nurse identifies desired outcomes. This might be to address any known or suspected complications following an invasive procedure. The patient may desire to be further evaluated in a face-to-face setting or the patient might prefer being able to better understand their situation and to be able to care for themselves at home unless further problems develop.

### 21.4.2.4 Plan of Care

The plan of care is how the nurse and patient have collaboratively agreed to achieve the desired outcomes. This might be represented as "seek care immediately," "observe extremity for signs of vascular compromise," or "continue home care unless situation deteriorates."

### 21.4.2.5 Intervention

As in other nursing encounters, the intervention is operationalization of the plan of care. This provides a detailed account of how the plan will be carried out. In looking at the plans of care identified above, the corresponding interventions might be "Hang up and dial 911" or

"Proceed to emergency department immediately with another adult to drive." In the second instance an intervention might be to educate the patient and/or caregiver on the signs of vascular compromise, explain the significance of such findings, and extract a commitment from the patient to call back or seek care immediately if any of those signs or symptoms develop. Finally, the patient whose plan is to continue home care should be instructed on what observations to make and with what frequency, and how to care for himself at home. The patient should always be encouraged to call back (including information of who and where to call) if any additional problems or questions arise. Don't forget to provide information of who and where to call.

#### 21.4.2.6 Evaluation
Finally, a decision must be made regarding how to evaluate the success of the encounter. This is based on progress toward achievement of the desired outcomes. Most simply, this can be an assessment of the patient's level of understanding of, or comfort with, the health education/information provided. Verbalization of understanding is of equal if not greater importance in the telehealth setting where nonverbal indications of understanding (such as the nodding head) are not available. If action was taken, whether the patient understood the need to "seek care immediately" and agreed to comply might be the extent of the evaluation. It is important to explore this step carefully because a plan without action is meaningless. If the patient is facing transportation challenges or financial concern, that might impact his ability to comply with the agreed upon plan of care. Once this secondary information has been gathered, the nurse might have to perform further interventions to collaborate with and guide the patient in problem solving.

### 21.5 Documentation

Use of the nursing process also provides a blueprint for excellent documentation. Using this process as a basis for documentation enables the nurse to systematically record patient data and express conversion of that data into clinical information that reflects critical thinking, clinical judgment, and clinical reasoning (if required). Further, documentation of the plan of care, how it is carried out, and the process utilized to evaluate the care rendered (i.e., achievement of desired outcomes) will provide complete documentation of the nursing care provided and serve as a basis for follow-up calls, should they be necessary. As a safety measure, timely documentation (communication) in the electronic health record (EHR) is essential in radiology where the radiologist, referring and or consulting provider, and all department team members access the information in the EHR [12].

### 21.6 Basic Skill Set for Telehealth Nursing

As has been demonstrated, nursing is nursing, and use of telehealth technology does not mitigate the nurse's imperative to comply with the standards of care. However, several clinical pitfalls have been identified which have been shown to negatively impact care in the telehealth setting. Although some were alluded to earlier in the chapter, they are worth specific mention in order to assure patient safety in a radiology telehealth encounter[7].

To illustrate and promote understanding of the importance of avoiding the pitfalls discussed, consider the following scenario.

A 70-year-old female had a femoral artery catheterization earlier today and was discharged home without incident. The nurse is tasked with the responsibility of making a follow-up call in the midst of a very busy workday. The patient states that she is "worn out" and admits to some vague back pain. However, when the nurse seeks clarification, the patient immediately discounts her symptoms, explaining that she already has a bad back and it was aggravated by having to lie on a hard table for an extended time prior to and following her procedure. She does mention, however, that it is unusual that this is radiating to her groin, but again, she is sure the pain is positional.

The nurse should review and recognize the potential for a bad outcome in this case in the context of the following precautions.

### 21.6.1 Speak Directly with the Patient Whenever Possible

Occasionally, especially when the patient is likely to be regarded as a poor historian for one reason or another (e.g., illness, age, health literacy), it is tempting to speak exclusively with a family member or caregiver. However, while these individuals can certainly participate in the interview, it is important to speak directly to the patient as well. Failure to do so may cause the nurse to overlook meaningful symptoms. While the family or caregiver may be a good source of information, the most accurate description of symptoms will come from the patient. Additionally, as discussed previously, direct auditory assessment of the patient by the nurse can provide meaningful, sometimes critical, information. In the scenario above, failure to speak with the patient might fail to disclose the nonspecific back pain.

### 21.6.2 Listen to the Patient

*Listen* to what the patient is saying. Research in telephone triage encounters has shown that nurses are occasionally poor listeners (and sometimes poor communicators as well) [13, 14]. Listening for subtle signs of distress or a report of unexpected findings may be the nurse's first clue that a problem exists. Actively listening to what the patient says and doesn't say may provide significant insight into what is going on with the patient or what the experience means to them. In the example of the patient with post-procedure back pain, she made an offhand comment that it is unusual for the pain to radiate to her groin. If the nurse hears this and follows up, it might lead to discovery that this is different than her usual back pain.

### 21.6.3 Anticipate Worst Possible

Although the vast majority of telehealth radiology patients will not experience unexpected problems, the potential risk associated with overlooking a potentially life-threatening problem does exist. An adage goes, "If you don't find it often, you often don't find it" (source unknown), and this certainly applies to telehealth nursing in the radiology and interventional radiology settings. Considering our patient scenario, although uncommon, rare complications such as retroperitoneal hematoma do occur. However, if the possibility is not even considered, it might not be recognized until the patient is compromised.

### 21.6.4 Err on the Side of Caution

One hard-and-fast rule of thumb to assure patient safety is to *err on the side of caution* if there is even a remote possibility that the patient might be experiencing a high-risk complication. In other words, telehealth nursing (especially telephone triage) is often based on the practice of *exclusion*. Unless able to comfortably rule out a potentially life, limb, or vision threatening problem (a "worst possible" scenario) the patient should promptly be evaluated in a face-to-face setting. In our case example, back and/or groin pain following interventional radiology (even if it involved an extended period on a hard surface) must be evaluated if the possibility exists and the nurse is unable to rule out a significant complication. Many have learned the parable of the little boy who cried wolf and feel their clinical competence may come into question if they "overreact" to a clinical situation. In telehealth nursing encounters, it is not necessary to be "right" but being "wrong" can prove fatal.

### 21.6.5 Use Caution in Accepting Patient Self-diagnosis

Consider the preceding example of the patient with the retroperitoneal hematoma. Even though she admits to back pain, it is possible to summarily discount the symptom if the patient explains that her back pain is due to the hard table that she laid on for an extended period prior to and following her procedure. Patients endeavor to find explanations for problems that occur which they did not anticipate. Although patients are often right in their conclusions, they can also be wrong. Their picture can further be obscured if they have consulted "Dr. Internet," and in so doing have diagnosed themselves.

### 21.6.6 Avoid Jumping to a Conclusion

Closely related to other pitfalls, jumping to a conclusion can lead to unfavorable outcomes. Every encounter must be carefully considered for possibilities other than the obvious. Stereotyping patients ("she's a frequent complainer"), assuming "most common" instead of "worst possible," and accepting patient self-diagnosis are all pitfalls that can lead to unfavorable outcomes.

### 21.6.7 Use Special Caution when Fatigued or Rushed and Avoid Being Multitasked

It is not unusual for nurses to have multiple priorities during the course of a shift. It is critical to be aware that fatigue, haste, and multitasking can all take their toll on a nurse's ability to concentrate. Interruptions and distractions, both internal and external, might interfere with capturing and processing key elements of the encounter. Performing follow-up calls during a time with competing priorities or when time is short at the end of the day should either be avoided or approached with extreme caution.

### 21.6.8 Assure Continuity of Care and Document all Calls

Although telehealth nursing encounters may seem episodic, it is critical to remember that they are but one step along the continuum of care. If not the starting point of care, they are an integral part of the course of the patient's medical experience. And they are almost never the final point along that route. Although much of the function of the nurse engaging in the practice of telehealth nursing is autonomous, it must be recognized that it represents a highly collaborative practice. Communication with other members of the team is of critical importance and requires careful attention to ensure safe transitions between clinical specialty areas and the community. This imperative can be facilitated by clearly documented nurse-patient communication which can be accessed by other members of the team. This is a way to close real and potential gaps in care and facilitate safe and appropriate follow-up or intervention if needed. This is especially important in that professionals from multiple disciplines or specialties are often involved in the patient's care and the information communicated between the nurse and the patient serves to keep all in the loop.

## 21.7 Conclusion

The primary communication tool utilized in telehealth nursing, the telephone, is often not recognized as a method of delivering complex nursing care to high-risk patients. The process of providing care utilizing telehealth technology is more than simply the exchange of information, and it is certainly more than a "phone call." Telehealth nursing is a meaningful form of communication and care delivery that helps ensure safe care, facilitate access, and enhance continuity. Without adequate training and recognition of the validity of telehealth nursing, nurses may fail to capitalize on the vast potential of this practice. These types of encounters, whether involving telephones or more sophisticated technology, have become common practice and provide an opportunity to "be there" for the patient in their own environment. Telehealth technology provides the radiology nurse with daily opportunities to provide patient-centered care and to identify and prevent real or potential problems, thereby improving the health and safety of the patients who depend on them.

## References

1. ItriJN. Patient-centered radiology. RadioGraphics. 2015[cited 2019 Apr 30];35(6):1835–46. Available from: http://search.ebscohost.com.libproxy.nau.edu/login.aspx?direct=true&db=ccm&AN=117075159&site=ehost-live&scope=site.
2. Jabin SR, Schultz T, Hibbert P, Mandel C, Runciman C. Effectiveness of quality improvement interventions for patient safety in radiology: a systematic review protocol. JBI Database Syst Rev Implement Rep. 2016;14(9):65–78. https://doi.org/10.11124/JBISRIR-2016-003078.
3. Institute for Healthcare Communication. Impact of communication in healthcare. New Haven, CT:Institute for Healthcare Communication; 2011[cited 2019 May1]. Available from: https://healthcarecomm.org/about-us/impact-of-communication-in-healthcare/.
4. Lang EV. A better patient experience through better communication. J Radiol Nurs. 2012[cited 2019 May 1];31(4):114–9. https://doi.org/10.1016/j.jradnu.2012.08.001.
5. Joint Commission on Accreditation of Healthcare Organizations. Joint Commission Center for Transforming Healthcare releases targeted solutions tool for hand-off communications. Jt Comm Perspect. 2012;32(8):1, 3.
6. Hannaford N, Mandel C, Crock C, Buckley K, Magrabi F, Ong M, Allen S, Schultz T. Learning from incident reports in the Australian medical imaging setting: handover and communication errors. Br J Radiol. 2013;86(1022):20120336. https://doi.org/10.1259/bjr.20120336.
7. Rutenberg C, Greenberg ME. The art and science of telephone triage: how to practice nursing over the phone. Hot Springs, AR: Telephone Triage Consulting, Inc.; 2012.
8. Rutenberg C, Greenberg ME. Telephone nursing in radiology: managing the risk. J Radiol Nurs. 2014[cited 2019 May 1];33(2):63–8. https://doi.org/10.1016/j.jradnu.2012.08.001.
9. American Academy of Ambulatory Care Nursing. The scope and standards of practice for profession telehealth nursing. 6th ed. Pitman, NJ: AAACN; 2018.
10. Greenberg ME. A comprehensive model of the process of telephone nursing. J Adv Nurs. 2009;65(12):2621–9. https://doi.org/10.1111/j.1365-2648.2009.05132.x.
11. Greenberg ME, Espensen M, Becker C, Cartwright JP. Telehealth nursing practice SIG adopts teleterms. AAACN Viewpoint. 2003;25(1):8–10.
12. Swift M. The impact of poor communication on medical errors. The doctor weighs in, 5 Dec 2017 [cited 2019 May 1]. Available from: https://thedoctorweighsin.com/impact-poor-communication-on-medical-errors/
13. Ernesäter A, Winblad U, Engström M, Holström IK. Malpractice claims regarding calls to Swedish telephone advice nursing: what went wrong and why? J Telemed Telecare. 2012;18(7):379–83. https://doi.org/10.1258/jtt.2012.120416.
14. Ernesäter A, Engström M, Winblad U, Holmström IK. A comparison of calls subjected to a malpractice claim versus 'normal calls' within the Swedish healthcare direct: a case-control study. BMJ Open. 2014;4(10):e005961. https://doi.org/10.1136/bmjopen-2014-005961.

# Health Literacy

**22**

Beth Ann Hackett

## 22.1 Introduction

Health literacy is defined as the knowledge and competency of persons to meet the complex demands of health processes [1]. Individuals must be able to evaluate one's own health, the health of one's family, and the community's health in order to understand which influencing factors lead to good health, as well as understanding how to address pertinent issues. Unfortunately, inadequate health literacy is a widespread problem in both non-industrialized and industrialized nations, and it is mostly related to deficient reading skills [2]. One must differentiate however between reading skills and understanding the health information put forth [1].

It is important to differentiate between literacy and health literacy. The term "health literacy" first appeared in peer-reviewed academic literature in 1974 [3]. However, by the author's own report it had nothing at all to do with the current understanding of the concept and was more an accident of English than an intentional representation of a singular concept. The term health literacy began appearing in the academic peer-reviewed literature in earnest in the early 1990s and has experienced nearly exponential growth since these efforts began [4]. In the 1900s research showed that there was a strong correlation between education and health. As the lack of health literacy has been documented as a realistic healthcare issue, there has been much research and publications to address this problem. Low health literacy is associated with poorer health outcomes and improper use of healthcare. People cannot achieve their fullest health potential unless they are able to take control and understand those things which determine their healthcare services.

In the Institute of Medicine (IOM) report, *Health Literacy: A Prescription to End Confusion*, health literacy is defined as the ability of an individual to obtain, process, and understand basic health information and services needed to make appropriate health decisions [5]. The Patient and Affordable Care Act of 2010 defined health literacy as the degree to which an individual has the capacity to obtain, communicate, process, and understand basic health information and services in order to make appropriate health decisions [6]. An individual's level of health literacy is determined and affected by a multitude of variants. A person must possess basic literacy skills that include the ability to read, write, speak, and compute and solve problems prior to being able to navigate the healthcare system [7]. Additionally, the individual must be able to communicate and listen during interactions.

According to the National Assessment of Adult Literacy only 12% of adults have proficient health literacy [7]. Thus, nearly nine out of ten

B. A. Hackett, DNP, APRN, CRN (✉)
Midstate Radiology Associates, LLC,
Meriden, CT, USA

adults may lack the skills needed to manage their health and prevent disease. Fourteen percent of adults (30 million people) have below basic health literacy. These adults were more likely to report their health as poor (42%) and are more likely to lack health insurance (28%) than adults with proficient health literacy [4]. Language barriers, socioeconomic status, and educational attainment influences explained that even people with high literacy skills might have difficulty using information [5].

Specific outcomes associated with low health literacy include, but are not limited to, poor adherence to medical regimes, poor understanding of the complex nature of their own health, a lack of knowledge about medical care and conditions, poorer comprehension of medical information, low understanding and use of preventive services, poorer overall health status, and earlier death [8]. Those with low health literacy tend to use emergency services more often, are hospitalized more often, are readmitted to the hospital over and over, have a hard time understanding numbers, such as cholesterol and blood sugar levels, and medication amounts, and die earlier[7].

## 22.2 Identification of Patients with Low Health Literacy

Providers and healthcare workers must be able to identify patients with low health literacy to provide optimum care to the full spectrum of their practice. Patients with low literacy have an inclination to present with particular tendencies. The AHRQ Health Literacy Universal Precautions Toolkit defines red flags for low literacy. Red flags for low literacy are listed in Table 22.1.

People with low health literacy are less able to: share health history, with providers, use preventive services, such as early disease screenings, or manage a chronic health problem, such as diabetes or high blood pressure. Low health literacy is linked to: low quality of care, high healthcare costs, poor health outcomes, and increased health disparities.

**Table 22.1** Red flags for low literacy

| |
|---|
| Frequently miss appointments |
| Submit incomplete registration forms and take a long time to complete forms |
| Are noncompliance with medication regimes |
| Are unable to name medications, explain purpose or dosing of their medication |
| Identify pills by looking at them, not reading the label |
| Are unable to give coherent, sequential medical histories |
| Lack follow-through on tests or referrals |
| Forget his or her glasses and state the need to read materials at home |
| Seek help only when illness is advanced |
| Have a tendency to not ask questions or have fewer questions |
| Have relevant documents related to their medical care tucked away in their purse |

## 22.3 Barriers to Health Literacy

According to the U.S. 2003 National Assessment of Adult Literacy (NAAL), limited health literacy affects some groups more than others. These include the elderly, individuals with limited education, members of minority groups who do not speak English as their first language, and the poor [7]. Additionally, even those individuals that possess good reading skills may still face low health literacy skills due to the fact that they are unfamiliar with medical terms and how the body works, are diagnosed with a serious disease and feel scared and confused, and might have disabilities that make it hard to access health services. Research demonstrates that increased age, low education, low socioeconomic status, and poor reading level are among the major barriers to health literacy [5]. Along with other socioeconomic issues, literature reveals that one of the barriers faced by people having low health literacy level around the world is due to misunderstanding of health information [9]. The ability to correctly read medical information declines with age [10]. Inadequate health literacy is strongly linked with education. Poor understanding of health-related information and ignorance leads to poor management of health among the less educated population, leading to early deaths [5]. A study conducted in 11 European Union countries concluded that secondary and tertiary education contributes in improving health-related knowledge among individuals [11]. The more a higher level of education is attained, the more health knowledge is improved, personal empowerment is gained, and self-worth is valued [12]. Furthermore, evidence supports cognitive impairment and dementia associated with the elderly leads to difficulty in information processing; however, these are not associated with a lower education level [4, 13]. Low-income populations usually possess low reading skills resulting in low health literacy [10]. A good level of earning contributes positively to managing health and taking proper self-care [11]. A high prevalence of chronic diseases like hypertension, diabetes, and hypercholesterolemia leading to cerebrovascular disease and stroke are among the major barriers to health literacy as all of these diseases affect mental abilities and disables the brain to function properly [4].

### 22.3.1 The Language of Healthcare

Healthcare professionals have their own culture and language. Many adopt the "culture of medicine" and the language of their specialty as a result of their training and work environment that may affect how health professionals communicate with the public. This communication may not meet the needs of their patients, especially those with low health literacy. For many individuals with limited English proficiency (LEP), the inability to communicate in English is the primary barrier to accessing health information and services. Health information for people with LEP needs to be communicated plainly in their primary language, using words and examples that make the information understandable.

### 22.3.2 Deficiency in Knowledge of Health Topics

In addition to basic literacy skills, health literacy requires knowledge of health topics. People with limited health literacy often lack knowledge or have misinformation about the body, as well as the nature and causes of disease. Without this knowledge, they may not understand the simplistic relationship between lifestyle factors such as diet and exercise and the health consequences. They lack the ability to implement self-care activities. In 2014 an American Society of Neuroradiology analysis found that the patient education resources on their web sites failed to meet the guidelines of the National Institutes of Health (NIH) and American Medical Association (AMA) [14]. Members of the public may fail to fully understand website resources and would benefit from revisions that result in more comprehensible information cast in simpler language.

## 22.4 Health Literacy in Radiology

Literature analysis of the effects of low health literacy in the radiology environment is limited. A movement is growing within radiology to adapt to the changing healthcare environment and focus on a patient-centered approach to improve patient satisfaction, quality, and safety [15]. Included in the pre-imaging or preintervention steps for some radiological examinations are preps or other instructions that must be followed. It is challenging for radiology patients with low health literacy to follow written instructions regarding the home preparation in order for examination completion [16]. In a study regarding bowel preparation for colonoscopies, it was found that patients with low health literacy presented for their colonoscopies without having followed the bowel prep leading to an inferior diagnostic quality of the examination, repeated radiation exposure, or cancellation of the examination [16, 17]. Frequently patients receive written materials for radiological examinations that are written at an elevated reading level and not well understood [14, 18–21]. In a study done on emergency room pediatric patients and the utilization of radiologic testing in this group, it was found that both a minority race and low health literacy were linked with less testing [22]. Failure to obtain the proper testing leads to improper diagnosis and treatment. A comparative analysis of online patient educational resources was conducted for health literacy in interventional radiology. Researchers found that due to lack of reading skills, online patient education materials are not understood by most which leads to poor examination preparation as well as interpretation of the result in the imaging report [19]. The consequences of unprepared patients undergoing imaging examinations may delay the imaging, as well as cause a delay in treatment[19]. According to research, there is a discrepancy between the level of readability of information provided on the internet and the literacy level of patients; thus, the information is not understood and interpretation is incomplete [23].

## 22.5 Interventions and Tools for Improving Health Literacy

There is a plethora of information available to assist in the development of educational tools for patients. There are, however, limited studies that examined the impact of different interventions for improving health literacy especially in specific populations [24]. The Centers for Disease Control and Prevention (CDC) website (https://www.cdc.gov)offers a multitude of resources to assist in developing health communication and social marketing programs [25]. The U.S. Department of Health and Human Services, National Resource Center for Health IT, offers a guide and checklist, "*Accessible Health Information Technology (IT) for populations with Limited Literacy: A Guide for Developers and Purchases of Health IT*" (https://healthit.ahrq.gov/sites/default/files/docs/page/LiteracyGuide), that can be used to develop and evaluate internet products for consumers on health information [26]. Additionally, the U.S. Department of Health and Human Services, National Cancer Institute, and National Institutes of Health outlines a process for developing publications for people with limited literacy skills called "Clear and Simple: Developing Effective Print Materials for Low-Literate Readers" [11]. A "*Quick Guide to Health Literacy*" is offered by The U.S. Department of Health & Human Services, Office of Disease Prevention and Health Promotion. The *Quick Guide to Health Literacy* is for government employees, grantees, contractors, and community partners working in healthcare and public health fields. The guide provides information on key health literacy concepts; techniques for improving health literacy through communication, navigation, knowledge building, and advocacy; examples of health literacy best practices; and suggestions for addressing health literacy in your organization [11].

Some guideline information targets specific populations, for example, the "*Quick Guide to Health Literacy and Older Adults*" guide provides background information on health literacy, strategies, and suggestions for communicating with older adults. This guide is published by the U.S. Department of Health & Human Services, Office of Disease Prevention and Health Promotion's [9].

The following tools have been developed for the evaluation of healthcare literacy. These are listed in Table 22.2.

Health finder® is an award-winning federal web site for consumers, developed by the U.S. Department of Health and Human Services and other federal agencies. Since 1997, Health

**Table 22.2** Tools for the evaluation of healthcare literacy

| Tool name | Source |
| --- | --- |
| Universal Precautions Toolkit | www.nchealthliteracy.org/toolkit/ |
| Optimizing Health Literacy and Access Process(Including health literacy needs, assessment, and intervention development) | www.ophelia.net |
| Building Health Literate Organizations: A guide book for Achieving Organizational Change (Includes excellent case studies and teach-back resources | www.unitypoint.org/healthliteracy-guidebook.aspx |
| "Always Use Teach-back" Training Toolkit | www.eteachbacktraining.org/ |
| Enliven Organizational Health Literacy Self-assessment Resource50 | www.enliven.org.au/library.html |
| Multidimensional health literacy measurement tools | www.ophelia.net.au16 |

**Table 22.3** Six levels of evaluation and potential purposes for measuring health literacy

| Levels | Potential purposes for measuring health literacy |
|---|---|
| Individual patients | To problem solve for complex patients, to train staff in responding to differing health literacy needs |
| Patient groups | To identify common factors that contribute to poor access and health outcomes to plan for services to respond to health literacy needs to inform advocacy activities |
| Individual health services | To diagnose health literacy strengths and limitations of the target population and how these strengths and limitations contribute to known inequalities of access, participation in health and health outcomes to develop specific strategies for responding to common health literacy limitations community and population settings |
| Local areas (both health and community services/authorities) | To plan marketing and education strategies across services to assess the ability of community members to participate in community-based health planning activities (critical health literacy) and develop suitable approaches to enable their participation |
| National surveys (to compare regions and groups) | To identify relationships between health literacy and access, equity and outcomes, in order to develop appropriate health service and public health policies and strategies; plan health education campaigns, or campaigns to support the introduction of new services, screening initiatives (e.g., bowel or skin cancer) or vaccination programs; assess regional "patient difficulty" for planning and funding purposes (assuming that it takes more intensive resources to improve health outcomes for people with low health literacy than it does for people with higher health literacy) |
| Countries (international comparisons) | Advocacy for governments in countries where there is systemic low health literacy; identify countries that are role models for how to improve health literacy levels of populations |

Adapted from: https://ppgenf.fen.ufg.br/up/127/o/Batterham_2016.pdf

finder® has been recognized as a key resource for finding the best government and nonprofit health and human services information on the Internet. Health finder® links to carefully selected information and web sites from more than 1500 health-related organizations [13].

According to Batterham et al. [27] health literacy is multidimensional and must be evaluated at varying levels. They suggest six levels of evaluation and potential purposes for measuring health literacy across the healthcare spectrum which are the following [27] (Table 22.3).

## 22.6 Improvement of Health Literacy

The healthcare providers across the spectrum must work together to ensure that health information and services can be understood and used by all. We must engage in skill building with healthcare consumers and health professionals. Adult educators can be productive partners in reaching adults with limited literacy skills. The National Institutes of Health (NIH) and the American Medical Association (AMA) recommend online patient education resources written at a third-to-seventh grade level. Plain Language (www.planlanguage.gov) is a technique to write clear and to the point. It is also a strategy we can use to improve health literacy. Presently, there is not a global organization for health literacy researchers, practitioners, and policymakers. Therefore, there is no known structure through which to contact practitioners, researchers, academics, and policymakers working with health literacy.

The "teach-back" method has been used to assess patient comprehension of medical instructions and has been shown to improve adherence [4, 15]. Literature review confirms that both written and verbal health information combined are necessary to improve the knowledge and level of satisfaction of caregivers at the time of discharging their patients as compared to provision of verbal information only [28]. Repetition reinforces the patient's knowledge.

The use of available trained professional medical interpreters should be used whenever there is a need and the resource is available. Using family or friends as interpreters is *not* recommended as the interpretation may not have the intended meaning. The International Medical Interpreters Association is one available resource (see https://www.imiaweb.org/resources/telephoneint.asp).

## 22.7 Conclusion

Low health literacy is known to be a "silent killer." This can be tackled by closing the gaps between health messages and health messengers by using simplified language and including cultural appropriateness [5]. A review of the literature confirms that both written and verbal health information combined are necessary to improve the knowledge and level of satisfaction of care givers at the time of discharging their patients as compared to provision of verbal information only [4, 12].

Despite the diligence worldwide to address low health literacy, it remains a prominent issue in the healthcare setting. Patients are not receiving proper health instructions due to lack of understanding of the information put forth, written and digitally. It has been suggested in the literature that needs based assessments should be performed in order to assist healthcare providers in providing the most comprehensive literature to promote health for patients [15].

There are many tools available to measure health literacy; however, we need to incorporate and evaluate the way healthcare information is presented. Low health literacy has been identified as an ongoing issue in the healthcare environment that must be collaboratively and collectively incorporated into our workflow. Professional societies can play a role in increasing health literacy through promotion of patient-centered care.

## References

1. Sørensen K, Broucke SV, Fullam J, Doyle G, Pelikan J, Slonska Z, Brand H. Health literacy and public health: a systematic review and integration of definitions and models. BMC Public Health. 2012;12(1):80. https://doi.org/10.1186/1471-2458-12-80.
2. Pleasant A. Health literacy: an opportunity to improve individual, community, and global health. Adult EducHealth Wellness. 2011;130(2011):43–54.
3. Simonds SK. Health education as social policy. Health EducMonogr. 1974;2:25.
4. Johnson A, Sandford J. Written and verbal information versus verbal information only for patients being discharged from acute hospital settings to home: systematic review. Health Educ Res. 2005;20(4):423–9.
5. Nielsen-Bohlman L. Health literacy: a prescription to end confusion. Washington, DC: National Academies Press; 2004.http://healthit.ahrq.gov/portal/server.pt/gateway/PTARGS_0_3882_803031_0_0_18/LiteracyGuideh.pdf.
6. Williams J. The patient protection and affordable care act meets the 'persistently uninsured'. Soc Pol Admin. 2016;50(4):452–66. https://doi.org/10.1111/spol.12238.
7. National Assessment of Adult Literacy (NAAL). n.d. Retrieved from https://nces.ed.gov/naal/health.asp,www.nci.nih.gov/cancerinformation/clearandsimple.
8. Institute of Medicine (US) Roundtable on Health Literacy. Measures of health literacy: workshop summary. Washington, DC: National Academies Press; 2009. Available from: https://www.ncbi.nlm.nih.gov/books/NBK45384
9. U.S. Department of Health and Human Services. Quick guide to health literacy and older adults. Washington, DC: U.S. Department of Health and Human Services; 2007.
10. Comprehensive Cancer Information.n.d.Retrieved fromhttp://www.nci.nih.gov/cancerinformation/clearandsimple. Accessed 20 Jan 2019.
11. Quick Guide to Health Literacy. n.d. Retrieved from https://health.gov/communication/literacy/quickguide/Quickguide.pdf13.
12. Zarcadoolas C. The simplicity complex: exploring simplified health messages in a complex world. Health Promot Int. 2011;26(3):338–50.
13. Health Literacy.n.d.Retrieved from https://healthfinder.gov/FindServices/SearchContext.aspx?topic=3798
14. Hansberry DR, Agarwal N, Gonzales SF, Baker SR. Are we effectively informing patients? A quantitative analysis of on-line patient education resources from the American Society of Neuroradiology. AJNR Am J Neuroradiol. 2014;35(7):1270–5.
15. Abujudeh HM, Danielson A, Bruno MA. A patient-centered radiology quality process map: opportunities and solutions. Am J Roentgenol. 2016;207(5):940–6. https://doi.org/10.2214/ajr.16.16803.
16. Goguen J. Health literacy and patient preparation in radiology. J Med Imag Radiat Sci. 2016;47(3):283–6. https://doi.org/10.1016/j.jmir.2016.06.002.
17. Nguyen DL, Wieland M. Risk factors predictive of poor-quality preparation during average risk colonos-

copy screening: the importance of health literacy. J Gastrointest Liver Dis. 2010;19:369–72.
18. Hansberry DR, John A, John E, Agarwal N, Gonzales SF, Baker SR. A critical review of the readability of online patient education resources from RadiologyInfo.Org. AJR Am J Roentgenol. 2014;202:566–75.
19. Hansberry DR, Kraus C, Agarwal N, Baker SR, Gonzales SF. Health literacy in vascular and interventional radiology: a comparative analysis of online patient education resources. Cardiovasc Intervent Radiol. 2014;37(4):1034–40.
20. McEnteggart GE, Naeem M, Skierkowski D, Baird GL, Ahn SH, Soares G. Readability of online patient education materials related to IR. J Vasc Interv Radiol. 2015;26(8):1164–8.
21. Shukla P, Sanghvi SP, Lelkes VM, Kumar A, Contractor S. Readability assessment of internet-based patient education materials related to uterine artery embolization. J Vasc Interv Radiol. 2013;24(4):469–74.
22. Morrison AK, Brousseau DC, Brazauskas R, Levas MN. Health literacy affects likelihood of radiology testing in the pediatric emergency department. J Pediatr. 2015;166(4):1037–41.e1. https://doi.org/10.1016/j.jpeds.2014.12.009.
23. McCray AT. Promoting health literacy. J Am Med Inform Assoc. 2005;12(2):152–63.
24. Madeeha M, Rubab ZZ, Azhar H. Health literacy as a global public health concern: a systematic review. J Pharmacol Clin Res. 2017;4(2):555632. https://doi.org/10.19080/JPCR.2017.04.555632.
25. Campaigns|Gateway to Health Communication|CDC. n.d. Retrieved from http://www.cdc.gov/healthcommunication/campaigns/index.html.
26. Whitten P, Nazione S, Lauckner C. Tools for assessing the quality and accessibility of online health information: initial testing among breast cancer websites. Inform Health Soc Care. 2013;38(4):366–81. https://doi.org/10.3109/17538157.2013.812644.
27. Batterham R, Hawkins M, Collins P, Buchbinder R, Osborne R. Health literacy: applying current concepts to improve health services and reduce health inequalities. Public Health. 2016;132:3–12. https://doi.org/10.1016/j.puhe.2016.01.001.
28. Sudore RL, Schillinger D. Interventions to improve care for patients with limited health literacy. J Clin Outcomes Manag. 2009;16(1):20–9.

# The Patient Experience in Radiology

**23**

Sanne H. Henninger

## 23.1 Introduction

Patient experience is increasingly recognized as one of the three pillars of quality in healthcare alongside clinical performance effectiveness and patient safety [1]. The growing body of research demonstrates meaningful links between clinical safety and focus on the patient experience. A summary of 55 studies indicates positive associations and recommendations for patient experience as a primary focus in safety and quality efforts [2]. The concepts of safety, medical errors, and harm have been of interest but were brought into focus when the Institute of Medicine's landmark report, *To Err is Human: Building a Safer Health System* (1999), revealed tens of thousands of patients die every year from medical errors [3]. This interest launched an increasing focus on understanding how the patient experience and safety are inextricably linked and have been elevated as the base for performance improvement efforts in healthcare. To be successful in this regard, healthcare facilities must have an integrative model with system designs and a culture that put the patient at the center of all decisions. It will require teams that perform at the highest possible level where performance improvement is continuous. Nursing plays a primary role in the success of patient experience, team functioning, and performance improvement.

## 23.2 Importance of Patient Experience and Alignment with Safety Culture and Performance Improvement

A healthcare system should affirm that patients are at the center of all decisions, teamwork focus, and improvement strategies. When patient experience efforts are in isolation from safety and performance improvement initiatives, the opportunities for teams to fully evaluate problems and solutions from a systems perspective is lost. For example, most diagnostic decisions come from the history-taking component of the patient experience with nursing and providers. This interaction requires comfortable and thorough communication between patient and healthcare staff, typically considered a patient experience tactic. If that interaction is poor because a healthcare worker is not perceived as caring or is not thorough, that information gathering, physical examination, lab evaluation, and final diagnosis may be compromised [4]. Careful listening is often considered a soft-skills domain of the patient experience but is as much about safety and clinical effectiveness as it is about

S. H. Henninger, Ed.D, MSW, LCSW (✉)
Duke Health—Private Diagnostic Clinic, PLLC, Durham, NC, USA

positive interactions with our patients. Studies show that patients are often interrupted and not provided the opportunity or time to tell their story leading to incomplete data upon which decision are made [5]. Research shows that enhanced patient experience is associated with better patient engagement and therefore greater adherence to treatment plans and follow-up [6, 7]. Additionally, patients with better care experiences have better health outcomes [8]. For example, studies of patients hospitalized for heart attack revealed that patients with more positive reports about their experiences with care had better health outcomes a year after discharge [9]. These are just a few examples of the importance of effective communication and relationships on the patient experience. Patient experience is also associated with patient loyalty, reduced likelihood of malpractice claims, and even healthcare staff personal resilience. Patient experience is more than soft-skills or kindness but includes all aspects of the patient experience and alignment with all patient quality and safety outcomes is critical. In summary, when patient experience efforts are in the forefront on strategy and integrated with safety and performance initiatives, patients have better outcomes.

## 23.2.1 Definitions and Key Drivers of Patient Experience

In order to direct efforts to the needs of our patients, developing patient experience definitions that best encompass those needs is a critical first step. To start, patient experience and patient satisfaction are often used interchangeably but they are not the same thing. The term patient satisfaction might be limited to soft-skills communication and pleasantries to make patients happy or satisfied with a healthcare event. The term patient satisfaction implies that the patient was satisfied with their care but potentially represents a mediocre standard. It does not embrace the many moments a patient may experience and is limited to a single emotion of "satisfaction." Patient experience encompasses the range of interactions that patients have with the healthcare system, including their care from health plans, and from doctors, nurses, and staff in hospitals, physician practices, and other healthcare facilities [10]. This broad concept should consider all of the moments a patient might experience to include ease of access, first encounters, feelings, safety, adherence to care, diagnosis, long-term health, communication, medical outcomes, and overall well-being. Definitions of patient experience and the components that drive patient experience have spanned a wide range of models with emerging themes. The Beryl Institute defines the patient experience as "We define the patient experience as the sum of all interactions, shaped by an organizations culture that influence patient perceptions across the continuum of care" [11]. The Mayo Clinic offers this definition: "An unparalleled patient experience is the result of inspired and dedicated employees demonstrating excellence, compassion and respect by partnering with patients, family and colleagues to continuously improve the healthcare service experience" [12]. From their definition of the patient experience, the Mayo Clinic provides these patient experience components of focus: first impressions, respect and diversity, rights and responsibilities, hospitality, professionalism and healthcare literacy [12]. In a review of studies, Mohammed and colleagues presented the top three key drivers of patient experience: communication, access, and shared decision-making [12]. Recent studies have found that the strongest overall key driver on patient experience is the care provider interaction with the patient [13]. In the case of radiation nursing, patients seek a close relationship with the clinical staff who often spend the most time with the patient and the patient would perceive the nursing staff to be a most important care provider. Identifying strategies for how to develop a relationship with patients will be important. Research shows that empathy leads to better exchange of information, partnership, increased perception of expertise, increased interpersonal trust, and a positive correlation with patient care [14]. A synthesis of the research on patient experience produced key determinants for positive patient experience: healthcare workers who are empathetic, respectful, timely, collaborative, compassionate, informed, active listeners, curious, and understanding [15]. Patients' reports of doctor communication are the strongest predictors of overall doctor ratings for both primary care physicians and specialists [16, 17]. Other important facets of the patient experience consistent in research include coordination of care, communication between referring and specialist practices, giving patients handouts that they are able to read and understand, close follow-up care instructions, quick access to care, pre-appointment communication if long waits are anticipated, and managing patient expectations before, during, and after the visit [18]. Recommendations for improving the patient experience in specialty encounters listed similar components and provided definitions of each as follows:

- *Expectations*: Providing an opportunity for the patient to tell their story.
- *Communication*: Patient satisfaction increased when members of the healthcare team took the problem seriously, explained information clearly, and tried to understand the patient's experience, and provided viable options.
- *Control*: Patient experience is improved when patients are encouraged to express their ideas, concerns, and expectations.
- *Decision-making*: Patient satisfaction increased when the importance of their social and mental functioning as much as their physical functioning was acknowledged.
- *Time spent*: Patient satisfaction rates improved as the length of the healthcare visit increases.
- *Clinical team*: Although it is clear that the patient first concern is their clinician, they also value the team for which the clinician works.
- *Referrals*: Patient satisfaction increases when they receive continuing care from the same healthcare provider(s).
- *Dignity*: As expected, patients who are treated with respect and who are invited to partner in their healthcare decisions report greater satisfaction [19].

Given the daunting number of communication interventions, researchers have suggested that a key strategy is focusing efforts on aspects of communication that are most important to patients in each specialty area [20]. For instance, Halkett and O'Connor offer this helpful quote regarding the specialty of radiation oncology: "In our previous research we also found that patients placed high importance on radiation clinical staff communicating effectively and were pleased when they were able to form a relationship with the radiation clinical staff who treated them regularly throughout their treatment. Much of our time is focused on patients; however, involvement of family members is also likely to improve the experience of patients and their loved ones" [21]. The point taken from this article is that understanding the specific needs of patients based on specialty areas is important to have in mind, and in the case of radiation nursing, the focus on the relationship will be most important.

### 23.2.2 The Patient Experience and Communication

Given that the key drivers for patient experience involves the relationship the patient perceives to have with the healthcare staff and the effectiveness of communication, this section will focus on best practices in these areas. It is important to note that any efforts to improve the patient experience will require that nursing works in close partnership with providers and physicians and those improvement efforts should be clearly defined and based on patient feedback and needs [22]. The teamwork section of this chapter will further discuss coordination among staff for the patient experience but with regard to communication, when clinical staff and providers coordinate their strategies around patient needs, service area priorities, low scoring patient experience components, or deficits in communication skills, everyone benefits. For instance, providers and clinical staff might discuss a difficult patient scenario or a special patient need and coordinate their language, timing, and messages to successfully support a patient. Perhaps the system workflow might be changed to allow for more personal interactions with clinical staff or if metrics reveal that patients need clear instructions (and are not perceiving to receive them), staff can coordinate to use words, handoffs, language, repetition in a coordinated and consistent way. Another key strategy relies on the personal improvement goals and skills of each nursing staff. Nursing staff are encouraged to identify personalized phrases, greetings, and responses that are not scripted but thought-out and natural. These personal formulas might be used for difficult situations or for improved ways of connecting with patients. In this way, staff can feel at ease and capable of managing a variety of interactions in a personal, natural, and effective manner. Often, clinical staff might even develop a list of difficult interactions with personalized phrases for reference. It is not necessary to develop exact or memorized phrases but it can be helpful to have a sense of how to manage situations that reoccur. While there are many communication techniques and scripting phrases to consider, there are best practices for communication with patients based on a synthesis of the research on communication. Communication priorities for patient experience improvement will include building rapport, listening, showing empathy and respect, and giving clear instructions. Healthcare workers can ensure patients feel attended to in a personal way by relaxing the appearance of any time urgency with a calm, caring demeanor particularly at the greeting. The greeting and opening moments and time together are critical in establishing psychological safety and comfort for the patient and in building rapport for a strong ongoing relationship. From the beginning, narrating care and the sharing of next steps reassures patients, provides a sense of structure to the conversation and offers them a sense of control when they are otherwise feeling uneasy. Techniques for reassurance include sharing confidence in the physician and facility by discussing credentials or offering personal phrases and styles of putting the patient at ease [23]. It is helpful to watch the facial expressions and body language of a patient to determine what kind of connection will make a patient comfortable. Patients feel more confident when the healthcare organization or caregivers have been praised with high regard. An example might be, "Dr J is an excellent doctor and he/she and I have worked together for many years. We are going to take great care of you." Patients are made more comfortable when they feel heard, listened to and understood, so we have to give clear evidence of both [24]. In order for patients to feel more comfortable, another important skill to develop is that of redirecting a patient without seeming dismissive. An example of supportive communication particularly if redirecting might be, "Thank you so much for sharing that. It is helpful that you are organized. I have another question I would like to ask you that is so important to your care." A helpful mnemonic for improved listening skills is the **Invite, Listen, and Summarize** sequence that can be applied to understanding a patient's reports of their ideas, feelings, and values and to ensure a display of understanding and empathy [25]. Empathy skills involve the acknowledgment and recognition of the journey or feelings a patient communicates directly or indirectly and then the communication of that recognition. A helpful mnemonic for acknowledgment of feelings is **NURS**; **Name** the feeling, **Understand** and legitimize it, **Respect** the patient's attempts to cope, and offer **Support** and partnership in the future. Clinicians are encouraged to invite the patient to offer corrections and incorporate them into the summary. Another consistent driver of patient experience is the show of respect by the healthcare worker. Based on research from the Learning Lab of the Studer Group, certain tactics have been identified as being most impactful on improving a patient's perception of respect [22]. Those are greeting with professionalism, demonstrating empathy, using direct phrases that indicate caring "I care about you and your health…;" and effective service recovery responses with an acknowledgement of feelings and then an apology. Research shows that patients forget 40–80% of the medical information patients receive by the time they leave the provider's office [26, 27] and nearly half of the information that patients retain is incorrect [28]. Providing clear instructions is a patient need listed in the literature that can occur with verbal explanations supplemented with written information [22]. There are three tactics to consider. The first is to notify patients in advance of the session that written information will be provided. A second method is the **Teach Back Method** which is as simple as asking the patient to repeat back what they understood about next steps and follow-up care. It also further engages patients in discussion and interest in their own care. The authors of The CG CAHPS Handbook [22] offer these helpful sentences to share with patients as part of the **Teach Back Method**: "Mrs. A, we are covering a lot of information today for this visit. I care that you walk away from this informed. You must have some questions for me. I am happy to answer." "I want to do a good job of explaining everything we are covering today during your visit, so please tell me when something I said isn't clear or if you have any questions." "To help me know if I did a good job of explaining…". In summary, it is important to identify the special needs of patients per service area and to recognize the needs of each patient. Then, learning skills for particular areas of communication using techniques or developing personalized phrases are ways to build a reassuring, empathetic relationship that supports patients many emotional and physical needs.

### 23.2.3 Domains of Patient Experience Models for Improvement

In order to improve patient care, pursuing a patient care-system design that gives full attention to the medical, emotional, and informational needs of patients and their families will have to involve focus areas that will reach of the growth and culture requirements of the healthcare entity. The Mayo Clinic provides the following common domains found in successful models: service recovery training, metrics with clear measures of success, staff accountability, consultation services, education and training, monitoring and recognition and reward [12]. Additional domains could include physician and clinical staff coaching, sustainment plans, patient advocacy for patient complaints and grievances, and learning resources for improving the patient experience.

### 23.2.4 Measurement of the Patient Experience

Healthcare organizations typically have access to or can easily gather various types of administrative data to determine which performance issues should be targeted. Examples of sources of administrative data include the CAHPS family of surveys. The Consumer Assessment of Healthcare Providers and Systems (CAHPS®) is an Agency for Healthcare Research and Quality (AHRQ) program that began in 1995 [29]. Its purpose is to advance our scientific understanding of patient experience with healthcare. The acronym "CAHPS" is a registered trademark of AHRQ.CAHPS surveys cover topics that are important to healthcare consumers and focus on aspects of quality that are best qualified to assess, such as the communication skills of providers and ease of access to healthcare services. All CAHPS surveys (and tools) and related documentation are free to anyone who wants to use these surveys to assess patients' experiences with care. Users of CAHPS survey results include patients and consumers, healthcare providers, public and private purchasers of healthcare, healthcare accreditation organizations, health plans, and regional improvement collaboratives. These individuals and organizations use the survey results to evaluate healthcare providers and to improve the quality of healthcare services [10].The following are key steps for improving the patient experience offered by AHRQ:

- Compare your scores to benchmarks.
- Compare your current scores to past performance.
- Assess which aspects of performance are most relevant to your members or patients.
- Review complaints and compliments, patients' comments, and administrative data [30].

## 23.3 Teamwork as a Part of Safety, Quality, and the Patient Experience

It has widely been established that organizational culture is related to performance [31]. There is also broad acceptance within the healthcare literature of the importance of culture on patient outcomes to include patient experience, safety, and medical outcomes [32]. Many organizations such as the Joint Commission (TJC), Institute for Healthcare improvement (IHI), the National Quality Forum (NQF), and the Accreditation Council for Graduate Medical Education(ACGME) have sited of the importance of teamwork and patient safety [33]. The saying by Peter Drucker, "Culture Eats Strategy for Lunch" [34], suggests and reminds us that no operational effort can succeed without a culture of employees that support it. In order for a patient experience effort to be successful, the coordination of the staff around that effort will be required. This is more likely to happen in a supportive environment that fosters psychological safety and has clearly defined communication protocols and meeting structures as well as team coping skills for stress management and conflict resolution. For instance, we cannot implement a process improvement strategy if the employees are not ready for change, are overworked, or if relationships are poor. When a culture is defined by stress, conflict, or poor communication, it is not possible for improvement efforts to move forward. On the other hand, it is possible to have a culture where employees are not stressed and have good communication and coping skills but who have no interest or structure by which to improve processes. In that case, the mission needs to be redefined and new team norms need to be established. In the wake of reports documenting the sources of medical errors, there is a belief and re-invigorated focus on the notion of culture change to include team coordination as a key element of health system redesign [3]. A healthcare system must fully embrace an integrative model that builds systems, processes, and a culture that puts patient experience and patient safety at the heart of all decisions and does so by engaging staff and fostering an environment where collaboration is a natural part of daily work. Nursing plays a primary role in the overall functioning of a healthcare system and its success in these areas. The following section will explore the importance and methods of teamwork, a program called TeamSTEPPS for building teams, culture, and strategies that lead to successful patient outcomes.

### 23.3.1 The Models and Domains for Building a Teamwork Culture in Organizations

A synthesis of research reveals themes of what comprises the healthy culture of an environment. Those would include leadership alignment among the leaders and with the mission values and goals, effective teamwork, mutual accountability, behavioral norms, support, performance management, reward systems, conflict management systems, role clarity monitoring, clear processes and procedures, and employee engagement. Davies (2002) offered practical steps and interventions for each of these areas [35, 36]. The next section will provide information about the most prominent healthcare teamwork program today, which is TeamSTEPPS (Team Strategies and Tools to Enhance Performance and Patient Safety).

### 23.3.2 TeamSTEPPS®

Given the necessity for cooperation among healthcare workers who are dependent on one another, it is critical that they are successful as a team. Teamwork requires an organization that is committed to sustaining a patient-centered culture as well as competencies and beliefs that become permanent mental models for how a healthcare facility functions as it relates to interactions beyond the process improvement domains previously discussed. The best and most widely known teamwork program is the Team Step Strategies and Tools to Enhance Performance and Patient Safety (TeamSTEPPS) [37]. TeamSTEPPS is a systematic approach developed by the United States Department of Defense and Patient Safety Program and the Department of Health and Human Services Agency for Healthcare Research and quality

(AHRQ). It works to improve the quality, safety, and the efficiency of healthcare [33]. The program was built on research conducted in healthcare that first determined the core mechanisms of teamwork that became the foundation for the TeamSTEPPS program. Those core mechanisms are communication, leadership, situation monitoring, and mutual support.

The AHRQ then designed tools to help healthcare staff members build skills around the core competencies. For communication, the commonly used acronym, **SBAR** stands for: situation, background, assessment, and recommendation. This tool organizes communication to be brief, timely, and clear in verbal conversation or as a written template in the variety of electronic communications. A nurse could use the format to organize personal conversation or as an electronic template with prompts added to ensure critical information is collected or provided. For handoffs between staff members during patient care, mental and verbal checklists can ensure all patient care information has been transmitted. An appropriate handoff also requires that the staff members receiving information ask the right questions for clarification to ensure a final handoff. AHRQ used the term "**Call-out**" for healthcare workers to point out a potential or real error. It is suggested that assertive communication should be clear, direct, and respectful. Healthcare workers are encouraged to practice phrases they are comfortable with when pointing out potential errors. Teams are encouraged to discuss communication patterns openly in staff meetings in order to establish ground rules for how best to phrase needs and recover from poor interactions. The management of meetings is another area addressed in the communication section of the AHRQ TeamSTEPPS [37] program. The **Brief** is a meeting that occurs between nursing staff and providers they support in preparation for a variety of events such as a difficult patient, a procedure, and early in the day organize patient flow. These meetings are most effective when they follow a standard checklist so that healthcare workers are prepared to ask questions or respond to predicted questions. It can be very effective for clinical staff and providers to brief to begin the day with a shared understanding of patients' needs as well as clarification of needs for one another. The **Huddle** is a meeting designed to be impromptu and to respond to changes or urgent situations. Huddles are a semi-structured kind of meeting designed to respond to urgent situations while quickly getting people organized. Finally, the **Debrief** is a meeting that follows an event such as the end of the day, the end of a week, or after an encounter with a difficult patient scenario. It is designed for staff members to recover, regroup, or to learn from an event and to bring people together. Learning from these meetings can often be tied to performance improvement efforts and tend to generate discussion around events as opposed to pointing out blame.

Conflict management is a critical component to TeamSTEPPS in that conflict and disagreements are a primary source of nursing turnover and sentinel events [38]. TeamSTEPPS provides this acronym for managing difficult conversations: **DESC** which stands for **Describe, Express, Suggest**, and **Consequences** and is used for organizing thoughts before having a difficult conversation. Feedback guidelines for communication suggest it should be timely, respectful, specific, directed, and considerate. Situation monitoring involves a team's commitment to watching the flow of work as it changes through the day and knowing how and when to assist one another. It is important that team members come to agreement for norms and ground rules around mutual support and task assistance. This may involve some discussion around role clarity, the changing demand of the workflow through the day, and ground rules for how to ask for help and how to gracefully decline. The developers of TeamSTEPPS are clear that embedding this program into a culture cannot be successful simply through training but must be embedded into orientation programs, ongoing training efforts, regular local meetings, customized interventions by clinical area and offered regularly to leaders. TeamSTEPPS is a widely used, evidenced-based program that has successes consistently supported in research.

### 23.3.3 Performance Improvement Models

Healthcare cultures, teamwork, and coordination have been associated with success in the implementation of continuous quality improvement practices [38].Patient communication and safety culture initiatives must be integrated with a systematic, structured performance improvement model that continuously focuses on problem solving and provides metrics on the progress of the patient experience. The AHRQ CAHPS Improvement Guide [10] lists these three main models: *The Institute for Healthcare Improvement's Model for Improvement, Lean* and *Six Sigma*. Key principles for operational excellence in healthcare are the development of a culture that sees problem solving as continuous with rapid cycles of experimentation. In this paradigm, engaged employees collaborate with leaders and problems are addressed immediately. If those problems lead to successful outcomes, improvements identified as best practices are then shared across the system. Problem solving follows a scientific process using the **PDSACycle** (Plan, Do, Study, Act) method and for larger improvement projects the **DMAIC model** is used (Define, Measure, Assess, Improvement opportunities and Control and sustain) [10].

From the May 2017, AHRQ Ambulatory Care Improvement Guide, steps for improvement are encouraged at the micro level: "To develop and refine such systems, healthcare organizations start by defining the smallest measurable cluster of activities" [10]. Healthcare organizations can take advantage of established principles and approaches to quality improvement, and should involve employees from a bottom-up approach with those closest to the problems, solving the problems. First, metrics are reviewed and clinical areas are identified as priorities for improvement goals, strategies, and interventions. A possible action plan is established with identified goals that should follow the **SMART model** (specific, measurable, achievable, realistic, and time bound) [10]. The guide offers this list of common features for improvement models:

- Emphasis on leadership to hold people accountable, communicate the vision and strategy, and eliminate cultural and other barriers to improvement.
- Clear goals.
- Use of measurement and analysis to identify issues and guide decisions.
- Emphasis on stakeholders as participants and audiences for the improvement processes.
- Use of structured, iterative processes to implement improvement interventions.
- Use of many of the same tools to support analysis and implementation.
- Monitoring of front-line clinical activity through observations and the collection and reporting of process data as feedback on the effect of changes or to track the progress of the implementation process.
- Transparent metrics.

## 23.4 Conclusion

Several key points have been made in this chapter. First, it is important to understand that patient experience, teamwork through safety culture, and performance improvement must be integrated into a single paradigm and jointly drive all decisions for patient care. It has also been established that key strategies should be developed based on the needs of patients by specialty area and personalized for each staff member. Many techniques are available for learning positive communication skills and several examples were offered. Improving patient communication is also a strategy for patient safety given that when patient communication is enhanced patient outcomes are improved. Patient experience outcomes cannot be improved without the coordination of the team members who rely on one another. A teamwork section was offered that focused on TeamSTEPPS, a widely used healthcare teamwork program. It is important that teams join together in regular discussion about norms for communication, positive interaction, handoffs, call-outs, meetings, briefs and debriefs, and for managing conflict and stress. Nursing is a critical component and central to the success of a healthcare organization. Nursing insights move beyond medical care of a patient to the medical, emotional, and cognitive needs of the patient. Nursing is also instrumental in the health of the organization as they play a key role in monitoring both patient well-being and the well-being of the culture around them.

## References

1. Institute of Medicine. Crossing the quality chasm: a new health system for the 21st century. Washington, DC: National Academy Press; 2001.
2. Doyle C, Lennon L, Bell D. A systematic review of evidence from many studies refer to the link between patient experience and patient safety and effective processes. BMJ Open. 2013;3:e001570. https://doi.org/10.1136/bmjopen-2012-001570.
3. Institute of Medicine. To err is human: building a safer health system. Washington, DC: National Academy Press; 1999.
4. Peterson MC, Holbrook J, Von Hales D, Smith NL, Staker LV. Contributions of the history, physical examination and laboratory investigation in making medical diagnoses. Western J Med. 1992;156:163–5.
5. The Impact of Communication in Healthcare. Institute for Healthcare Communication. 2019. BEST.
6. ButterworthS, SharpA. Part 2: A happy patient: what drives patient satisfaction? From our blog: Improving quality through satisfaction: a four-part series. 2018. http://qconsulthealthcare.com.
7. Zolnierek KB, Dimatteo MR. Physician communication and patient adherence to treatment: a meta-analysis. Med Care. 2009;47(8):826–34.
8. Stewart MA. Effective physician patient communication and health outcomes: a review. CMAJ. 1995;152(9):1423–33.
9. Fremont AM, Clearly PD, Hargraves JL, et al. Patient-centered processes of care and long-term outcomes of acute myocardial infarction. J Gen Intern Med. 2001;14:800–8.
10. InternetCitation: Section 5: Determining where to focus efforts to improve patient experience (page 1 of 2). Rockville, MD: Agency for Healthcare Research and Quality. Content last reviewed Jan 2018. http://www.ahrq.gov/cahps/quality-improvement/improvement-guide/5-determining-focus/index.html.
11. Internet Citation: The definition of the patient experience. Nashville, TN: The Beryl Institute. Content last reviewed 2019. https://www.theberylinstitute.org/page/CopyofDefiningPati.
12. PruthiS, VerNessC, StevensS. The Beryl Institute patient experience conference 2015. Service recovery in healthcare: movement from reactive to proactive presented at Mayo Clinic.
13. Johnson DM, Russell RS. SEM of service quality to predict overall patient satisfaction in medical clinics: a case study. Qual Manag J. 2015;22(4):18–36.
14. Kim SS. The effects of physician empathy on patient satisfaction and compliance. Eval Health Prof. 2004;27(3):237–51.
15. WeinackerA. Press Ganey Again? Strategies for improving the patient experience. Stanford Health Care. Accessed on 20 May 2019.
16. Ruiz-Marol R, Perez Rodriguez E, Perula De Torres LA, De la Torre J. Physician-patient communication: a study on the observed behaviors of specialty physicians and the ways their patients perceive them. Patient Educ Couns. 2006;64(1–3):242–8. https://doi.org/10.1016/j.pec.2006.02.010.
17. Sofaer S, Crofton C, Goldstein E, Hoy E, Crabb J. What do consumers want to know about quality of care in hospitals? Health Serv Res. 2005;40(6 Pt 2):2018–36. https://doi.org/10.1111/j.1475-6773.2005.00473.x.
18. Golda N, Beeson S, Kohli N, Merrill B. Analysis of the patient experience measure. J Am Acad Dermatol. 2018;78:645–51.
19. Thiedke CC. What do we really know about patient satisfaction? Fam Pract Manag. 2007;14:33–6.
20. Quigley D, Elliott M, Farley D, Burkart Q, Skootsky S, Hays R. Specialties differ in which aspects of doctor communication predict overall physician ratings. J Gen Intern Med. 2013;29(3):447–54. https://doi.org/10.1007/s11606-013-2663-2.
21. Halkett G, O'Connor M. What is the best way to support patients undergoing radiation therapy? J Med Radiat Sci. 2015;62(1):3–5. https://doi.org/10.1002/jmrs.100.
22. Morris J, Hotko B, Bates M, Studer Group LLC. The CGCAHPS handbook: a guide to improve patient experience and patient outcomes. Pensacola, FL: Fire Starter Publishing; 2015.
23. 5-Step patient-centered interviewing adapted by FortinAH VI, SteinJ from: SmithRC. Patient centered interviewing. 2nd ed. Philadelphia, PA: Lippincott Williams & Wilkins; 2002.
24. Platt F, Gordon G. Field guide to the difficult patient interview. 2nd ed. Philadelphia, PA: Lippincott Williams & Wilkins; 2004.
25. Myers S. Empathic listening: reports on the experience of being heard. J Hum Psychol. 2000;40:148–74.
26. Kessels RP. Patients' memory for medical information. J R Soc Med. 2003;96(5):219–22.
27. Anderson JL, et al. Patient information recall in a rheumatology clinic. Rheumatology. 1979;18(1):18–22.
28. Negarandeh R, Mahmoodi H, Noktehdan H, Heshmat R, Shakibazadeh E. Teach back and pictorial image educational strategies on knowledge about diabetes and medication/dietary adherence among low health literate patients with type 2 diabetes. Prim Care Diabetes. 2013;7(2):111–8. https://doi.org/10.1016/j.pcd.2012.11.001.
29. Internet Citation: About CAHPS. Rockville, MD: Agency for Healthcare Research and Quality. Content last reviewed Apr 2019. https://www.ahrq.gov/cahps/about-cahps/index.html.

30. Your business strategy and improvement goals guide your benchmark choices. Internet Citation: Section 5: Determining where to focus efforts to improve patient experience (page 1 of 2). Rockville, MD: Agency for Healthcare Research and Quality. Content last reviewed Jan 2018. http://www.ahrq.gov/cahps/quality-improvement/improvement-guide/5-determining-focus/index.html.
31. Westrum R. A typology of organizational cultures. Qual Safe Health Care. 2004;13:22–7.
32. Davies H, Nutley S, Mannion R. Organizational culture and quality of healthcare. Qual HealthCare. 2000;9:111–9.
33. King H, Battles J, Baker D, Alonso A, Salas E, Webster J, Toomey L, Salisbury M. TeamSTEPPS: Team strategies and tools to enhance performance in Public Safety. Mayo Clin Proc. 2017;92(1):129–66. https://doi.org/10.1016/j.mayocp.2016.10.004, www.mayoclinicproceedings.org.
34. Drucker P. Management: tasks, responsibilities, practices. London: Butterworth-Heinemann; 1973.
35. Davies H. Understanding organizational culture in reforming the National Health Service. JRSoc Med. 2002;95(3):4–6.
36. McAleese D, Hargie O. Five guarding principles of culture management: a synthesis of best practices. J Commun Manag. 2004;9(2):155–70.
37. Internet Citation: About TeamSTEPPS. Rockville, MD: Agency for Healthcare Research and Quality. Content last reviewedMar2019. http://www.ahrq.gov/teamstepps/about-teamstepps/index.html.
38. Shortell S, O'Brien J, Carmen J, et al. Assessing the impact of continuous quality improvement and total quality management: concept versus implementation. Health ServResour. 1995;30:377–401.

# Children and Young People in Radiology

**24**

Joan Turner

## 24.1 Introduction

Radiologic imaging is an example of a common yet potentially complex medical experience requiring children and young people (CYP) and families to engage with the healthcare system for a relatively time-limited but potentially stressful event. Used to diagnose, monitor and screen, or treat a condition the range of available imaging procedures often place CYP in the unusual position of entering a strange environment where the expectation to cooperate and participate is high and the individual's ability to cope is challenged. Views on what makes a pediatric imaging procedure a *success* are dependent on the differing goals and values of all of the stakeholders, including the CYP. Prepared from the viewpoint of a child life specialist, the best interests of CYP are at the center of the discussion presented in the chapter. Ideas of ways in which to plan environments that align with the experience of the CYP as a competent and capable participant are emphasized.

Application of an ecological model draws attention to the nature of the interactions of the CYP *with* existing systems, particularly highlighting the status of the individual as an active agent. While the present discussion will deal primarily with factors in the immediate context of an imaging procedure, acknowledgement of the advocacy role of pediatric radiology nurses to advance the interests of the CYP through policy and procedural change is also offered. Therefore, approaches for appreciating the potential strengths of the CYP undergoing an imaging procedure will be outlined followed by a presentation on ways to engage their competence and capacity through welcoming relationships, inviting collaboration, and recognizing success. Ultimately, the goal of fostering a successful outcome that also acknowledges the best interests of the CYP will be the focus of the chapter.

## 24.2 Ecological Model

In viewing the experience of the child from an ecological perspective, we are encouraged to look beyond the immediate context of the developing CYP. If we can pause to observe the CYP within the larger context and attend to the environmental interconnections that impact CYP, we can consider that the healthcare system has a unique influence. Bronfenbrenner's ecological model [1] is a useful lens to examine the experience of the CYP and family as they are guided into the domain of radiologic procedures within the larger system of healthcare. For as we view the individual within a set of interacting systems, the ways the systems ultimately interact with the

J. Turner, PhD, CCLS (✉)
Child and Youth Study Department,
Mount Saint Vincent University, Halifax,
Nova Scotia, Canada

CYP become visible. The role of the radiology nurse in supporting a CYP and family includes the establishment of supportive relationships, health promotion, teaching and advocacy, coordination and collaboration, as well as engagement with policy and procedure activities of the larger healthcare system. A framework for care that places the CYP at the center can result in policies and practices that ultimately result in optimizing a positive experience for the individual while attaining a clinically relevant result.

Briefly, Bronfenbrenner's ecological model [1] illustrates five layers of interrelated systems. The microsystem, where the CYP is an active participant while undergoing a radiological procedure, represents an interplay of the CYP and family's individual characteristics with the physical and social environment of the setting. The mesosystem refers to the *process* of interrelationships with the exosystem—represented by practices, procedures, and policies that result from staff and CYP's experience and ultimately impact the CYP's experience. An example of a feature of the exosystem is the quality, availability, and uptake of information and resources to engage families and CYP prior to a radiology appointment. The macrosystem refers to overarching attitudes, beliefs, and ideals of a society, in this case relating to health and healthcare. These interact with the mesosystem processes and affect a CYP and family's experience, for example, relating to the expectations that CYP have before engaging with pediatric radiology procedures. Finally, the chronosystem represents the whole system as it moves through time and historical change. Respect for the rights of CYP is an example of an attitudinal change over decades affecting the whole healthcare system including serving the best interests of the child, children's right to be involved in decisions, education and the right to play [2].

## 24.3 Perceptions of the Radiology Environment

Children and young people are distinct from adults in many ways including the lens through which they perceive the environment. Entering a radiology department for the first time exposes CYP and their caregivers to unfamiliar sights, sounds, and experiences [3]. Technological in nature, the human elements of a radiology space can be overlooked by adults whose attention is focused on managing the procedural requirements of imaging. Imaging staff, as well as caregivers, have their own expectations that may or may not align with that of a CYP. In placing the CYP at the center of this discussion, the aim is to point out features of the environment that may influence CYP's reactions to the radiology environment and the imaging experience.

The state-of-the-art technology of X-ray, ultrasound, MRI, CT, and other imaging modalities can be both fascinating and intimidating at the same time. Consideration of the features of technology as seen through the eyes of CYP requires attention to the size, shape, color, placement, and even the lighting of the equipment. The theory of affordances [4] suggests that CYP immediately perceive the potential actions and functions of materials and that this perception influences how they respond. In nature environments, for example, a tree stump may be valued for its affordance for jumping and balancing; the angles of a tree branch may represent a wild animal or a sword. Imagine what CYP may perceive upon their first encounter with imaging technology, when lying prone or when the lights are dimmed? Many pediatric facilities incorporate child-friendly design into the imaging spaces such as paint colors, images, music, and even virtual reality goggles. However, where these features are not supported, CYP may be left to their own imagination and influenced by additional elements of the environment or past experiences.

The sensory elements of spaces can also influence a CYP's response. For children, the passage of time, particularly when unoccupied, is relative. Exposure to smells from cleaners and alcohol swabs, sounds like beeps, voices and footsteps, changes in temperature, shifts between bright and dim lighting can bombard a young person. Chairs that are too big, counters and sinks too high and adult oriented media and materials overlook the range of interests, particularly of small children. Young people may be expected to adapt to adult dimensions and sometimes intentionally childish design features too. However, for youth, their interests and needs are distinctive relative to younger children and require additional consideration. The adequacy of environmental accommodations for both children and youth, although commonly featured in pediatric facilities, may be deficient in adult spaces or disregard the interests of mature pediatric patients.

The behavioral expectations of imaging procedures primarily include the ability to hold still for a period of time. When this request follows a sequence of requirements in preparation for the procedure, the CYP's tolerance for the demands of the procedure can be compromised. Changing out of clothes and into an examination gown, ingesting substances or fluids, enduring the insertion of an intravenous line or urinary catheter, perhaps donning a lead apron while interacting with many unfamiliar people, and waiting for an undetermined amount of time all play into the reaction of children undergoing an imaging procedure. Additional expectations align with the specifics of the procedure—tolerating gel for an ultrasound, lying in the frog-legged position, and exposure to loud sounds of an MRI are examples of features of radiology environments in need of attention in order to meet the needs and interests of a pediatric population. Further, the identification of specific strengths and stressors for individuals and their family must be explored for their influence on reactions and responses in radiology environments.

Stepping away from an adult perception of the environment and everyday interactions requires the intentional invitation of CYP's voices and perspectives into the healthcare environment. Recognition that adult perceptions and expectations are likely to differ from a CYP is one component of this discussion. Another is accepting that we may need to follow the CYP's lead in order to accomplish the task at hand. Bröder et al. [5] suggest we give credit to CYP as active players in their own health and allow for a movement toward the inclusion of CYP as collaborators in healthcare decisions.

## 24.4 Placing the Child or Young Person at the Center

Appreciation for the interests and needs associated with individual patients seen in pediatric settings is complicated due to the wide range of developmental abilities observed in CYP presenting for radiologic procedures. A message often communicated in the pediatric literature reminds us that children are not small adults [6]. Most relevant to this discussion is that individual CYP should not be reduced to the catch-all *age equals developmental ability* and should be approached for their unique interests, needs, and abilities too. Upon initial encounters with CYP, the manner in which you greet and interact with individuals does affect the reception you will experience in return. At the very least, enhanced awareness of the importance of exploring the capacity and competency of individual children and youth is warranted in anticipation of a successful procedure. Three related ideas—image of the child, child agency, and health literacy friendly—are introduced as ways of thinking about healthcare environments that are respectful of the CYP as an essential player in health promotion (Fig. 24.1).

### 24.4.1 Image of the Child or Young Person

The image of the CYP that one favors related to competence and capacity to actively participate does have an influence on the ways that a CYP is

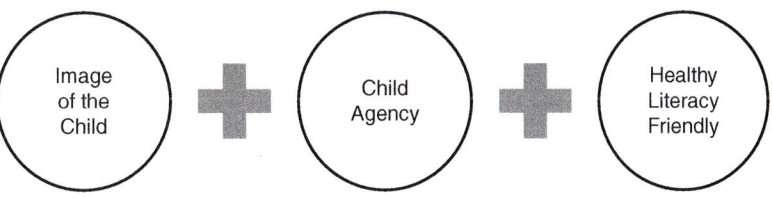

**Fig. 24.1** Thinking about children and young people as essentials players in health promotion

approached, engaged in communication, and included in health-related activities. Strict adherence to a developmental perspective, for example, can limit our view of CYP to be in a constant state of development—perhaps never quite as capable as we might want them to be—particularly within the context of complex medical experiences. Whether we view a CYP as competent and capable (or not), reflects the level of social agency we attribute to individuals, the level of participation we are willing to offer, and ultimately our propensity to collaborate with CYP throughout an imaging process. To see CYP as partners in healthcare can position the power of the relationship away from adult-directed and toward a collaborative approach to practice with CYP.

In describing child life specialists (CLS) as a key member of the team in pediatric radiology, Metzger et al. [7] demonstrate an attitude of the competent and capable child through a case study of an evaluation of 8-year-old *Michael* preparing for an arthrogram and MRI. Clearly, the evaluation is conducted to assess the child's potential to tolerate the procedures without sedation. Through a systematic process of building rapport, exploring interests and concerns, and gathering additional background information, the CLS determines Michael understands the procedures and what is expected of him. Notably, because of the CLS propensity to collaborate, she is also able to pinpoint Michael's personal perspective of success: attending a football game that evening. "He is nervous but motivated to not receive sedation by the desire to go to a football game that evening, something he cannot do if he is sedated today [7, p. 154]."

## 24.4.2 Child or Young Person Agency

Montreuil and Carnevale [8] conducted a concept analysis of children's agency within the healthcare literature. Application of the term agency as referring to children as agents who have the capacity to act was found to have changed over time, vary by discipline and by paradigmatic orientation. Early reference to child agency was identified as related to "one's ability to engage in self-care in order to enhance treatment and prevent illness" [8, p. 506]. Seen through a developmental lens, children were viewed as transitioning from being the recipients of care toward greater abilities for self-care that developed along with a greater sense of self. Later, constructivist or participatory views included children as contributing to or having the right to participate and be involved as developers and evaluators of interventions (particularly related to health research). Due to the inconsistent use of the term found by Montreuil and Carnevale, the authors put forth a tentative definition of agency as follows: "Children's capacity to act deliberately, speak for oneself, and actively reflect on their social worlds, shaping their lives and the lives of others" [8, p. 510].

In the case of Michael mentioned earlier [7], he was invited to ask questions, suggest his preferred methods for coping (e.g., sitting up and watching the IV start, play a football trivia game during the arthrogram, watch a movie during the MRI), and rehearse coping behaviors as the CLS walked with him through the step-by-step process of the demanding and time-consuming series of procedures. Reflection on the Montreuil and Carnevale [8] understanding of agency relative to healthcare in general allows for additional consideration of ways in which CYP, like Michael, express their knowledge and understanding of health and healthcare-related information and behaviors.

## 24.4.3 Health Literacy Friendly

Health literacy in CYP is just beginning to receive attention in the literature [5]. Usually, child health literacy is derived from adult concepts of health literacy, including basic reading, writing, and numeracy skills and a combination of health-related knowledge, competencies as well as motivation; as such, the unique character and life situations of young people may be overlooked. In systematically reviewing the literature, Bröder et al. [5] have documented this gap and encourage opportunities for CYP that acknowledge the active role they do play in their health. Bröder et al. [5] introduce a suitable phrase,

# 24 Children and Young People in Radiology

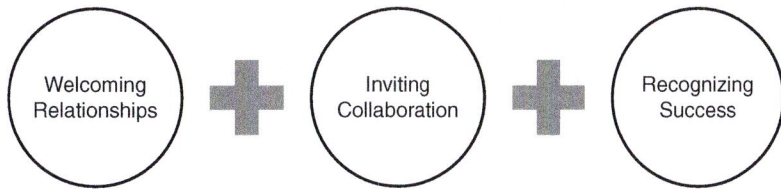

**Fig. 24.2** Collaboration with children and young people

"health literacy friendly services," in reference to ways in which the role of CYP in developing their health literacy can be acknowledged and supported through inclusive and collaborative approaches. By prioritizing the viewpoint of the CYP, we are better able to focus on what is important to the individual as they progress through a complex system of care.

Again, we can refer to the case of Michael [7] and recognize his interest and ability (competence and capacity) to engage in a complex process of preparation and planning to increase his health-related knowledge, understanding and ability to participate in his healthcare. The health-literacy friendly initiatives provided by the radiology team supporting Michael throughout the experience demonstrate an inclusive and collaborative approach that allow for the recognition of his motivation to succeed in order to meet a personal goal for the day. Patient and family education and support that intentionally invites the unique motivations of the CYP into the process can seize both the attention and trust of the CYP and increase the chances of achieving a successful procedural outcome and positive experience. Approaches discussed in the following section highlight the value of welcoming relationships, inviting collaboration, and recognizing success in the development of collaborative approaches to radiological practice (Fig. 24.2).

## 24.5 Collaboration with Children and Young People

Together, the three concepts—image of the child, child agency, and health literacy friendly—were introduced to encourage a movement toward considering the CYP as an essential player in healthcare procedures. Looking at the individual as a subject who holds the capacity to engage with procedural processes, rather than an object for radiologic examination, starts at the moment of relationship. The teaching, advocacy, coordination, and collaboration processes can occur to support a successful imaging experience and outcome when the CYP is welcome as a partner in health promotion. Upon consideration of policy and procedural practices from a collaborative framework, radiology nurses can examine and modify existing procedural practices to position the voices and perspectives of children explicitly in the forefront of practice.

The timing of the initiation of the relationship among the CYP, family, and radiology professionals is dependent on the specific context of the referral for a radiologic procedure. Additionally, each imaging modality features its own idiosyncratic processes that cannot be fully addressed in this brief chapter. However, the underlying thesis of the necessity of consulting with and informing CYP is supported when attention to the establishment of trust and communication in relationships with young people is embraced. Whether the discussion features *this* radiology modality or *that* imaging modality, consideration of the CYP as an essential player in their healthcare procedures who is capable and competent requires experienced radiology professionals prepared to appreciate the perspectives of the CYP upfront: "Clinical decision-making must be based on the requirements of each patient, guided by the latest sources of information available, including local guidelines and newly published trial data" [9, p. 2]. In order to create this positive experience, we must incorporate all we know about the CYP and caregiver experiences into the clinical decision-making process [10].

### 24.5.1 Welcoming Relationships

Whether initiated by a primary care physician, clinical specialist, or emergency room team, the introduction of the caregivers to the forthcoming procedure should include a conversation underscoring the importance of inviting the CYP into the preparation and planning for a successful experience. Bates [10] suggests the referring physician begin to educate the caregivers through the provision of the particulars of the imaging procedure beyond the diagnostic label. When general details of the process of the preparation and procedural requirements are shared upfront, ideally supported with appropriate educational materials, then adequate time for caregivers to prepare questions, raise concerns, and consider the implications of the procedure on their CYP's capacity to participate is provided.

Follow-up contact initiated by a radiology nurse equipped to address questions, concerns and initiate the inclusion of the CYP as an active participant in the procedure is a next step. The CYP will be included in this process when caregivers are comfortable that the existing supports will allow the CYP to demonstrate their interest and ability to participate. Following the introduction of the planned procedure, radiology nurses can be proactive in building a relationship with the CYP through an intentional exploration of who the individual is apart from their medical concerns. The establishment of a positive relationship begins as the radiology nurse explores existing interests and knowledge held by the CYP. Conversation around the CYPs interpretation of the purpose, process, and meaning of the procedures can uncover existing and potential strengths and stressors. Ultimately, the capacity of the radiology nurse to recognize and employ the potential motivation of the CYP relative to the achievement of a successful experience is fundamental.

Although child life specialists (CLS) are not available for all radiology centers, lessons shared can support practice across professions. CLS have offered the following perspectives to account for their ease in establishing meaningful relationships even during brief encounters with CYP [11]. Showing genuine interest, creating a sense of connection, and offering real opportunities for choice and control are all part of the approach of CLS as they initiate relationships [11]. They carry materials with them to convey a sense of who they are to the CYP and family and to support an ongoing interaction. Bubbles, books, interactive games, and multi-media materials and models are some tools the CLS may use to facilitate a relationship. Ideas for hands-on materials, gadgets, and images can be found using search terms such as *interesting gadgets in radiology* on Google or *medical/health care play* on Pinterest.

### 24.5.2 Inviting Collaboration

With some effort, materials introduced early to capture CYP attention provide a welcoming environment that allows for a collaborative interaction to advance. As with CLS, radiology nurses may also select an intriguing collection of materials that can be used as an invitation into an interaction. As mentioned earlier, imaging modalities can be fascinating as well as intimidating. In early childhood education the term *provocation* is used to reference the deliberate invitation of children into thinking about something or experimenting with ideas and materials [12]. Similarly, from the field of educational psychology, placing abstract learning concepts into meaningful and interesting contexts, personalizing learning, and offering choices serves to increase CYP sense of control and self-determination [13]. In making the process of preparation for a radiology procedure collaborative to CYP, the radiological nurse has a role in making the whole process meaningful for the CYP.

When introducing the radiology environment, the interests and exploration behavior (curiosity) of the CYP can be observed and combined with open-ended dialogue to provide opportunities for offering choice and control relative to the play activities or in preparation for the procedure. Callery and Coyne suggest familiar educational principles are applied in approaches to interventions to engage CYP in decisions: "appropriate, structured and based on active rather than passive learning" [14, p. 606]. Initially, exploring a basket of play imaging models with people figures, materials and devices with moveable parts, or books with images can take the pressure off direct interactions by shifting attention off the CYP and onto the materials. Additionally, as nurses progress through an explanation or tour of the radiology environment they may enter into the preparation process. The aim is to facilitate an understanding of ways in which the process can be presented to spark the interest, motivation, and need for control of the individual.

### 24.5.3 Recognizing Success

Through conversations exploring who the CYP is you can discover the values, beliefs, interests, and ambitions of the individual and make determinations regarding the potential behavioral response that may occur during a radiological exam. However, the competence of the radiology nurse relative to the recognition of the potential motivations of CYP is fundamental. Recall the case of Michael [7]. Although he had limited familiarity with hospital environments and was observed as anxious, he took on the challenge of learning about the procedure and his role in achieving his goal of no sedation in order to attend a football game that evening. In an effort to encourage radiological nurses to think about the *why* behind the observed behavior of CYP undergoing challenging radiology procedures, a social-cognitive approach to achievement motivation is reviewed [15]. In reviewing this model, an experienced radiology nurse will no doubt recall specific experiences that speak to patterns of the behavior CYP experienced in the radiology environment; think of those individuals who maintain a posture of curiosity and an eagerness to learn throughout a procedure in contrast to individuals who present unprepared to face the complex expectations of the environment.

From a social-cognitive approach, Dweck and Leggett identify two patterns of cognition-affect-behavior in which they describe how goals influence the interpretation and reaction of individuals to events [15]. A *performance-oriented* individual is characterized as showing a pattern of seeking positive judgements and avoiding negative judgements on their competence. The goal is about *proving* their ability. However, when facing what they perceive to be obstacles, their competence becomes compromised due to maladaptive thinking, affect, and behaviors. In sum, their adaptive and competent behaviors deteriorate into helplessness. In contrast, a *learning-oriented* individual has the goal to improve their competence. When faced with obstacles, they pursue mastery through increasing effort and generating strategies to reach a solution to challenges. Whereas performance-oriented individuals attribute difficulties to their lack of ability to succeed, learning-oriented individuals see challenges to be solved through increased effort [15]. It seems the performance-oriented individuals see threat in challenge where learning-oriented individuals see opportunity. Therefore, in recognizing success, the maintenance of CYP dignity and advancing mastery through learning are two elements of success to keep in mind as relationships with CYP are established.

Given the many opportunities for challenge inherent in the processes involved in preparing for and undertaking a radiological procedure, radiology nurses need to be equipped to present the best options to match the underlying needs of individuals in order to attain the successful experience for the CYP. When each CYP is approached with the belief in their competence and capacity, then the radiology nurse opens the door to creating conditions for collaboration and the identification of pathways leading to a successful experience. Increasing a CYP sense of control and self-determination involves sensitivity to the goal orientation of the individual by placing the radiological experience into meaningful and interesting learning contexts, personalizing learning, and offering choices within a collaborative relationship.

## 24.6 Summary

The primary question of how we can make the radiology experience of children and young people a positive one is complex. This chapter was written from a child life perspective noting that the responsibility of the CLS lies primarily with the child and family. Therefore, an explicit acknowledgement that radiology nurses have the additional responsibility of managing complex radiology procedures is necessary: The combination of nursing responsibilities includes both the technical and human elements of a radiology procedure. This suggests that in order to collaborate with children and young people, planning to intentionally include their voice is required. Wyatt et al. conducted a meta-analysis and determined that shared decision-making in pediatric interventions rarely targeted children and focused on parents [16]. Indeed, there is work to be done to establish practices that allow radiology nurses to present the best options to CYP matched to their specific needs in order to attain the successful experience for the CYP.

Application of an ecological model draws attention to the nature of the interactions of the CYP *with* existing systems, particularly highlighting the status of the individual as an active agent.

Suggested approaches to addressing current and future policy and practices arising from this discussion include the following.

1. A movement toward considering the CYP as an essential player in healthcare procedures is encouraged. Quality improvement projects to capture current ways that concepts such as image of the child, child agency, and health literacy friendly are interpreted may reveal a diverse response and opportunities to engage in transformative learning events that align, for example, with the rights-based principles in the CRC [2] that acknowledge the rights of children to be involved in decisions, education, and play.
2. Recognition that adult perceptions and expectations are likely to differ from a CYP is one component of this discussion to be examined by radiology nurses at all levels. Reflection and critical examination of the values, beliefs, and attitudes held toward CYP that impact approaches to advocacy for the CYP may highlight ways to enhance efforts to support successful radiology experiences.
3. Examination of current practices on ways to engage children and young people's competence and capacity through welcoming relationships, inviting collaboration, and recognizing success may result in the development of new policies and procedures targeting greater attention to these particular aspects of pediatric services.
4. The capacity of the radiology nurse to recognize and employ the potential motivation of the CYP relative to the achievement of a successful experience is fundamental. In making the process of preparation for a radiology procedure collaborative, the radiological nurse has a role in making the whole process meaningful for the CYP. The prospect of assessing the competence of radiology nurses in addressing questions, concerns and initiate the inclusion of the CYP as an active participant in the procedure is likely an area for future investigation.
5. Health literacy friendly services should be included to support the needs of all users of the radiology environment. Radiology teams can complete an environmental scan of the area and a review of educational documents and media from the viewpoint of the user from a range of developmental stages. Acknowledgement of the diverse and changing needs and interests of growing children and youth can be made visible through the provision of developmentally appropriate approaches to the environment and learning.

## References

1. Bronfenbrenner U. The ecology of human development. Cambridge: Harvard University Press; 1979.
2. The United Nations. Convention on the Rights of the Child Treaty Series 1577, Nov 1989, p. 3.
3. Alexander M. Managing patient stress in pediatric radiology. Radiol Technol. 2012;83(6):549–60.
4. Gibson J. The theory of affordances. In: Shaw R, Bransford J, editors. Perceiving, acting and knowing. Hillsdale, NJ: LEA; 1977.
5. Bröder J, Okan O, Bauer U, Bruland D, Schlupp S, Bollweg T, et al. Health literacy in childhood and youth: a systematic review of definitions and models. BMC Public Health. 2017;17:1. https://doi.org/10.1186/s12889-017-4267-y.
6. Linder J, Schiska A. Imaging children: tips and tricks. J Radiol Nurs. 2007;26:23–5.

7. Metzger T, Mignogna K, Reilly L. Child life specialists: key members of the team in pediatric radiology. J Radiol Nurs. 2013;32:153–9.
8. Montreuil M, Carnevale FA. A concept analysis of children's agency within the health literature. J Child Health Care. 2016;20(4):503–11.
9. Bhargava R, et al. Contrast-enhanced magnetic resonance imaging in pediatric patients: review and recommendations for current practice. Magn Reson Insights. 2013;6:95–111.
10. Bates DG. VCUG and the recurring question of sedation: preparation and catheterization technique are the key. Pediatr Radiol. 2012;42(3):285–9.
11. Turner J, Fralic J. Making explicit the implicit: child life specialists talk about their assessment process. Child Youth Care Forum. 2009;38(1):39–54.
12. Parnell EC. Making space: designing the classroom environment for movement. PhysHealth EducJ. 2013;78(4):26–8.
13. CordovaDI, LepperMR. Intrinsic motivation and the process of learning: beneficial effects of contextualization, personalization, and choice. J Educ Psychol. 1996 [cited 2019 Mar 30];88(4):715–30.
14. Callery P, Coyne I. Supporting children and adolescents inclusion in decisions and self-management: what can help? Patient Educ Couns. 2019;102:605–6.
15. DweckCS, LeggettEL. A social-cognitive approach to motivation and personality. Psychol Rev.1988 [cited 2019 Mar 30];95(2):256–73.
16. Wyatt, et al. Shared decision making in pediatrics: a systematic review and meta analysis. Acad Pediatr. 2015;15(6):573–83.

# Forensic Patients in the Healthcare Setting

## 25

Debra S. Holbrook

## 25.1 Introduction

According to the World Health Organization millions of patients are being victimized by interpersonal violence and presenting to hospitals and clinics daily [1]. Healthcare providers (HCP), including those working in departments of radiology, are uniquely positioned to interact with patients in a safe and private setting and view physical wounds. Encouraging HCPs to become aware of the signs of abuse, neglect, and maltreatment offers victimized patients a safety net, creating a proactive workplace and giving a voice to victims of egregious crimes of abuse.

The purpose of this chapter is to provide an overview of interpersonal violence, describe commonly visualized wounds, offer suggestions for screening patients for abuse, evaluate attitudes regarding patient disclosures, develop multidisciplinary collaboration and referral of these patients as victims, and create an environment where patients are believed and provided safety and improved healthcare outcomes.

D. S. Holbrook, MSN, RN, SANE-A, FNE-A/P, FAAN(c) (✉)
Mercy Medical Center, Baltimore, MD, USA

## 25.2 Wounds Commonly Seen in Patients Victimized by Violence

Patients experiencing interpersonal violence are subjected to acts that may cause wounds often seen in various stages of healing. The most common wounds assessed are defined in Table 25.1.

## 25.3 Intimate Partner Violence

Intimate partner violence (IPV), a form of interpersonal violence, is defined as physical, sexual, or psychological harm caused by a former or current partner or spouse [7]. With an estimated 35% of emergency department visits annually and 21% of injuries requiring surgical intervention, IPV is the most frequently committed violence against women [7, 8]. With the knowledge that IPV is increasing, and that only a small percentage of victims report their abuse to medical care providers or law enforcement, IPV is a worldwide public healthcare crisis.

Implausible histories that are inconsistent with the mechanism of injury in wounds visualized by the HCP are a red flag that a patient may be experiencing IPV. Often patterned wounds, bruising in protected areas such as beneath the breast, medial thighs, medial upper arms, and behind the ears are regions injured by intent rather than by accident.

**Table 25.1** Common types of wounds

Bruising (also contusion)—is caused by blunt or squeezing force trauma resulting in superficial discoloration due to a hemorrhage into the tissue from ruptured blood vessels beneath the surface, without the skin being broken. Bruises may take days or weeks to come to the surface, or, in some cases, may never be visualized with the unaided eye. Visualization of bruising is subject to: age, amount of escaped blood, body location, depth, skin pigmentation, velocity of the object, exposure to cold, and medications. There is no valid scientific study validating the practice of dating bruising [2–4].

Abrasion—a wearing, grinding, or rubbing away by friction. Abrasions are often referred to as scratches or scrapes, and may be described as linear, as in fingernail abrasions [5].

Central clearing—area of lighter color with surrounding bruising caused by blunt force trauma; also known as sparing [6] (see Fig. 25.1).

Laceration—a tearing of the skin caused by blunt force trauma, often characterized by irregular borders.

Incision—a cut to the skin, often characterized by even borders [5].

Fracture—the cracking or breaking of a hard object or material [5].

\*\*It is important to note that injuries also present as bite marks, branding, burns, and patterned wounds that reflect the impression of the mechanism that caused the injury.

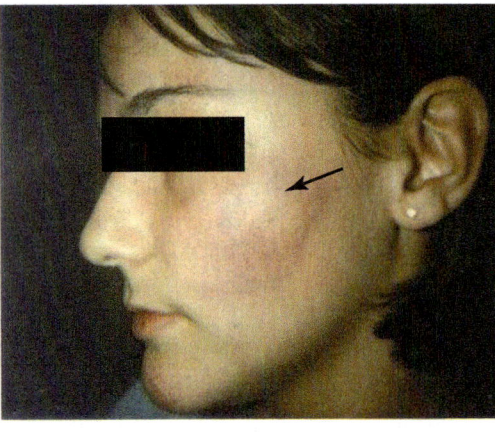

**Fig. 25.1** Central clearing. (Photo courtesy Debra Holbrook)

While physical abuse and injury may be obvious signs of an assault, screening for IPV is difficult as secondary illnesses manifest in a variety of presenting symptoms such as headaches and migraines, gastrointestinal maladies, neurologic complaints, sleep disorders, cardiac illnesses, and mental health issues including depression [1]. Patients who may be experiencing IPV often demonstrate:

- Frequent visits to HCPs for seemingly unrelated symptoms, but delaying visits for physical wounds and fractures
- Not speaking for themselves with hovering family members or care takers
- Being brought by partners or family members who are adamant about not leaving the patient alone in a room with a HCP
- Expressing an urgency to leave as soon as possible or the need to sign out against medical advice
- Distress regarding the need to wait for radiology procedures or lab results
- Eating disorders
- Recurrent sexually transmitted infections [1]

### 25.3.1 Strangulation

One of the most violent and intentional acts committed by abusers is strangulation which is defined as "a form of asphyxia characterized by closure of the blood vessels or air passages of the neck as a result of external pressure" [9]. There are two common ways that strangulation trauma is inflicted. *Manual strangulation* via a one-handed, two-handed, or chokehold mechanism and is also known as throttling. *Ligature strangulation* uses a cord, rope, or clothing to compress the neck and is also known as garroting[10]. Ligature injuries are further separated into hanging strangulations (using the body weight to compress a ligature) and autoerotic strangulations (self-induced asphyxiation for sexual gratification)[11].

Small blunt-force trauma, such as fingertips, generally causes bruising that can be seen by the unaided eye. This is due to energy directed to a small focal area similar to what happens when one bumps their shin on the corner of a table resulting in a painful bruise or contusion. Conversely, when an equal amount of energy is directed to a broad focal area, such as bumping the upper arm against the broad surface of a wall,

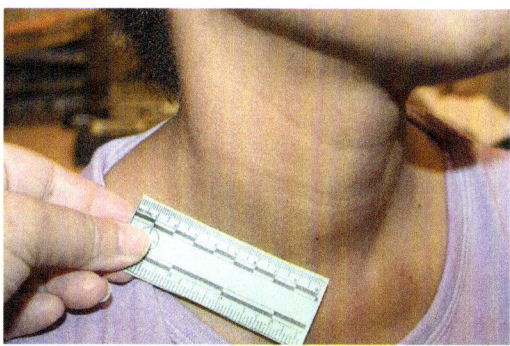

**Fig. 25.2** Strangulation with no visible injury. (Courtesy Debra Holbrook)

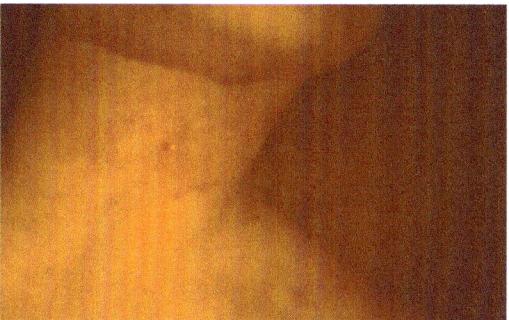

**Fig. 25.3** Same strangulation under ALS 450 wavelength orange goggles. (Courtesy Debra Holbrook)

intradermal bruising may be present but is rarely seen due to the dispersing of energy. As most patients are not strangled by fingertips, when the mechanism of injury is an arm or hand exerting pressure on the neck, intradermal capillary beds under the skin may be disrupted that are not visible to the naked eye[12]. It is important to recognize that the absence of bruising does not mean that an assault did not occur as described by the patient (see Figs. 25.2 and 25.3).

### 25.3.2 Detection of Bruising

Many communities have developed proactive Forensic Nurse Examiner (FNE) and Law Enforcement Investigative Programs (which will be examined further in this chapter). These programs have begun to utilize alternate light source technology (ALS) to visualize bruising and other injury intradermally. An ALS consists of a powerful lamp that emits ultraviolet, visible, and infrared wavelengths. It filters the light into individual color bands (wavelengths) that enhance the visualization of evidence by light interaction techniques: fluorescence (evidence that glows), absorption (evidence that darkens), and oblique lighting (small particle evidence that is revealed). These light sources can reveal bruises and patterned wound details that are invisible under normal white-light illumination[12]. ALS offers FNEs and investigators the ability to identify broad focal trauma by revealing intradermal bruising/absorption.

A HCP in the radiology setting may be perplexed as to why a patient is being seen for computerized tomography (CT) with angiography or magnetic resonance imaging (MRI) when the patient has no marks visible on their neck, no petechial hemorrhaging to the sclera of their eyes, and no untoward symptoms such as hoarseness, voice changes, coughing, difficulty breathing, or pain. Oftentimes when an FNE has visualized darkened areas beneath the skin during an ALS assessment, especially when these areas are patterned consistent with the mechanism of injury described by the patient, the FNE will alert the physician to the ALS findings, yielding a request for radiologic procedures. Understanding that many patients are strangled by several mechanisms, edema in the neck may present immediately, "or be delayed for up to 36 hours after the initial injury leading to airway compromise and arterial occlusion" [7]. A thorough assessment is critical for patients who report strangulation due to the severity of the development of these later symptoms, including death. (For more information related to recommendations for medical care and intervention post strangulation see https://www.strangulationtraininginstitute.com/.)

## 25.4 Elder Neglect, Abuse, and Maltreatment

The prevalence of interpersonal violence in the form of elder abuse, neglect, and maltreatment affects more than 1 million persons in the United

States (US) annually, with an estimated 25% of these persons experiencing physical assault. While in some cultures respect for elders is taught at an early age, that cultural aspect does not exist everywhere and many factors can affect this type of abuse. Elder abuse may be physical, financial, or in the form of neglect and is most often perpetrated by family members due to stress, burnout as care takers, or financial burdens [7]. Elder abuse is often unrecognized with an estimated 10% of older US adults experiencing maltreatment annually and less than 1 in 24 of these adults being identified and reported to Adult Protective Services (APS) or law enforcement [13]. HCPs often miss critical opportunities to identify elder abuse because it is so offensive to believe that caretakers would commit such egregious actions upon their elderly and most vulnerable family members. Poor physical health, disability, and mental deterioration such as dementia and depression are risk factors for elder abuse [14]. Additionally, many older adults are limited in their activities outside of the home, isolated from society, and dependent both physically and financially upon their family or caretakers. These assaults are seen in healthcare settings more often during evenings and weekends related to an increase in social interaction with abusers during these hours. Older adults are often reluctant, afraid, and embarrassed to admit that their trusted family members would demonstrate such cruel actions against them in the form of physical abuse and financial crimes.

While it may be difficult to discern between accidental versus intentional injury in older persons due to osteoporosis, fragility in skin and vascular integrity, and generalized weaknesses, the literature supports some distinctions [7]. Elder abuse is more likely to present with bruising of the posterior torso including high-energy injury such as rib fractures. Bruising is also common from intentional injury to the ulnar forearms—likely from the victim defending themself against the abuser [15]. Mechanisms of injury may include grabbing and use of restraints which may leave fingertip-like or circumferential bruising to the wrists and lateral aspects of the arms. Injuries to the lower extremity, inner thigh, or dorsal/plantar surface of the foot are also indicators of intentional abuse and are not accidental in nature [16]. Fracture of the distal ulnar diaphysis is also suggestive of intentional injury and is uncommon in accidental injury [7]. Wounds and bruises in various stages of healing are also red flags alerting healthcare providers to the possibility of maltreatment.

## 25.5 Child Abuse

"Child abuse is an international epidemic" and, although HCPs are more informed than ever before in history, the numbers continue to grow [17]. Nurses should remember that in order for an infant or toddler to bruise themself accidentally, they must be ambulatory in some way; otherwise the injury is inflicted upon them. As much is published regarding child abuse this section seeks to provide an overview of child abuse from the perspective of a nurse in a radiology setting.

Second to soft tissue injuries such as bruises and abrasions, fractures are considered the leading causes of injury, primarily in younger and nonverbal children who cannot offer a verbal explanation for causation of the injury. When there are concerns regarding physical abuse of a child, the nurse should consider mechanism of injury, plausibility of injury occurring as described by a caretaker, time elapsed between time of injury and time of treatment, and findings from radiologic studies [17]. Most fractures do occur accidentally in children; however, abuse must be considered in children younger than 2 years of age [18]. Common fractures seen in child abuse include: diaphyseal fractures in a non-ambulatory child, posterior rib fractures—especially when there are squeeze-like demarcations to the torso, and corner bucket-handle fractures (growth plate disconnected from the shaft). Baby-grams or skeletal survey films of the child's body are frequently ordered to assess the presence of healing fractures within a child's body.

CT may be requested to assess head, spinal, rib, and abdominal injuries resulting from intentional as well as accidental injuries. The most common injuries to solid organs resulting from blunt force trauma are to the liver, spleen, pancreas, and bowel. Lacerations and hematomas to solid organs of the torso are not uncommon in intentional injury. CT is also useful in demonstrating skull fractures and intracranial injuries such as subdural hemorrhage. Trauma to the brain via shaking of a child is widely published and includes anoxic brain injuries including diffuse axonal trauma [19]. It is imperative that a HCP procures a detailed history, including mechanism of injury, in order to develop an informed basis for conclusion in determining intentional versus accidental causation of radiologic findings.

## 25.6 Human Trafficking

Few can imagine the suffering of being sold for sex with strangers, working 18 or more hours every day, being beaten and humiliated, and yet dependent on the cruel abuser who owns you for the drugs for which you are dependent. This is the face of a victim of human trafficking. Human trafficking has been referred to as "modern day slavery," and is defined as being hired to work by force, fraud, or coercion, and HCPs are caring for these victims of sex and labor trafficking daily. *Minors who are induced into commercial sex trades are considered victims regardless of whether force, fraud, or coercion is present* [20]. Global estimates are that there are 20.1 million people trapped in forced labor in both sex and labor trafficking [1]. Trafficking is tied with illegal arms trading as the second largest criminal industry in the world, and in 2015 it was estimated that $50 billion was generated from forced labor and sexual exploitation [21].

The money that these victims make is never their own, they wear tracking devices, and are often branded and tattooed with the abusers name or a bar code as his property. Many of these victims are abducted from the streets as children, chosen for their innocence or vulnerability, and sold into slavery where they are forced to perform as many as 50 sex acts a day [22]. Patients who are trafficked might migrate from one healthcare facility to another with complaints and/or symptoms of: strangulation, bruises in various stages of healing, scars, pelvic inflammatory disease, frequent urinary tract infections, signs of malnourishment, foot pain/neuropathy, and chemical dependence/withdrawal [21]. They are most often guarded by another female known as the "bottom" girl who is most trusted by the trafficker and are moved from city to city—sometimes weekly. The victim will not be left alone with a HCP, will not speak for him/herself, will rarely display eye contact with another individual, may not know their name, address, birth date, or social security number, and is coached to answer questions [21].

**Table 25.2** Sample screening questions for human trafficking patients—recommended in conversational format

1. Have you been physically or verbally abused, raped, threatened, or made to feel physical pain for working slowly or trying to leave your current location or residence?
2. Have you been in a situation in which you are being held against your will, had your documents taken, or forced into situations that do not make you feel safe or comfortable?
3. Have you been forced to perform sexual acts for housing, money, food, or to pay off a debt?

Courtesy Debra Holbrook

HCPs are key first responders to the signs of trafficking (see Table 25.2) and should become familiar with the language of trafficked people such as: stable (where the victim stays), daddy (the trafficker), bottom girl (daddy's most trusted trafficked victim), folk or family (others in the stable), johns (the buyers of sex), and stroll (the area where the victim walks to solicit johns) (see https://sharedhope.org/the-problem/trafficking-terms/ for more information on language used).

## 25.7 Forensic Nurse Examiners

In an effort to provide state-of-the-art forensic medical care to patients who are victims of crime, healthcare facilities across the world are embracing forensic nursing programs. Some programs may care for only patients victimized by sexual assault and are known as Sexual Assault Nurse Examiners (SANE). Forensic nurse examiner programs care for patients across the life span victimized by crimes including, but not limited to, sexual assault, interpersonal violence, elder abuse, child abuse, human trafficking, dating violence, non-accidental gunshots, stabbings, burns, poisonings, and suspects of persons crimes. These advanced practice nurses, known as Forensic Nurse Examiners (FNEs), are specially educated in forensic medical assessments, forensic medical interviews, and crisis intervention (see info@academyofforensicnursing.org to request information on becoming a forensic nurse and regional FNE programs). FNEs use state-of-the-art technology to conduct nonjudgmental, sensitive, medical evidentiary examinations in the care of patients victimized by bodily crimes [23]. In the state of Maryland (US) the state board of nursing oversees an FNE's practice and education requirements for advanced practice (see https://mbon.maryland.gov/Pages/forensic-nurse-examiner.aspx for an example and listing of available programs). The outcomes of these FNE-driven evidentiary examinations may be analyzed by crime lab technicians, and findings may be used in judicial proceedings where the FNE may be deemed either a fact or expert witness. As a result, FNEs have become a best practice standard and have become leaders in the education of medical and nursing staff, and many groups within the community. The Academy of Forensic Nursing (AFN) supports the specialty of nursing caring for victims of interpersonal violence across the life span (see www.academyofnursing.org).

## 25.8 Victimization and Believing a Patient's History

Healthcare professionals would never think to respond to a victim of a fall or a motor vehicle collision with disbelief; however, that is exactly how many victims of sexual assault and interpersonal violence are treated in hospitals daily. Terms such as "alleged sexual assault" and "alleged abuse" are commonly used diagnostic terms that are assigned to patient reports implying doubt and skepticism regarding the patient's history. This perpetuates a culture of shame and self-blame that often leads to a decrease in reporting rates and a reluctance for a patient to share the history of some of their darkest moments with medical and nursing staff. End Violence Against Women International (EVAWI; https://www.evawintl.org) and their *Start By Believing* awareness initiatives support the knowledge that when a victim of crime is not believed by caretakers, family, healthcare providers, law enforcement, and the community at large—that one failed response equals 5 more assaults [24]. Healthcare providers are uniquely qualified to care for victims as *patients* who in turn entrust their histories, medical care, and healthcare to these providers. A single negative reaction may have devastating results which may lead to a decline in a patient's health, well-being, and safety. It is imperative that healthcare providers consider how they would react and respond to a patient disclosure of assault *prior to* such a disclosure.

### 25.8.1 Screening of Patients Suspected of Being Abused

It is imperative that the HCP isolates the victim patient of IPV or trafficking from anyone that is suspected of guarding them. HCPs in radiology settings are uniquely positioned to speak to a patient alone due to the nature of the unit. Nurses routinely justify having visitors leave a patient suspected to be abused by stating that the patient may need to go to have X-rays. Another approach to isolating a patient for safety is to request that the "visitor" sign forms out of the department and yet another is to request that the patient be assisted by the HCP to a private restroom. It is important to remember that a patient who is being abused will almost never disclose when the abuser or their designee is in hearing distance of their conversation. That includes triage, interactions with nurses and physicians, during procedures or when speaking with technologists or lab technicians.

Screening questions work best when weaved into a conversation with a patient and not asked in a line item format [25]. Consider these two interview scenarios:

- A HCP is facing the computer and asks: "What brings you into the emergency department today? Did you put ice on the wound? When was your last tetanus shot? Does anyone harm or control you in your home? Do you smoke?", versus
- A HCP is facing the computer and asks: "What brings you into the emergency department today? Are you up to date on your tetanus shots? Did you put ice on the wound?" At the end of the encounter the HCP turns to the patient (with whom they are alone) and says, "I care about you, you are safe here, and I believe you. I see you have some serious wounds that do not look like you fell down. Can you tell me more about these wounds? I would like to help you."

Use of a more conversational screening technique engages the patient and builds trust. Sitting at or below eye level also conveys a nondominant position and is less threatening than looking down at the patient[21].

As with other forms of abuse, victims of trafficking are afraid or reticent when being screened by HCPs. Tips for speaking candidly with these patients revolve around gaining their trust, being kind and nonjudgmental. Asking open-ended questions such as "Can you tell me more?" and assuring them that you want to keep them safe may be helpful. Remember that victims may not disclose their abuse the first time that they are asked. It is important to share mandated reporting requirements with the patient if you are required to call law enforcement, Adult or Child Protective Services. In those instances when reporting is *not* required, a patient has learned that you cared enough to ask about their safety and well-being and may remember that you are safe haven when they *are* ready to report [25].

## 25.9 Referrals and Collaborative Practices

So what do hosts of forensic leaders recommend that a HCP do when they have identified a patient/victim of abuse, neglect, maltreatment or trafficking and screening questions have been confirmed? Table 25.3 lists appropriate interventions once the victim has been identified.

**Table 25.3** Actions to consider when a victim has been identified

1. Keeping the patient safe is a primary consideration. This may include notifying your manager or agency's security department.
2. Discuss discreetly with the patient's care team the suspicions, disclosure from the patient, and other pertinent signs and symptoms that may require additional medical intervention or radiologic procedures.
3. Know the laws regarding reporting of abuse in a state or region and take the time to review agency protocols regarding mandated reporting. In the USA this generally includes 24/7/365 contact information for law enforcement, Child Protective Services and Federal Bureau of Investigation (FBI) or other relevant agencies. As discussed, mandated reporting varies greatly from jurisdiction to jurisdiction. There should be a designated person within an agency or unit who is defined as the contact to make these calls. The forensic nurse or other forensic examiner may make these referrals when called for a consultation.
4. Contact appointed advocacy from either social work or a host of strong patient advocates within the community. This resource is essential as advocates are the voice of the patient and have extensive training in appropriate referrals, safety planning, lethality assessments, emergency admission protocols, and answers to patient concerns. Advocates give patients options and are their voice in the medicolegal system [25].

## 25.10 Documentation

It is widely regarded that nurses are the most trusted profession for ethical standards and honesty [26] and it is not uncommon for patients to disclose intimate details of an abusive relationship with their nurse. Documentation is a key component to assuring that statements made by a patient or their family are immortalized in such a manner as to share with other members of the healthcare team. Excited utterances—the first statements made by the victimized patient after an assault—are often crucial to beginning an investigation which includes deployment of protective services, law enforcement, and a forensic nursing team.

Any statement made directly by a patient should always be documented in quotations. This practice protects the nurse from accusations of misinterpretation of the patient's statements and may be the only disclosure that is shared with a HCP. It is generally not recommended that a HCP other than a forensic nurse or other forensic discipline document details describing the assault. Differing details recorded from provider to provider may be interpreted as a patient telling multiple versions of a history rather than HCPs offering differing versions of that history. This in turn may affect prosecution outcomes. It is recommended that a nurse within the radiology department always consult with their healthcare team and risk management department regarding the proper procedures governing documentation of neglect, abuse, and maltreatment of patients within a particular institution.

## 25.11 Conclusion

HCPs in radiology and other medical specialty units are ideally positioned to interact with patients in a safe and private setting and view physical wounds. Encouraging HCPs to become aware of the signs of abuse, neglect, and maltreatment offers victimized patients a safety net, which creates a proactive workplace giving a voice to victims of egregious crimes of abuse. As HCPs become more comfortable with screening and assessing *all* patients for abuse, neglect, and maltreatment, they will become more comfortable with the screening process. Additionally, as HCPs assure that healthcare facilities are well versed in multidisciplinary team collaboration, patients are given a voice and experience significant improvement in their health outcomes.

## References

1. World Health Organization. Responding to intimate partner violence and sexual violence against women.2013.Retrieved from:https://books.google.com/books?hl=en&lr=&id=q7IXDAAAQBAJ&oi=fnd&pg=PP1&dq=world+health+organization+violence+statistics&ots=luz3Gv1mld&sig=sUJoItdlaaNy2P0cLR_cneGi0OM#v=onepage&q=world%20health%20organization%20violence%20statistics&f=false.
2. Sheridan DJ, Nash KR. Acute injury patterns of intimate partner violence victims. Trauma Violence Abuse. 2007;8:286–9.
3. DiMao VJ, DiMao D. Chapter 4: Blunt trauma wounds. In: Forensic pathology. 2nd ed. Boca Raton, FL: CRC Press; 2001. p. 91–116.
4. Scafide KR, Sheridan DJ, Campbell J, DeLeon VB, Hyatt MJ. Evaluating change in bruise colourimetry and the effect of subject characteristics over time. Forensic Sci Med Pathol. 2013;18(4):561–9.
5. Merriam-Webster. n.d. Retrieved from:https://www.merriamwebster.com/dictionary/abrasion, http://www.merriam-webster.com/dictionary/fracture, andhttps://www.merriam-webster.com/dictionary/incision
6. Holbrook D. Documentation of wounds in a forensic medical assessment: an interactive learning module. Forensic Nurse Examiner Adult Adolescent Curriculum. Baltimore, MD: Mercy Medical Center; 2018.
7. Russo A, Reginelli A, Pignatiello M, Cioce F, Mazzei G, Fabozzi O, Parloto V, Cappabianca S, Giovine S. Imaging of violence against the elderly and the women. Semin Ultrasound CTMRI. 2019;40:18–24. https://doi.org/10.1053/j.sult.2018.10.004.
8. Regueira-Dieguez A, Perez-Rivas N, Munoz-Barus JL, et al. Intimate partner violence against women in Spain: a medico-legal and criminological study. J Forensic Leg Med. 2015;34:119–26.
9. McClane GE, Straek GB, Hawley D. A review of 300 attempted strangulation cases part II: clinical evaluation of the surviving victim. J Emerg Med. 2001;21:311–5.
10. Iserson K. Strangulation: a review of ligature, manual and postural compression injuries. Ann Emerg Med. 1984;13:179–85.
11. Ernoehazy W Jr. Hanging injuries and strangulation. Updated 16 Jul 2008. Available at: emedicine.medscape.com/article/826704-overview. Accessed on 5 Mar 2012.
12. Holbrook DS, Jackson MC. Use of alternative light source to assess strangulation victims. JForensic Nurs. 2013;9(3):140–5.
13. Huecker MR, Smock W. Domestic violence. Treasure Island, FL: StatPearls Publishing; 2018.https://pearlpublishing.net.
14. Vandeweerd C, Paveza GJ, Fulmer T. Abuse and neglect in older adults with Alzheimer's disease. Nurs Clin North Am. 2006;41(1):43–55.
15. Switzer JA, Michienzi AE. Elder abuse: an update on relevance, identification, and reporting for the orthopaedic surgeon. J Am Acad Orthop Surg. 2012;20:788–94.
16. Breckman R, Burnes D, Ross S, et al. When helping hurts: non-abusing family, friends, and neighbors in the lives of elder mistreatment victims. Gerontologist. 2018;58(7):719–23.

17. Karakachian A, Eichman A, Sekula K. Understanding the importance of radiology screening when suspecting child abuse. J Radiol Nurs. 2017;36:70–8.
18. Flaherty EG, Perez-Rossello JM, Levine MA, Hemrikus WI, Christian CW, Crawford-Jakubik JE, et al. Evaluating children with fractures for child physical abuse. Pediatrics. 2014;133(2):477–89.
19. Tun K, Choudhary AK, Methratta S, Boal DK. Radiological features of nonaccidental injury. J Radiol Nurs. 2013;32(1):3–9.
20. Department of Homeland Security. Blue Campaign.n.d. Retrieved from:https://www.dhs.gov/blue-campaign.
21. Polaris Project. n.d. Retrieved from:https://polarisproject.org/.
22. StackT.What does a victim of human trafficking look like? Maryland law enforcement training symposium presented 2Apr2019, Ocean City, MD. 2018.
23. Linden JA, Young JS. Overview in adolescent and adult sexual assault. In: Giardino AP, Datner EM, Asher JB, editors. Sexual assault victimization across the life span. St. Louis, MO: GW Medical Publishing; 2004.
24. End Violence Against Women International. Start by believing.2018.Retrieved from:www.startbybelieving.org/whattosay.
25. HolbrookDS. Forensic documentation and reporting in Sigma Theta Tau Forensic Nurse Examiner Online Curriculum Modules.2019.
26. Forbes Magazine. America's most and least trusted professions. 2018. Retrieved from: https://www.forbes.com/sites/niallmccarthy/2018/01/04/america.

# Section V

# Professional Topics

# Cybersecurity: Cyberspace Wars—The Unseen Enemy

## 26

Thomas Hough and Kathleen A. Gross

## 26.1 Introduction

What is more important; knowing your bank balance at an automated teller machine (ATM) in a distant gas station or having the ability to view your most recent computed tomography (CT) scan and report at your doctor's office in your town? The banks appear to have this figured out reasonably well. What is holding up healthcare? Is it money or priorities? As more and more of healthcare events are migrated to have more and more relevant data digitally transferred, managed, and stored, the chances of someone hacking into patient healthcare records increases exponentially. Why would hackers want this information? This chapter will reveal this as part of the challenges in keeping unwanted visitors out while giving permissions to view to wanted visitors. The effect of breaches is to "reduce patient trust, cripple health systems, and threaten human life" [1]. More research on cybersecurity has focused on technology but all aspects (human, organization, management, and strategy) need to be researched [2].

---

T. Hough, CMC (✉)
True North Consulting & Associates Inc.,
Mississauga, ON, Canada

K. A. Gross, MSN, BS, RN-BC, CRN
Owings Mills, MD, USA

## 26.1.1 Intranet Versus Internet

If we could create an intranet (a closed network within the boundaries of the enterprise), then it would be much easier to maintain security and grant permissions to who gets to see what information. The Internet and the need to use its digital pathways for cost-effective sharing of data is what creates the opportunity for unwanted visitors to break into the closed networks within healthcare systems. Examples of threats to security are listed in Table 26.1.

**Table 26.1** Threats to security come in the following forms

- Identity Information Theft
- Ransomware
- Spy Ware
- Computer Viruses seeking private information
- Trojan Horses
- Malware
- Hackers seeking databases to exploit
- Data Leaks—software created with backdoors
- Data Leaks—through healthcare laptops stolen with PHI databases on them
- Phishing—trickery to get you to log into a false web site to harvest User Identification (UID) and Password(s) and security questions
- Cyberattacks—on servers and data centers to view function to exploit; enterprise control systems
- Manipulation or theft of social media accounts
- Harvesting your Internet travels and preferences to target you for marketing
- Plus, hundreds if not thousands of other security breaches too numerous to mention

For all the threats listed above, antidotes are developed as quickly as possible and new security protocols are deployed, in the never-ending cat and mouse game of digital security.

As we get up each day and go about our lives, there are hundreds of thousands of criminals who are spending 24 h day working and developing new ways to compromise our digital life. It is this counter culture that has waged a war on our digital lives which causes us to have to implement complex and very complicated barriers to entry.

## 26.2 Why Is Protected Health Information (PHI) Critical?

Consider if a new diagnosis of a disease was shared from a hacked information source with an insurance company. The insurance company could then deny or cancel coverage even before the patient is told of the diagnosis. Here insurance companies could profit from the misfortune of others who they collect premiums from up until the disease is known. Alternatively, imagine a professional level athlete having the magnetic resonance imaging (MRI) results on his or her knee leaked to the press as they enter into contact negotiations with a team. It could cost the athlete millions and disrupt the normal sequence of events for the team, the athlete, and the fans. It would feel like an injustice has been done.

Hackers are increasingly targeting healthcare providers because of the high price they can command for sensitive patient data and for the recent success from ransomware attacks. In the United States, in the past year, there has been more than one hospital held up with ransom payments to extortionists in order to regain the use of their computers back from the ransomware. Aside from this driving up the already high cost of healthcare imagine if all computers are compromised at a time of a national emergency and hundreds of thousands of lives are lost due to a ransomware event designed to bring a country to its knees by a corrupt organization attempting to leverage their beliefs over another.

## 26.3 Is Cybersecurity Important?

Clinical care has become dependent on equipment using information technology (IT) [2]. Cybersecurity is much more important because it affects not only money and who get it or does not get it but the natural course of people's lives. Compromised PHI determines if they can live with dignity or shame and disgrace because the wrong people accessed information.

Within a healthcare enterprise there can be hundreds, thousands, or tens of thousands of devices on the network—most are high technology healthcare applications designed to do specific healthcare functions built by vendors who are not aware of the invading enemies. Should the IT department do their jobs well then there is no problem. Smaller health centers often do not have the staff nor budgets to defend the enemy with all the current state-of-the-art tools required. As seen in Fig. 26.1, the classic IT configuration is to create a "De-Militarized Zone" (DMZ) where devices known to the enterprise can approach the protected network and permutate the firewall to gain access remotely as require. Clinicians and administrators who have extended responsibilities to access the hospital network during off-hour situations are often given special permissions for this.

The challenge is to prevent or intercept cyberattacks. A mechanism which can detect malicious activity within devices and data transfer into or out of the enterprise while not interfering with the daily operations is essential. Larger healthcare providers most likely have more resources to address cybersecurity. The availability of tools that can protect a range of devices without requiring individual device vendor software changes will significantly reduce cyber threats.

One of the greatest vulnerabilities comes with image sharing. Images are a key part of healthcare operations. Compact disc (CD)/digital versatile disc (DVD) based image sharing applications are being replaced with cloud-based applications. Server-side viewing and rendering technologies employing internal cloud-type services where all data is on a single server that

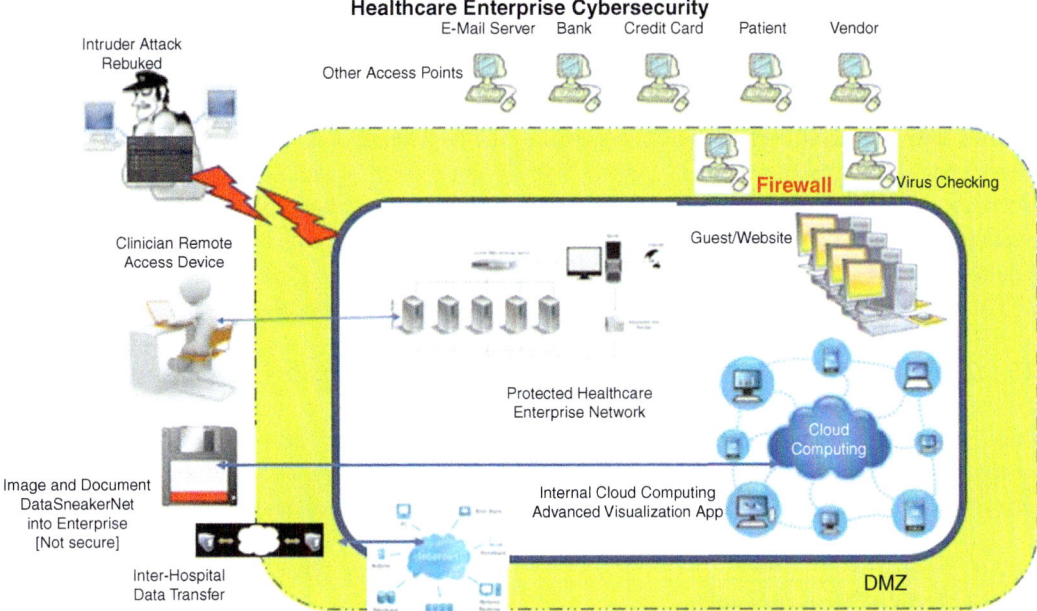

**Fig. 26.1** Configuration drawing of a Healthcare Enterprise Security system with access ports to known devices and access blocking to intruders. Yet this is not enough as there are a number of work-arounds to harvest PHI and other valuable data or inject ransomware to bring the enterprise to a halt

performs the image rendering as opposed to many devices around the enterprise limit the risk of image manipulations by corrupted applications providing non-uniform images resulting in a misdiagnosis.

## 26.4 Medical Device Cybersecurity

As medical devices have become more sophisticated so have the challenges to guard and secure protected health information. Coronado and Wong have defined two distinct cybersecurity threats to devices as affecting the operation of a medical device and tampering with the integrity of the information [3]. Researchers have recently shown how an attacker can remove or add evidence of disease conditions from volumetric (3D) medical scans by using deep learning [4]. In 2014, a provider in the United States (US) faced misdemeanor charges related to theft of PHI belonging to about 97,000 patients [5]. In the USA PHI theft falls under federal law.

Threats to cybersecurity may also impact the operation of medical equipment. Many newer models of physiologic monitoring equipment are capable of transferring collected data directly to the electronic medical record (EMR), as well as notifying providers via personal mobile devices. Staff with cell phones or pages can be instantly alerted to patient alarms. This interoperability and interconnectivity leads to new cybersecurity issues that are very challenging [3].

## 26.5 Preventing Cyberattacks

As hackers have gained expertise in their craft, preventing cyberattacks has become more difficult. Authentication and encryption are two strategies to reduce attacks.

### 26.5.1 Authentication

Authentication, which is the way an individual is identified before entering a system, is one method to reduce unauthorized access [6]. A single-factor authentication (SFA) involves the use of a username and password. Users of SFA find it challenging to create unique passwords and then to comply with frequently changing these passwords. Multifactor authentication (MFA) has emerged to remedy this situation [6]. MFA requires the user to complete at least two authentication methods.

### 26.5.2 Encryption

Data can be protected through encryption. Encryption can be divided into transparent data encryption and column-level encryption [6].

### 26.5.3 Role of Management

According to a recent IBM study "For the 9th year in a row, healthcare organizations had the highest cost of a breach—nearly $6.5 million on average (over 60% more than other industries in the study)" [7]. Cybersecurity insurance is available; however, that does not restore trust.

Cybersecurity needs to be an organizational priority. This may involve a culture change within an organization to include education and training for staff on ways to protect information, as well as to identify any problems that may surface. Backup and safe storage of data and an annual security audit are recommended [8]. Maintenance and updates including antivirus and antimalware protections should be current. Virtual private networks (VPNs) should be used when working offsite; these use a safe encrypted connection for authorized users [8].

Guidance documents on the subject of cybersecurity are available from The National Electrical Manufacturers Association (NEMA) [9]. (See https://www.nema.org/Standards/Pages/Cybersecurity-for-Medical-Imaging.aspx for the document Cybersecurity for Medical Imaging and others.) United States federal guidance on cybersecurity is found in publications from the National Institute of Standards and Technology (NIST) [10].

Available research papers on incident recovery and legality are scarce as most research related to cybersecurity is focused on privacy and compliance [2]. Financial penalties and harm to the healthcare organization's reputation are consequences of a data breach [11]. Assessing if a reportable breach has occurred should follow the institution's policies and procedures and regulatory standards.

## 26.6 Conclusion

Cyberattacks are not limited to financial or healthcare institutions. They are omnipresent in the cyber-world as the enemy can attack from anywhere in the physical world. The inability to achieve a secure cyber-world costs us collectively billions each year. When a breach happens to us, we expect someone else to pay for it regardless of whose fault it was.

In healthcare, we can only do our very best to prevent cyberattacks. The odds are in the favor of the enemy; sooner or later one of them will get though. They will compromise the patient and their privacy or will bring an enormous healthcare enterprise to an instant halt, thus possibly compromising the health of thousands of others. The world's financial institutions who have been at the information technology cybersecurity game for more than 20 years ahead of healthcare still do not have this figured out yet. Therefore, we will need to accept this threat of an attack as a daily risk and do our best to protect institutions and our patients as best we can till cybersecurity is perfected.

## References

1. Coventry L, Branley D. Cybersecurity in healthcare: a narrative review of trends, threats and ways forward. Maturitas (Eur Menopause J). 2018;113:48–52.
2. Jalali MS, Razak S, Gordon W, Perakslis E, Madnick S. Health care and cybersecurity: bibliometric analysis of the literature. J Med Internet Res. 2019;21(2):e12644. https://doi.org/10.2196/12644. https://www.jmir.org/2019/2/e12644/.
3. Coronado AJ, Wong TL. Healthcare cybersecurity risk management: keys to an effective plan. Adv Saf

Health Technol. 2014;48(S1):26–30. https://www.aami-bit.org/doi/full/10.2345/0899-8205-48.s1.26.
4. Mirsky Y, Mahler T, Shelef I, Elovici Y. CT-GAN: malicious tampering of 3D medical imagery using deep learning. Published in the 28th USENIX Security symposium (USWENIX Security2019). https://arxiv.org/pdf/1901.03597.pdf.
5. Long Island radiologist arrested over HIPPA violation. HIPPA Journal. 9Dec2014. https://www.hipaajournal.com/long-island-radiologist-arrested-hipaa-violation/.
6. The future of health care cybersecurity. J Nurs Regul. 2018;8(4):S29–31. https://www.journalofnursingregulation.com/article/S2155-8256(18)30025-5/fulltext.
7. IBM study shows data breach cost on the rise; Financial impact felt for years. 23Jul 2019. https://newsroom.ibm.com/2019-07-23-IBM-Study-Shows-Data-Breach-Costs-on-the-Rise-Financial-Impact-Felt-for-Years.
8. Young R. How secure is that scanner. Radiology Business Journal. 25 Jun 2019. https://www.radiologybusiness.com/topics/privacy-security/how-secure-scanner.
9. Zagoudis J. Building a cybersecurity team in radiology. Imaging Technology News (ITN). 6 Nov 2017. https://www.itnonline.com/article/building-cybersecurity-team-radiology.
10. National Institute of Standards and Technology (United States Department of Commerce) (NIST). https://www.nist.gov/cyberframework.
11. Knudson J. Data breach: what's at stake for hospitals. Radiology Today, vol.16(2), p.18, 2015. https://www.radiologytoday.net/archive/rt0215p18.shtml.

# Nursing Research and Outcomes

## 27

Kathleen Shuey
and Marygrace Hernandez-Leveille

## 27.1 Introduction

Radiology nurses and advanced practice providers are in the perfect clinical setting to raise awareness and have a high level of clinical inquiry in order to meet the needs of the patients that are in their care while in the radiology suite. It is imperative that care and radiology clinical practice are established on evidence-based practices and benchmarks which have been determined by radiology nurses. The radiology nurse should also be mindful of patient outcomes after a radiologic procedure, as well. Who knows your practice better than you? Who can present the unique radiology nursing body of knowledge to the forefront other than the radiology nurse? Clinical practice is the main source of clinical inquiry. Hedges [1] describes a three-legged stool whereby nursing practice sits on a stool-supported research, evidence-based research, and quality improvement, the three legs of the stool. As part of daily nursing practice, the radiology nurse is continually monitoring the patient's vital signs and other physical assessment indicators and documenting all of the data being collected before, during, and after a radiologic procedure. All of this work can potentially be transformed into a research project, evidence-based practice project, or a quality improvement initiative. Data is everything. "In God we trust; all others bring data" [2].

### 27.1.1 The First Nursing Research

Since the 1800s, when Florence Nightingale, the founder of nursing and a statistician, established nursing as a profession, nurses have worked diligently to promote the principles of hygiene, healthy living, safe environments, and preventative care to all people. Throughout her work during the Crimean war, and in the various hospitals in London and military barracks, Nightingale adhered to a daily practice of assessing a problem by clinical observation utilizing her five senses (sound, touch, sight, taste, and smell), implementing a change process and evaluating the outcomes by using statistical analyses of the data generated from the patients being cared for [3]. Nightingale is also revered as the first nurse scientist as she asked simple questions about the effects of personal hygiene, the transmission of communicable diseases, and

K. Shuey, RN, ACNS-BC, AOCN (✉)
Department of Nursing,
Baylor University Medical Center,
Dallas, TX, USA

M. Hernandez-Leveille, PHD, RN, ACNP-BC
UT Southwestern Office of Advanced Practice Providers, Dallas, TX, USA

UT Southwestern Medical Center,
Dallas, TX, USA

the importance of hand hygiene to prevent the spread of illness. Her studies were dedicated to promoting a safe and healthy environment to enhance the patients' physical and mental well-being. As a fledgling nurse scientist, Nightingale wrote: "It is not for the sake of piling up miscellaneous information or curious facts, but for the sake of saving life and increasing health and comfort" [4]. Nightingale was instrumental in research, evidence-based practice, and quality improvement through *clinical inquiry*. What distinguishes these three forms of clinical inquiry in the daily practice of a radiology nurse? The purpose for conducting research, evidence-based practice (EBP), and quality improvement (QI) is to improve patient care, clinical care, administrative infrastructure, and educational outcomes. "All three approaches have an important, yet different relationship with knowledge: Research generates it; EBP translates it; and QI incorporates it" [5].

## 27.2 Research

Research is a rigorous systematic investigation or scientific process that validates and refines existing knowledge and develops new knowledge that is generalizable. Research is considered to be the most rigorous form of scientific appraisal and the highest level of evidence. Research provides evidence for EBP and QI. All research requires the approval of an institutional review board (IRB) in an effort to provide ethical and regulatory oversight of research that involves human subjects. Nursing research generates new knowledge about patient outcomes, nursing practice, nursing education, and nursing administration and can influence nursing practice and healthcare organizations [5, 6]. The benefits of nursing research includes better patient outcomes, cost efficiency for patients and healthcare organizations, and nurses can prove that the nursing profession can make a difference in people's lives, nationally and globally. Nursing research can demonstrate the effectiveness of nursing interventions [7].

### 27.2.1 Role of Nurses

Nurses can assume a variety of roles in the research process such as principal investigator (PI), member of the team conducting the research, member of the statistical analyses team, and/or member of the dissemination of findings team. As a member of the research team, the nurse has the opportunity to participate in writing the research protocol, recruiting subjects, consenting the subjects, conducting the actual components of the research process, analyzing the data, and presenting the data, either as a manuscript or by presentations at conferences and healthcare organizations, locally, nationally, or internationally.

## 27.3 Research Approach

New nursing knowledge can be generated from either quantitative research, qualitative research, mixed methods research, and outcomes research (Fig. 27.1).

**Types of Quantitative Research**

Descriptive Research

Experimental Research

Quasi-experimental Research

Correlational Research

**Types of Qualitative Research**

Phenomenological Research

Grounded Theory Research

Exploratory-descriptive Research

Ethnographic Research

**Mixed Methods Research**

**Outcomes Research**

**Fig. 27.1** Research methods

### 27.3.1 Quantitative Research

Quantitative research uses formal, tightly controlled objective systematic measurements which can have the ability to produce generalizable findings [7]. Measurement is a primary method of quantitative examination in research. Typically, quantitative research uses numerical data to perform statistical analyses to answer the research question or hypotheses [8]. Quantitative studies usually have a minimum of two groups involved and may test for differences between and within the groups. Types of quantitative research include descriptive, experimental, quasi-experimental, and correlational research. Radiology nurses may want to assess and measure the vital signs such as blood pressure, heart rate, respiratory rate, or pulse oximetry during a particular procedure or after a particular medication has been given to the patient to evaluate a potential cause and effect of a particular variable. Additionally, quantitative research can test for effectiveness of interventions and patient outcomes, as well.

### 27.3.2 Qualitative Research

There are four types of qualitative research: phenomenological, grounded theory, exploratory-descriptive, and ethnographic research. Qualitative research is not as tightly controlled as quantitative research because it is more subjective. Qualitative research centers more on the meaning of experiences to the patient. In this case, the radiology nurse would be conducting interviews and observing the patients' experiences. Instead of producing analytical numerical results, emerging themes and phrases would be the end result of a qualitative study [9]. Radiology nurses who conduct interviews or focus groups and attempt to capture the lived experience of a patient who had undergone a radiologic procedure is an example of a qualitative study. The radiology nurse would then be able to cluster the themes and phrases derived from the interview or focus groups and report the findings.

### 27.3.3 Mixed Methods

Mixed methods research is the use of both quantitative and qualitative components in a research study, and it is frequently utilized in healthcare because of the complexity of the ever-changing healthcare system. When conducting a nursing mixed methods research project in a radiology suite, the radiology nurse is able to use numbers (quantitative) and words (qualitative) to answer the research question [7]. Mixed methods research offers the unique ability to explain a phenomena or a patient outcome objectively and subjectively based on the data received from the patient.

### 27.3.4 Outcomes Research

Outcomes research is a rigorous scientific method that concentrates on the outcomes of patient care. With regard to nursing outcomes research, the focus pertains to how a patient's health status changes as a result of care provided by nurses [10]. As healthcare systems, providers and nurses assess the importance of patient-centered outcomes to drive best practice and healthcare cost reduction. The Agency for Healthcare Research and Quality (AHRQ) supports the endeavor of patient-centered outcome research (PCOR). This type of outcomes research allows for the identification of gaps in healthcare delivery, research to provide answers and rationale, and the dissemination of findings. This cyclical process, endorsed by AHRQ, ensures that outcomes research findings are known, understood, and properly utilized [11]. Outcomes research is known for developing processes to improve quality of care.

## 27.4 Evidence-Based Practice

Evidence-based practice (EBP) usually starts, again, with clinical inquiry. Once a thorough review of the literature has been completed and sufficient evidence is presented to support a practice change, an EBP project can be implemented [5]. However, if a review of the literature and critical appraisal of the literature does not yield sufficient evidence to conduct an EBP practice change, then a research study is required. EBP is an unequivocal interdisciplinary process that empowers clinicians to seek out the best current scientific evidence to determine best practices. Scientific evidence is in the form of existing research, particularly randomized controlled trials (RCTs). Usually, reviews of the evidence are performed by experts in the field and are published as national guidelines and practice protocols [1]. EBP is the application of findings from research to inform nurses and clinicians of clinical decision-making skills at the point of care. EBP promotes change from practicing because of "tradition" to practicing based on scientific evidence. EBP projects generally do not require IRB approval. Wolf and Greenhouse [12] identified five trends that emphasize the necessity of an evidence-based approach to promote effective healthcare delivery for the future: changes in the patients' knowledge level, changes in the types of clinicians and settings required, advances in medicine, advances in information technology, and changes in reimbursement. The implementation of EBP projects has shown a reduction in healthcare cost and the increase in patient satisfaction.

### 27.4.1 EBP and the Radiology Nurse

Radiology nurses are well positioned to develop skills for finding scientific evidence to support their nursing practice. Patients, who are consumers of the healthcare system, are much more knowledgeable regarding their health and the healthcare delivery system than previous generations. With the assistance of the internet, patients are able to query any symptom, any drug, any treatment, any disease, and any treatment plan with the stroke of a few keys. Nurses, advanced practice providers, and physicians are expected to be apprised of the current trends and best practices especially because patients now have accessible knowledge. For example, patients may come to a consult session with their own idea of a test or procedure desired and may request a computed tomography examination for lower back pain as they believe this would be the best test per their own investigation of the problem via public magazine articles or searching internet sources (all types). The practitioner who gathers information from the history and performs a physical exam may determine that a magnetic resonance imaging examination is the preferred diagnostic test.

The practitioner can locate information on many databases such as PubMed, Ovid, CINAHL, and Medline[13–16]. In late 2018, the ECRI Guidelines Trust™ initiated access to clinical practice guidelines after the Agency for Healthcare Research and Quality (AHRQ) National Guideline Clearing House™ site was discontinued due to lack of funding [17].

### 27.4.2 Cochrane Database

In the 1970s, Archie Cochran, MD, challenged the practice of physicians and suggested that physicians were not using the best evidence to deliver appropriate care. As a result of his tenacious work, the Cochrane Database was established in 1993 [18]. This database is a warehouse of medical research to facilitate evidence-based options for healthcare providers. This global network is not only available to healthcare providers but also to patients and people interested in healthcare. The Cochrane Database of Systematic Reviews (CDSR) database offers systematic reviews, which summarize large bodies of evidence and protocols prepared by established Cochrane Review groups who have conducted critical appraisal of the scientific evidence. As a result of this systematic review process, a best practice or evidence-based practice change can be established.

### 27.4.3 Joanna Briggs Institute

Another database that supports clinicians in providing evidence-based practice information is the Joanna Briggs Institute (JBI) which is established in South Australia [19]. Since 1996, when the institute was established, JBI has identified many healthcare evidence-based protocols to promote effective healthcare practices.

### 27.4.4 Models for Clinical Decision-Making

EBP projects are usually guided by a variety of models to offer a systematic process for clinical decision-making (see Table 27.1).

EBP projects start with a clinical or organizational issue which then leads to the development of a question. Any of the EBP models will guide the implementation of the project. Crafting a specific question guides the multidisciplinary team towards a more detailed literature review. Many EBP projects start with a PICO question (**P**atient, population or problem; **I**ntervention; **C**omparison with other interventions and **O**utcomes) (Fig. 27.2).

Once the team has refined the PICO question and the literature review has revealed a best practice change, then the team proceeds to the implementation stage. The team will assess the outcomes and re-evaluate the process, and if the desired outcomes have not been achieved, a redesign of the intervention may be required. Once the desired outcome has been achieved, sustainability is monitored. Continued surveillance of the intervention and outcomes are essential in order to ensure the desired initial outcome.

## 27.5 Quality Improvement

Quality improvement (QI), sometimes referred to as process improvement (PI), is another modality to improve healthcare delivery that can be championed by radiology nurses and a multidisciplinary team. QI is an internal systematic process of change that does not require IRB approval unless the data are presented outside of the institution[1].

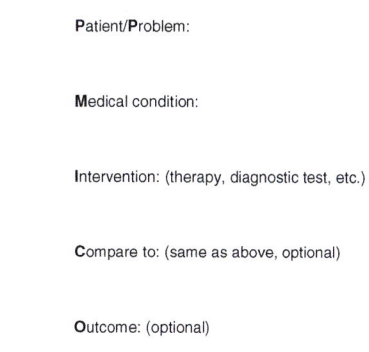

**Fig. 27.2** PICO format [28]

**Table 27.1** Models for clinical decision-making

| Model title | Authors | Website |
|---|---|---|
| Iowa Model [20] | Titler and colleagues | https://uihc.org/iowa-model-revised-evidence-based-practice-promote-excellence-health-care%C2%A9 |
| Advancing Research and Clinical Practice through Close Collaboration Model (ARCC) [21] | Melnyk and Fineout-Overhol | |
| The Johns Hopkins Hospital EBP Model [22] | Poe and White | |
| Academic Center for EBP Star Model of Knowledge Transformation (ACE) [23] | Stevens | |
| Stetler Model [24] | Stetler | https://www.nccmt.ca/knowledge-repositories/search/83 |
| PRISM Model [25] | Feldstein and Glastow | https://www.nccmt.ca/knowledge-repositories/search/135 |
| Rosswurm and Larrabee Model [26] | Rosswurm and Larrabee | |
| Promoting Action on Research in Health Services Framework (PARIHS) [27] | Kitson, Harvey, and McCormack | https://www.nccmt.ca/knowledge-repositories/search/85 |

QI improves workflow processes which can lead to cost containment and increased staff satisfaction and patient satisfaction[5]. Similar to research and EBP, QI requires the use of a problem statement or question, some type of protocol, and collection of data. A unique attribute to QI is that the change process is considered to be rapid and cyclical in nature which allows for the rapid evaluation of the process and results. If the desired outcome has not been achieved, the process is changed and additional evaluation of the process is later required. Once the desired effect has been achieved, sustainability is achieved by continued monitoring of the data and re-evaluation. Parallel to research and EBP, QI has a variety of methods to accomplish successful QI projects. These methods include Lean Six Sigma, Six Sigma, Plan-Do-Check-Act (PDCA) model, and the Plan-Do-Study-Act (PDSA) model.

Tools utilized to conduct a QI project include benchmarking, field analysis, and checklists. Unlike research, QI projects are institution specific and the results cannot be considered generalizable. Results from a QI project can be disseminated through publication and presentations internally and externally at a variety of conferences.

## 27.6 Nursing Research Studies in Radiology

Nurse-driven research in radiology falls into four major categories: clinical practice, patient experience, safety, and nursing education. Additionally, joint research with colleagues, including physicians and radiology technologists, provides nurses an opportunity to collaborate on a wide range of topics. In large departments there may be a designated radiology research nurse.

Research studies evaluating clinical practice have focused on a variety of clinical issues including, for example, sedation and patient safety, music therapy, nursing diagnosis, staff satisfaction, role, and competence [29–37].

Selection and management of procedural sedation relies on assessment of the patient's medical history, allergies, current condition, and previous experience with sedating medications. Collaboration with the radiologist enhances patient selection and appropriate level of sedation. A review of 727 adverse events experienced in the pediatric population showed inadequate sedation, agitation and delirium was found to occur in 196 cases; desaturation below baseline occurred in 173 cases [29]. An evaluation of a radiology specialist nurse-led unit assessed patient outcomes over a 10-year period in 401 angiography procedures [30]. Patients referred to the clinic were assessed by a specialist nurse before, during, and after angiography procedures. A low incidence of major complications was observed. Patients indicated a high level of satisfaction with nursing. Cost savings were approximately $187–$500 per patient.

Studies in clinical areas outside of radiology and/or nursing utilize a variety of techniques to decrease patient stress [38–44]. In the pediatric population, play therapy specialists used age-appropriate language to explain magnetic resonance imaging (MRI) procedure [45]. Children were provided with photographs of children or a teddy bear undergoing a MRI. A 2010 study used mock MRI scanners prior to pediatric procedures [46]. Patient education was provided by a pediatrician and child life specialist. Results showed an increase in quality of scans. Children as young as three participated in the observational study.

Music therapy has also been employed to decrease stress. A review of 13 studies [32] indicated that music interventions lower blood pressure and reduce the need for medication during interventional radiology studies. Further studies are needed to determine the benefits of stress-relieving techniques in radiology. Collaborative efforts with physicians, child life therapist, and radiologic technologist provide an opportunity to expand non-pharmacologic options.

A 2012 Swedish nurse interview study analyzing the nurse's experience in caring for patients undergoing radiologic interventions [34] identified four themes: creating a trusting atmosphere, creating a dialogue, dealing with unpredictable outcomes, and dealing with pain and agony. The first patient encounter was identified as essential to patient perception; if the encounter "turns out badly in the beginning, it is very hard to reverse" [34]. Establishing a trusting atmosphere is a crucial step for the nurse to achieve when dealing with unpredictable outcomes and pain that the patient may be experiencing. Additionally, forming a caring relationship with the patient can increase the nurse's satisfaction with work. BroBrask's study [35] supports the earlier work of Lunden [34] and broadens the scope supporting the concept that care is more than just the relationship between patient and nurse.

Patient experience is defined as "the sum of all interactions, shaped by an organization's culture, that influence patient perceptions, across the continuum of care" [47, 48]. Studies focusing on patient experience and quality of care demonstrate an absence of consistent definitions and use of nonvalidated satisfaction surveys [49]. An early phenomenological study indicated information provided on the radiology exam and interactions with staff influenced patient experience [50]. Nineteen participants who underwent MRI described problems dealing with the environment and isolation inside the scanner. Breathing exercises, music, and use of a buzzer to contact staff allowed participants to feel in control. Additionally, participants indicated an increased need for staff support when the individual experienced greater stress due to the procedure.

A cross-sectional study evaluated 698 participant's perception of quality of care [51]. The relationship between quality of care and demographic factors was also explored. A questionnaire was mailed to participants 2–3 days following the radiology procedure. Thirty-one percent of participants completed education post high school, 41% completed high school, and 28% did not complete high school. Over 50% of the participants indicated they were employed. Wait time in the radiology department varied from less than 15 minutes to greater than 1 hour. Perceived low quality of care was associated with longer wait times, low level of education, and female participants.

A culture of safety promotes evidence-based care, a positive work environment, and commitment to improvement [52]. Core values and behaviors illustrate an organizations dedication to safety and improved patient outcomes [53]. Key features of a culture of safety include acknowledgment of the high-risk nature of activities, establishment of a blame-free environment, collaboration across disciplines, and commitment to address safety concerns [54]. Medical emergencies in radiology were the focus of 2012 study [55]. A retrospective review of records indicated that 60% of patients experiencing an event were from a non-ICU area and 43% of events occurred on the initial day of hospitalization. Post event, 70% of patients required a higher level of care. The highest number of events occurred on weekdays between 8 AM and 12 PM. Results indicated that patients in radiology were at an increased risk of care escalation and death compared to patients in the inpatient area. A follow-up study indicated that patients who require transport may be at greater risk for instability [56].

Education specific to radiology is lacking in undergraduate nursing programs [57]. Skills required by nursing in radiology cover a wide variety of clinical specialties including operating room, post anesthesia/recovery care, ambulatory nursing, and even critical care when the patient condition deteriorates. Many facilities do not have educational support for the specialty of radiology and rely on clinical experts within nursing and radiology to facilitate orientation of staff. Assessment of competency may be based on observation of care, chart reviews, or demonstration of skills [58]. Research has not focused on educational techniques such as simulation, virtual reality/gaming technology, and journal clubs [59–61]. Although literature is available on these methods, studies have not been conducted to determine effectiveness in nursing.

A specific education topic that is crucial to both patients and nursing is radiation safety. A 2006 study in Kuwait utilized a self-administered questionnaire to investigate nurses awareness of radiation risks and safety procedures [62]. Thirty-five nurses completed the survey. Results indicated nurses were not aware of the "as low as reasonably achievable (ALARA)" principle [63].

A Korean study examined nurses' knowledge and compliance with radiation safety procedures [64]. The study evaluated data from the Korea Nurses' Health Study, the Korean version of the United States Nurses' Health Study. Fifty percent of nurses received no safety training and 14.4% received sporadic training. Education was observed to increase compliance with radiation safety efforts. A tool that could be used to guide education efforts, The Healthcare Professional Knowledge of Radiation Protection self-evaluation (HPKRP) tool was developed to assess knowledge and understanding of ionizing radiation and protection from effects [65]. The validated HPKRP tool could provide direction in the development of educational offerings specific to knowledge of radiation and radiation safety, thereby impacting compliance.

## 27.7 Conclusion

Research by nurses in radiology encompasses a broad range of topics. Additional study is needed for many of the topics presented. Research with physician and technologist colleagues offers an opportunity to collaborate on clinical topics that require a team approach. Nursing input into future trials can enhance patient experience and ultimately provide improved patient outcomes. Areas for future research are listed in Table 27.2.

**Table 27.2** Suggested areas for future research

- Optimal sedation and pain management
- Stress management in the peri-procedure time
- Best designs for clinical areas to enhance patient experience
- Patient and family amenities (e.g., waiting rooms, parking, communications)
- Management of peripheral contrast media extravasation
- Management of unique populations, e.g., pediatric population
- Education of the radiology nurse and advanced practice provider, including alternative education methods such as simulation, virtual reality, and gaming technology
- Peer review and evaluations
- Cost of services and ways to reduce costs

## References

1. Hedges C. Research, evidence based practice, and quality improvement. AACN Adv Crit Care. 2006;17:457–9.
2. W. Edwards Deming Quotes. AZ Quotes [cited 2019 Feb 17]. Available from:https://www.azquotes.com/author/3858-W_Edwards_Deming.
3. Clements PT, Averill JB. Finding patterns of knowing in the work of Florence Nightingale. Nurs Outlook. 2006;54:268–74.
4. Nightingale F. Notes on nursing: what it is and what it is not [cited 2019 Feb 22]. Available from: https://en.wikisource.org/wiki/Notes_on_Nursing:_What_It_Is,_and_What_It_Is_Not/Chapter_XIII.
5. Shirey MR, Hauck SL, Embree JL, et al. Showcasing differences between quality improvement, evidence based practice and research. J Contin Educ Nurs. 2011;42(2):57–68.
6. Grove SK, Gray JR. Understanding nursing research: building an evidence based practice. 7th ed. St Louis, MO: Elsevier; 2019.
7. Durepos P, Orr E, Ploeg J, et al. The value of measurement for development of nursing knowledge: underlying philosophy, contributions and critiques. J Adv Nurs. 2018;74:2290–300.
8. LoBiondo-Wood G, Haber J. Nursing research: methods and critical appraisal for evidence based practice. 8th ed. St Louis, MO: Mosby Elsevier; 2014.
9. Nieswaidomy RM, Bailey C. Foundations of nursing research. 7th ed. Pearson: New York; 2018.
10. Moorhead S, Johnson M, Maas ML, et al. Nursing outcomes classification (NOC): measurement of health outcomes. 5th ed. St. Louis, MO: Elsevier Mosby; 2013.
11. Agency for HealthCare Research and Quality. Dissemination of patient centered outcomes research[cited 2019 Feb 22]. Available from:https://www.ahrq.gov/pcor/dissemination-of-pcor/index.html.
12. Wolf AC, Greenhouse PK. Blueprint for design: creating models that direct change. J Nurs Adm. 2007;37:381–7.
13. PubMed[cited 2019 Feb 22]. Available from:https://www.ncbi.nlm.nih.gov/pubmed/.
14. Ovid[cited 2019 Feb 22]. Available from:https://www.ovid.com/site/index.isp.
15. CINAHL[cited 2019 Feb 22]. Available from:https://www.ebscohost.com/nursing/products/cinahl-databases/cinahl-complete.
16. Medline [cited 2019 Feb 22]. Available from:https://www.nlm.nih.gov/bsd/pmresources.html.
17. ECRI Institute[cited 2019 May 22]. Available from: https://www.ecri.org/press/ecri-institute-opens-access-to-clinical-practice-guidelines.
18. Cochrane Database[cited 2019 Feb 22].Available from: https://www.cochranelibrary.com/.
19. Joanna Briggs Institute[cited 2019 Feb 22]. Available from: http://joannabriggs.org.

20. Iowa Model Collaborative. Iowa model of evidence based practice: revisions and validations. Worldviews Evid Based Nurs. 2017;14:175–82.
21. Melnyk BM, Fineout-Overholt E. Evidence-based practice in nursing and healthcare. Philadelphia, PA: Lippincott, Williams & Williams; 2005.
22. Poe SS, White KM. Johns Hopkins nursing evidence based practice: implementation and translation. Indianapolis, IN: Sigma Theta Tau International; 2010.
23. Stevens K. The impact of evidence based practice in nursing and the next big ideas [cited 2019 Feb 22]. Available from: http://ojin.nursingworld.org/MainMenuCategories/ANAMarketplace/ANAPeriodicals/OJIN/TableofContents/Vol-18-2013/No2-May-2013/Impact-of-Evidence-Based-Practice.html.
24. Settler CB. Updating the Stetler model of research utilization to facilitate evidence-based practice. Nurs Outlook. 2001;49(6):272–9.
25. Feldstein AC, Practical GREA. Robust implementation and sustainability model (PRISM) for integrating research findings into practice. Jt Comm J Qual Patient Saf. 2008;34(4):228–43.
26. Rosswurm MA, Larrabee JH. A model for change to evidence-based practice. Image J Nurs Scholarship. 1999;31(4):317–22.
27. Kitson A, Harvey G, McCormack B. Enabling the implementation of evidence based practice: a conceptual framework. Qual Saf Health Care. 1998;7:149–58.
28. National Library of Medicine. PICO Search [cited 2019 May 22]. Available from:https://pubmedhh.nlm.nih.gov/nlmd/pico/piconew.php
29. Crego N. Pediatric sedation: using secondary data to describe Registered Nurse practice in radiology. J Radiol Nurs. 2014;33(4):166–80.
30. Huang Y, Ong C-M, Walters HL, et al. Day-case diagnostic and interventional peripheral angiography: 10-year experience in a radiology specialist nurse-led unit. BJR J Radiol. 2008;18:537–44.
31. Hall JM. Procedural sedation by Registered Nurses in the Interventional Radiology setting: incorporating evidence-based practice regarding medication selection, fasting, and mitigating cardiorespiratory complications. J Radiol Nurs. 2005;24(4):63–8.
32. Vanderboom T. Does music reduce anxiety during invasive procedures with procedural sedation?An integrative research review. J Radiol Nurs. 2007;26(1):15–22.
33. Viegas L, Turrini RNT, Cerullo JA. An analysis of nursing diagnoses for patients undergoing procedures in a Brazilian Interventional Radiology suite. AORN J. 2010;91(5):49–52, 544–57.
34. Lunden M, Lundgren SM, Lepp M. The Nurse Radiographers' experience of meeting with patients during Interventional Radiology. J Radiol Nurs. 2012;31(2):53–61.
35. BroBrask K, Birkeulund R. "Patient care in radiology"—the staff's perspective. J Radiol Nurs. 2014;33(1):23–9.
36. Harding M. Effect of nurse navigation on patient care satisfaction and distress associated with breast biopsy. Clin J Oncol Nurs. 2015;19(1):e15–20.
37. Andersson BT, Fridlund B, Elgán C, et al. Radiographers' areas of professional competence related to good nursing care. Scand J Caring Sci. 2018;22(3):401–9.
38. Kim HS, Kim EJ. Effects of relaxation therapy on anxiety disorders: a systematic review and meta-analysis. Arch Psychiatr Nurs. 2018;32(2):274–84.
39. Aguilar BA. The efficacy of art therapy in pediatric oncology patients: an integrative literature review. J Pediatr Nurs. 2017;36:173–8.
40. Alexander M. Managing patient stress in pediatric radiology. Radiol Technol. 2012;83(6):549–60.
41. Standley J. Music therapy research in the NICU: an updated meta-analysis. Neonatal Netw. 2012;31(5):311–6.
42. Loprinzi CE, Prasad K, Schroeder DR, et al. Stress management and resilience training (SMART) program to decrease stress and enhance resilience among breast cancer survivors: a pilot randomized clinical trial. Clin Breast Cancer. 2011;11(6):364–8.
43. Anastos JP. The ambient experience in pediatric radiology. J Radiol Nurs. 2007;26(2):50–5.
44. Schupp CJ, Berbaum K, Berbum M, et al. Pain and anxiety during interventional radiologic procedures: effect of patients' state anxiety at baseline and modulation by nonpharmacologic analgesia adjuncts. J Vasc Interv Radiol. 2005;16(12):1585–92.
45. Pressdee D, May L, Eastman E, et al. The use of play therapy in the preparation of children undergoing MR imaging. Clin Radiol. 1997;52:945–7.
46. de Bie HMA, Boersma M, Wattjes MP, et al. Preparing children with a mock scanner training protocol results in high quality structural and functional MRI scans. Eur J Pediatr. 2010;169(9):1079–85.
47. Wolf JA, Niederhauser V, Marshburn D, et al. Defining patient experience. Patient Exp J. 2014;1(1):7–19.
48. Beryl Institute [cited 2019 Feb 2]. Available from: https://www.theberylinstitute.org/page/DefiningPatientExp.
49. Werthman A. Patient satisfaction, nursing, and radiology: a review. J Radiol Nurs. 2018;37(4):255–9.
50. Rörnqvist E, Månsson Å, Larsson E-M, et al. It's like being in another world—patients' lived experience of magnetic resonance imaging. J Clin Nurs. 2006;15:954–61.
51. Blomberg F, Brulin C, Andertun R, et al. Patients' perception of quality of care in a radiology department: a medical-physical approach. J Radiol Nurs. 2010;29(1):10–7.
52. Barnsteiner J. Teaching a culture of safety. Online J Issues Nurs. 2011;16(3):5.
53. American Nurses Association. Culture of safety[cited 2019 Feb 2]. Available from: https://www.nursingworld.org/practice-policy/work-environment/health-safety/culture-of-safety/.
54. Agency for Healthcare Research and Quality (AHRQ). Culture of safety [cited 2019 Feb 2].

Available from: https://psnet.ahrq.gov/primers/primer/5/culture-of-safety.
55. Ott LK, Pinsky MR, Hoffman LA, et al. Medical Emergency Team calls in the radiology department: patient characteristics and outcomes. BMJ Qual Saf. 2012;21(6):509–18.
56. Ott LK, Pinsky MR, Hoffman LA, et al. Patients in the radiology department may be at increased risk of developing critical instability. J Radiol Nurs. 2015;34(1):29–34.
57. Sousa MF. Management and leadership: educating and orienting the radiology nurse of the future. J Radiol Nurs. 2011;30(3):135–6.
58. Hagler D, Wilson R. Designing nursing staff competency assessment using simulation. J Radiol Nurs. 2013;32(4):165–9.
59. Nesbitt J, Barton G. Nursing journal clubs: a strategy for improving knowledge translation and evidenced-informed clinical practice. J Radiol Nurs. 2014;33(1):3–8.
60. Titzer JL, Swenty CF, Hoen WG. An interprofessional simulation promoting collaboration and problem solving among nursing and allied health professional students. Clin Simul Nurs. 2012;8(8):e325–33.
61. Reiner B. The potential for gaming techniques in radiology education and practice. J Am Coll Radiol. 2008;5(2):110–4.
62. Alotaibi M, Saeed R. Radiology nurses' awareness of radiation. J Radiol Nurs. 2006;25(1):7–12.
63. Hendee WR, Edwards FM. ALARA and an integrated approach to radiation protection. Semin Nucl Med. 1986;16(2):142–50.
64. Kim O, Kim MS, Jang HJ, et al. Radiation safety education and compliance with safety procedures—The Korea Nurses' Health Study. J Clin Nurs. 2018;27:2650–60.
65. Schroderus-Salo T, Hirvonen L, Henner A, et al. Development and validation of a psychometric scale for assessing healthcare professionals' knowledge in radiation protection. Radiography. 2019;25:136–42.

# Interprofessional Education and Collaboration

28

Wendy Manetti

## 28.1 Introduction

Over the past 20 years, the Institute of Medicine (IOM) released three reports sounding the alarm about the quality and safety of healthcare in the United States. On a much larger scale, the World Health Organization [1] reiterated the same concerns. The overarching message was that health professionals are unprepared to effectively communicate and collaborate as part of a team leading to poor outcomes including medical errors, patient safety issues, lack of patient and provider satisfaction, and higher costs [2]. In the United States, this turmoil is compounded by the fact that the healthcare system is undergoing major changes in delivery from a fee-based to value-based system [3]. Radiology as a specialty area has also undergone significant changes in the recent past due to advances in imaging technology, increased use of interventional procedures, and newly emerging roles such as radiology and imaging nursing [4, 5].

W. Manetti, PhD, CRNP (✉)
Department of Nursing, University of Scranton, Scranton, PA, USA

## 28.2 Calls for Change

In response, interprofessional education (IPE) and collaboration has come to the forefront as one solution. Expert consensus supports the notion that effective interprofessional collaborative practice leads to better patient outcomes [6]. Quality and Safety Education for Nurses (QSEN) developed competencies for nursing set forth by the IOM; patient-centered care, teamwork and collaboration, evidence-based practice, quality improvement, safety, and informatics [7]. According to QSEN, team members possessing proficient knowledge, skills, and attitudes of teamwork and collaboration encourage open communication, mutual respect, and shared decision-making to ensure delivery of high-quality patient care. Some of the main team premises include gaining knowledge of roles and responsibilities of all team members, demonstrating shared commitment to patient-centered goals, proficient skills in communication techniques to foster safe handoffs, and a positive attitude toward team functioning and appreciation of all team members [7].

Most accreditors for healthcare professional schools require IPE in the curriculum. Schools of nursing seeking accreditation from the American Association of Colleges of Nursing (AACN) must meet a minimum set of competences as provided in The Essentials of Baccalaureate Education for

Professional Nursing Practice, Essentials of Masters' Education in Nursing, and Essentials of Doctoral Education for Advanced Nursing Practice) [8–10]. Collectively, the Essentials challenged nurse educators to prepare future nurses for interprofessional teamwork at the appropriate level. For instance, the baccalaureate-prepared nurse should possess an understanding of the roles and responsibilities of professionals on the healthcare team and use effective communication techniques and collaboration skills to facilitate the delivery of evidence-based, patient-centered care. The master's-prepared nurse must possess skills to build and lead interprofessional teams with a focus on improving patient and population health outcomes by leading, communicating, collaborating, and consulting with other members of the healthcare team. The doctoral prepared nurse is expected to serve as an effective team leader when appropriate, overcome impediments to interprofessional practice, develop and implement practice models, health policy, and evidence-based standards of care, analyze complex practice and organizational issues, and serve as a change agent in the complex healthcare system.

Momentum for change continues, in 2017 The National Organization of Nurse Practitioner Faculties (NONPF) set forth nurse practitioner core competencies and offered content areas for the curriculum [11]. The nurse practitioner is expected to assume leadership roles and guide change to foster collaboration among the healthcare team in the delivery of quality care. Likewise, the American Association of Nurse Anesthetists (AANA) (2019) Standards for Nurse Anesthesia Practice *Standard 14: A Culture of Safety* calls for collaborative interdisciplinary engagement in practice conjoined by shared goals and decision-making [12]. The Association for Radiology and Imaging in Nursing (ARIN) expects the registered nurse in the imaging setting to serve as a role model with leadership abilities, effective communication skills, and a facilitator of teamwork focused on personalized care of the individual patient [13]. Additionally, one component of the American Nurses Credentialing Center's (ANCC) Magnet® Recognition model calls for exemplary professional practice within nursing that entails being an integral part of the interdisciplinary team [14].

As a result of these recommendations, IPE has been embedded into most health professions' curriculums. Operationalizing IPE requires extensive collaboration among champions at each school, in addition to time and resources. Operationalizing IPE in practice settings can be even more challenging. Slanetz and Mullins [5] support the need for IPE in radiology to promote collaborative practice in an effort to ensure better patient care in today's complex healthcare system [5]. The authors list team-based interprofessional experiences as key curricular components for diagnostic radiologists as per the Accreditation Council for Medical Education (ACGME).

## 28.3 Culture Change

Interprofessional collaboration must be preceded by interprofessional education. This education can occur in a variety of settings. Interprofessional education "occurs when two or more professions learn with, about, and from each other to enable effective collaboration and improve healthcare outcomes [1]. The ultimate goal is that IPE will lead to interprofessional collaboration which is "a type of interprofessional work involving various health and social care professionals who come together regularly to solve problems, provide services, and enhance health outcomes" [2].

In an ongoing effort to prepare future healthcare professionals for team-based patient care and improved individual and population health outcomes, the Interprofessional Education Collaborative (IPEC) published the National Core Competencies for Interprofessional Collaborative Practice [6]. The competences: values/ethics of interprofessional practice, rules/responsibilities, interprofessional communication, and teams and teamwork fall under one overarching domain of interprofessional collaboration. The goal is that the competencies will be embraced across all health professions because there is an expectation that healthcare providers enter the practice setting ready to engage in collaborative practice. No longer can health profession students be educated in silos. It is unrealistic to expect optimal team performance in the practice setting when students have never had the chance to work together previously. Along the same line, in clinical practice valuable input from colleagues in other disciplines is missed when work is carried out in silos.

Many barriers exist to effective change because change is difficult. For instance, seasoned nurse educators and nurses may not have the knowledge, skills, or training for teamwork. In addition, limited resources including time, space, equipment, and funding can restrict educational efforts [15]. Strategies to overcome barriers require champions to lead the effort to gain buy-in from key stakeholders in order to make this model a reality.

A culture change and new outlook in healthcare delivery is needed. Traditions must be challenged. In addition to training novices differently as they enter the profession, experienced practitioners will need to be retrained to think and act differently as well. Hierarchal leadership models must become a thing of the past. The culture of the unit is a critical factor in the overall success of the team. Each team member should be treated with kindness and respect. A positive attitude can be contagious. It is the responsibility of each individual to display these admirable qualities on a daily basis. This type of team cohesiveness will be sensed by patients. In addition to making the work environment a pleasant one, patients are entitled to be cared for by a happy, confident, proficient healthcare team.

## 28.1 Development and Implementation of a Plan

The goal is to offer a simple plan that can be used by everyone no matter their background. In order to make this meaningful, practical, and easy to use, the following is a suggested plan for embedding IPE into an educational curriculum or practice setting offering continuing education.

First, the learners must be identified as well as their level of knowledge and experience. Second, a curriculum is developed to address one topic or concept. An IPE curriculum might include a series of one IPE lessons per month. Third, a lesson plan is devised for each monthly session. "The one-sentence lesson plan" is an easy means of doing this [16]. The breakdown is as follows. Identify *"the what"* you want the learners to know or be able to do following the lesson. Determine *"the how"* this learning will be achieved or what teaching strategies or activities you will utilize to allow the learners time to apply or experience the content hands-on. Explain *"the why"* or the rationale for learning the content to the learners [16]. According to Eng, this step is critical because it creates learner buy-in by attaching a meaningful purpose [16].

A template for *the final "one-sentence"* might read: After this lesson, the learners will be able to *do x* by using y method, *so that they will be helped in z way*.

The following is an example of Eng's method applied to radiology [16]. The immediate radiology team includes the following healthcare professionals: a radiologist or proceduralist, a nurse, a radiology technologist and an anesthesiologist or a certified registered nurse anesthetist (CRNA). However, there are other professionals outside this intimate team that team members interact with such as: patients, families, transporters, and nurses on medical-surgical units. Thus, depending on the lesson the exact learners may change but can include anyone on the team.

When implementing a new IPE curriculum for radiology, scaffolding material might be helpful. Lessons could begin with learning roles and responsibilities of team members, then move on to teamwork strategies during procedures, and finally crisis management. Twelve sessions can be further defined from these categories. In planning a single monthly IPE lesson, "the one-sentence lesson plan" is written.

Team Strategies and Tools to Enhance Performance and Patient Safety (TeamSTEPPS®) is an evidence-based framework to optimize team performance across the healthcare delivery system [17]. TeamSTEPPS® framework consists of team structure and four skills: communication, leadership, situation monitoring, and mutual support. TeamSTEPPS® can guide the development of the learning activities for teamwork strategies lessons [17]. This framework can provide the tools to carry out "the one-sentence lesson plan" with the radiology team. For example, "the one-sentence lesson plan" might read: After this simulation, learners will be able to *effectively communicate* by using TeamSTEPPS® skills, *so that they function better as a team with the end goal of delivering high-quality, safe, patient-centered care.*

The following steps are taken in the implementation of the "the one-sentence lesson plan." *Open* the lesson with "*the why*" to allow learners an opportunity to contextualize the topic [16]. One might ask the learners, what experiences they have had in a crisis situation requiring clear communication and efficient teamwork. Then during the *Mini-lesson* introduce TeamSTEPPS® communication strategies (Table 28.1).

**Table 28.1** TeamSTEPPS® key principles and strategies

| Key principles | Strategies | |
|---|---|---|
| Communication | SBAR | Template used to communicate critical information requiring immediate attention. *Situation:* What is currently happening with the patient? *Background:* What is the relevant clinical background? *Assessment:* What is the perceived problem? *Recommendation and request:* Suggestions to correct the problem. |
| | Call-Out | Reporting critical information aloud for entire team to hear. |
| | Check-Back | Expecting and demanding "parroting" of requests. |
| Leadership | Brief | Short session prior to starting case, team roles and plan of care agreed on. |
| | Huddle | Ad hoc planning, often around a single patient or event. Establishes/reestablishes situational awareness. Reinforces plan already in place. Assesses need to adjust the plan. |
| | Debrief | Informal information exchange session designed to improve team performance and effectiveness through lessons learned and reinforcement of positive behaviors. |
| Situation monitoring | STEP | **STEP**: a tool for monitoring situations in the delivery of care. S—*Status of the patient:* history, physical exam, vital signs, medications, plan of care, psychosocial factors. T—*Status of team members*: fatigue, workload, task performance, skill, stress level. E—*Environment*: human resources, equipment, triage acuity, facility. P—*Progress toward goal*: patient status, goals/actions of team, is plan still appropriate. |
| Mutual support | Two-challenge rule | Empowers any member of the team to "stop the line" if he/she senses a safety breach. <br> – This action requires immediate cessation of the process and resolution. <br> – If initial assertion ignored, it is responsibility of team member to assertively voice concern at least two times to ensure it has been heard <br> – The team member being challenged must acknowledge <br> – If the outcome is still not acceptable: take a stronger course of action and utilize supervisor or chain of command |
| | CUS | – I am Concerned! <br> – I am Uncomfortable! <br> – This is a Safety Issue! "STOP" |
| | DESC Script | A constructive approach for managing and resolving conflict. <br> – Describe the specific situation or behavior, provide concrete data <br> – Express how the situation makes you feel/what your concerns are <br> – Suggest other alternatives and seek agreement <br> – Consequences should be stated in terms of impact on established team goals; strive for consensus |

Adopted and adapted from United States Department of Health and Human Services, Agency for Healthcare Research and Quality. TeamSTEPPS course management guide. Available from: https://www.ahrq.gov/teamstepps/index.html[17]

*Guided practice* could include watching video clips on the TeamSTEPPS® website. The brief clips demonstrate the same clinical scenario twice, when team members use the communication strategies and when they do not, thus highlighting the significance of the strategies in enhancing team performance. A simple simulation *activity* with trained actors or staff to serve as standardized patients could follow. This allows the team to apply the communication skills during a simulated scenario and serve as a rehearsal for an actual procedure as well. Since interventional radiology teams are performing many computerized tomography (CT)-guided percutaneous lung biopsies, this might provide the simulation scenario. In *closing the lesson*, debrief the team's performance, the communication strategies used, opportunities missed, and what could be done differently to improve team functioning in the future. The closing should reflect back on "*the why*" the learning experience was important in the first place. In this scenario, a complication such as a pneumothorax could occur requiring recognition and prompt reporting of the findings to the radiologist and mobilization of the team for chest tube insertion. Utilization of TeamSTEPPS® communication skills in managing the crisis can improve the patient's outcome.

Much of IPE and collaboration occurs at the point of care. Ideally, prior to diagnostic testing or a procedure, ordering providers such as nurse practitioners or residents would have phone consultations with the radiologist so that clinical findings could be discussed. This affords the radiologist the opportunity to suggest the best study or procedure to explore differential diagnoses. This collaborative exchange between providers offers an opportunity to learn from each other, increase patient safety, and decrease costs so that the most cost-effective test is performed. In addition, a nurse or radiology technologist interacts with the patient and/or the unit nurse caring for the patient on an inpatient unit. This would ensure the patient is appropriately prepped and educated beforehand.

Prior to the initiation of any surgical and nonsurgical invasive procedure, the Universal Protocol for Preventing Wrong Site, Wrong Procedure, and Wrong Person Surgery™ should occur with active involvement of all team members [18]. During a procedure, the ARIN asserts that there must be "consistent, reliable and competent nursing presence in procedure rooms and peri-procedure areas always." Therefore, most often a registered nurse is staffed per procedure room. If sedation is administered, the nurse or nurse anesthetist's sole responsibility is to monitor the patient and administer medication. Early identification and prompt intervention of an adverse event reaction is critical.

Post procedure, the team collaborates and develops a patient-centered plan for post procedure care. The nurse provides a thorough handoff to foster smooth transition and to ensure appropriate monitoring and patient education is given [19]. TeamSTEPPS® communication techniques should begin with a pre-brief, continue throughout the procedure, and close with a debrief [17].

### 28.4.1 Adult Learning Theory or Andragogy

Strong theory should dictate appropriate teaching strategies for the adult learner. It is important to understand and consider the characteristics of adult learners when developing a teaching plan. According to Knowles, adults are intrinsically motivated, self-directed learners who reflect on their performance and readily make assessments as to their inherent strengths and weaknesses [20]. Adults learn best through experiential learning activities that require collaboration in problem solving. A student-centered, active learning approach is critical. Adult learners need to apply new learning to real-life circumstances with the opportunity to see the consequences of their actions [20].

### 28.4.2 Teaching Strategies

Teaching strategies must be carefully devised and should align with the fundamental principles of andragogy. There is robust data to support IPE to promote interprofessional collaboration. Reeves et al.'s systematic review assessed studies based on a modified Kirkpatrick model and concluded learners respond well to IPE, their attitudes and perceptions of one another improve, and there is a reported increase in collaborative knowledge and skills [21]. The researchers also report a small but growing body of literature to support changes in behavior, organizational practices, and benefits to patients from IPE [21].

### 28.4.2.1 Team Building
Many teaching strategies foster teamwork. The following activities can be utilized to create the 12-month IPE curriculum. Team building strategies range from icebreakers to escape rooms. Something as simple as competing with other teams to build the longest paper chain in 5 min can be effective. This activity strengthens communication skills and enhances problem solving and creative thinking. In "the blindfold game" a blindfolded team member must rely on colleagues to navigate through a room of obstacles. This game can help teams build trust and improve communication and listening skills. Escape rooms are the new craze. Participation can be fun as team members work together using sound communication, critical thinking skills, and conflict management techniques to reach the common goal which is to solve the room's mystery in order to escape. Escape rooms have been used with nursing students [22], nurses [23], and interprofessional teams [24] as an active learning strategy to improve team skills.

### 28.4.2.2 Case Studies
Case studies can be done in an asynchronous format online. A discussion board or blog can be the platform. A team leader can be assigned weekly or monthly, depending on the frequency chosen. The leader finds a case study relevant to radiology and posts it for discussion. All team members must contribute to the discussion until the case is resolved. At that time the leader posts the answer. This can also be done in an unfolding case study format in which details of the case are revealed at different points in the discussion. The leader can use professional journals to find cases of various difficulty to challenge the team based on their background knowledge and experience. Strang Zook et al. used unfolding case studies in a virtual simulation format using SecondLife (Linden Lab, San Francisco, California) with health profession graduate students [25]. This and other IPE activities were integrated over three semesters. The researchers found over time participants reported increased self-perceived ability to work with others and increased comfort in doing so [25].

### 28.4.2.3 Radiology Grand Rounds
Grand rounds can engage the radiology team via discussion and brainstorming interesting or challenging cases they recently encountered or are currently handling. Team members learn from each other by listening and working together to resolve the problem. This can also be done in a weekly topic format with case-based presentations by members on the radiology team or other healthcare professionals the team can learn from. Topics and cases are selected based on a needs assessment to provide learner-centered, up-to-date knowledge about timely issues that impact patient outcomes in radiology [26]. Presentations should be brief and end with time for questions from learners. An interactive question-and-answer component could be utilized to foster engagement of the learners. Poll Everywhere® and Kahoot Polling® are two polling systems available to engage the audience in discussion.

Grand rounds is not a new pedagogical method. Medicine has been utilizing this teaching strategy for many years. More recently the idea has been reinvented with an interprofessional focus. Matamoros and Cook's innovative approach to a collaborative multidisciplinary grand rounds was well received in a pediatric practice setting [27]. Poore et al. used a simulated case for interprofessional grand rounds in a university setting including students from eight disciplines and received positive feedback from learners [28].

### 28.4.2.4 Friday Night at the ER®
Friday Night at the ER® game is an experiential learning tool that uses simulation to engage learners to develop organizational thinking skills

and improved team performance. The game requires game boards and is ideally played by a group of 24, divided among 4 to 6 tables. The teams compete by collaborating and making data-driven decisions in an emergency room (ER) setting and are charged with delivery of high-quality, safe, cost-efficient patient care. Bacon, Trent, and McCoy found undergraduate nursing students had significantly higher scores on the Systems Thinking Scale and self-reported proficiency with the quality improvement QSEN competency after playing the game [29].

A sense of urgency is created by the ER setting and time limit of one hour to play. Afterward, teams debrief evaluating performance measures: cost and quality and reflecting on two questions, "What felt real?" and "What strategies were used during the game?" [30]. A game such as this can give the radiology team a chance to become more fiscally aware in the context of a larger healthcare system while practicing teamwork skills.

### 28.4.2.5 High Fidelity Simulation

High-fidelity simulation (HFS) with patient simulators could offer a safe yet effective way for radiology teams to engage in IPE. Simulation is not a new teaching strategy for the specialty, for many years task trainers have been employed to allow learners the opportunity to practice skills before performing the procedure on an actual patient [31]. Interactive high-fidelity simulators add an entirely new dimension to their lower fidelity counterparts. High-fidelity patient simulators have the ability to bleed, breathe, sweat, seize, and speak and are equipped with audible heart, lung, and bowel sounds. These simulators can be pre-programmed to mimic specific conditions and will respond physiologically to medications, treatments, and procedures. HFS has been used for many years in healthcare professional schools.

More recently, acute care institutions have begun to use the evidence-based teaching-learning strategy. HFS allows for experiential learning, so the team can practice in a simulated but life-like setting prior to actual patient care [32]. It is a safe, realistic way to practice techniques, procedures, interpretive skills, crisis management, professionalism, communication, and collaborative practice. The addition of standardized actors to play the role of patients, family members, or ancillary staff can add realism. The roles can be played by theatre majors or by individuals hired from the public and trained accordingly.

Potential complications in the radiology setting should be anticipated and planned for. High-fidelity simulation could be utilized to prepare teams for such emergencies like anaphylaxis to contrast media or respiratory depression during the delivery of sedation and analgesia. Practice makes perfect. Scenarios can be designed to allow the team to practice for such adverse events ahead of time. Institutions could partner with local colleges or universities who have simulations if needed. This could foster future collaborative events between the two.

Medical students, undergraduate nursing and nurse anesthesia students' attitudes and behaviors toward interprofessional practice in an operating room setting were improved after HFS focusing on teamwork [33]. Wang et al.'s study with a radiology team found that HFS was more effective than computer-based training for the management of contrast reactions [34]. Niell et al. stated participants in their study reported significant improvement in teamwork and management of anaphylaxis after IPE using HFS [35]. Both contrast reaction management and team work skills can be taught and should subsequently be practiced. Retrieval of these skills on a regular basis is important to assure ongoing proficiency.

### 28.4.2.6 Sharing Applications

Team meetings can offer a chance for colleagues to engage in meaningful conversation and sharing of professional resources. Sharing applications (Apps) for cell phones that can be used as a resource at the point of care can build relationships among team members. Some Apps are free or available at low cost; yet, others can be expensive. Radiology Assistant by BestApps BV received the "Best Radiology Mobile App" award at the Radiological Society of North America (RSNA) 2018 in Chicago. Other useful Apps include: Radiology Rounds-Radiologists by Daily Rounds Inc., Radiology CT viewer by Ca Nguyen, and Medications in Radiology and Medications in Interventional Radiology by Murthy Chamarthy. Numerous drug references are available; IV Medications Gahart (2018) by Skyscape Medpresso Inc. is devoted specifically to intravenous medication administration.

#### 28.4.2.7 Interprofessional Conferences

Interprofessional conferences are an excellent venue to share IPE research and showcase what the radiology team has learned from IPE events. Participation does not have to be researched based, sharing IPE experiences can also serve as welcome information that others are interested in.

#### 28.4.2.8 IPE Book Club

An IPE book club for the team can be useful. Books on teamwork and leadership offer good topics. This might be an opportunity to engage colleagues outside the radiology team from other practice areas.

#### 28.4.2.9 Telehealth

Telehealth is becoming increasingly more common. Ciro et al. describe an IPE telehealth experience with graduate students facilitated by a university affiliated clinic [36]. Standardized patients were used to play the patient role. An interesting finding was that the students at the remote site stated they felt establishing a relationship with the patient was more challenging. However, teamwork may have been enhanced by detailed communication and reliance on each other especially for those students not on site with the patient.

### 28.5 IPE Resources

Resources are readily available online to support teaching and assessment efforts to transform the delivery of healthcare. Websites provide a wealth of information to aid in the initiation or advancement of IPE in any setting. Many are free, a few require membership fees. Information included on the sites include, but are not limited to, webinars, training courses, publications, conferences, funding opportunities, links to additional resources, and "how to" toolkits. The following is not intended to be a complete list of sites but is offered as a good starting point.

- Agency for Healthcare Research and Quality (AHRQ), Team Strategies and Tools to Enhance Performance and Patient Safety (TeamSTEPPS®) https://www.ahrq.gov/teamstepps/index.html
- American Interprofessional Health Collaborative (AIHC) https://aihc-us.org/
- Canadian Interprofessional Health Collaborative (CIHC) http://www.cihc.ca/
- Centre for the Advancement of Interprofessional Education (CAIPE) https://www.caipe.org/
- Institute for Healthcare Improvement (IHI) http://www.ihi.org/education/ihiopenschool/Pages/default.aspx
- Interprofessional Educational Collaborative (IPEC) https://www.ipecollaborative.org/
- Interprofessional Professionalism Collaborative (IPC) http://www.interprofessionalprofessionalism.org/
- *MedEdPORTAL* https://www.mededportal.org/collection/interprofessional-education/
- National Center for Interprofessional Practice and Education (Nexusipe) https://nexusipe.org
- Quality and Safety Education for Nurses (QSEN)http://qsen.org/
- Transforming Interprofessional Groups through Educational Resources (TIGER), by The University of Leicester, De Montfort University and The University of Northampton http://tiger.library.dmu.ac.uk/
- University of Washington, Center for Health Sciences Interprofessional Education Research and Practice https://collaborate.uw.edu/
- World Health Organization (WHO) https://www.who.int/hrh/resources/framework_action/en/

## 28.6 Evaluation of the Plan

Evaluating an educational program overall and individual lesson is needed no matter the teaching-learning strategy. This constructive feedback process informs changes in the program or lesson.

### 28.6.1 The Modified Kirkpatrick Model

The Modified Kirkpatrick Model offers a guide to evaluate outcomes [37]. Kirkpatrick and Kirkpatrick delineated four outcome levels: *Level one*: Reaction or satisfaction of the learners in the program [38]. This information can be ascertained via an anonymous survey at the conclusion of each lesson. This feedback informs the teacher and should be taken into consideration to improve the lesson in the future. *Level two*: Knowledge gained by the learners. A pre-test, post-test is an effective method to determine if learning occurred as a result of the lesson. *Level three*: Behavior changes in the learner. Long-term effects of the lesson might best be assessed months to years afterward or at various intervals. To accomplish this, a questionnaire could be sent to all the learners via email using an anonymous format such as Survey Monkey®. The addition of open-ended questions might provide robust information. For example, please describe *changes* to your daily routine providing patient care as a result of *xyz* IPE. *Level four*: Change in organizational practices or care delivery and benefits to patients as a result. In radiology, the success of this outcome could be measured by assigning a radiology team member to an observer role during a procedure where the individual's sole responsibility is to monitor use of specified communication techniques or lack thereof using a standardized tool. Anonymous surveys can be used to ascertain patient and family satisfaction.

### 28.6.2 Assessment Tools

Valid and reliable research instruments are needed to advance the science of interprofessional education. According to a multi-methods project by Blue et al. there is a lack of assessment methods and valid and reliable tools in IPE [39]. Blue et al. conducted interviews with IPE program leaders, a literature review, and an expert meeting with leaders from the United States and Canada and concluded there were valid and reliable tools available to assess attitudes and readiness of learners but tools to assess individual and team performance were scarce. The researchers called for longitudinal assessment that include multiple data sources to measure knowledge, skills, and behaviors of the learners in various settings. Furthermore, they stressed the need for formative feedback for learners to promote growth and development of their IPE skills. In addition, the researchers cited the need for behavioral assessment tools to evaluate competences of the individual and team. Objective structured clinical exams (OSCE) could provide the mechanism to achieve this. Finally, Blue et al. highlighted the need for frameworks and associated tools that connect learner or team performance and patient outcomes [39].

Blue et al. [39] and Rogers et al. [40] endorsed the *Interprofessional Collaborator Assessment Rubric (ICAR)* which assesses a learner's performance of the Canadian IPE competencies [41]. Subscales of the ICAR are communication, collaboration, roles and responsibility, collaborative patient/client-family centered approach, team functioning, and conflict management/resolution. Each subscale is divided into dimensions. For example, the collaboration subscale is divided into three dimensions: collaborative relationship, integration of information from others, and information sharing. These competencies are measured on a developmental trajectory. The developmental stages range from minimal, developing, competent, to mastery.

Rogers et al. endorsed the *Individual Teamwork Observation and Feedback Tool (iTOFT)* to assess a learner's performance [40]. Thistlethwaite et al. developed two versions of the tool: basic for junior level students and advanced for senior level students and novice healthcare professionals [42]. The Basic Tool lists 11 observable behaviors in two categories: shared decision-making and working in a team. The Advanced Tool includes 10 additional observable behaviors from two more categories: leadership and patient safety. The items are graded: not applicable, inappropriate, appropriate, and responsive. No matter which tool or method is used for assessment, it is imperative to remember that feedback should be ongoing. The learner should receive formative feedback from an assessment in order to improve where needed prior to summative evaluation.

Lockeman et al. shared a *refined IPEC Competency Self-Assessment Survey* [43]. This tool originally developed in 2012 was intended to assess outcomes related to collaborative practice [44]. According to Lockeman et al. the refined tool is shorter and easy to use while it retains sound reliability and validity [44]. The revised tool contains two domains: one linked to interprofessional interaction, the other interprofessional values. The revised self-assessment tool is a 5-point Likert scale with 16 items intended to measure the IPEC competencies.

## 28.7 Future Research Goals

The IOM challenged researchers to move beyond examining the impact of IPE on learners' knowledge, skills, and attitudes and instead to focus on the link between IPE and performance in practice, including the impact of IPE on patient and population health and healthcare delivery system outcomes [2]. Outcome research is needed to establish a link between IPE and patient safety, patient and provider satisfaction, quality of care, health promotion, population health, and healthcare costs [3].

The Triple Aim developed by Berwick, Nolan, and Whittington from the Institute for Healthcare Improvement (IHI) describes an approach to optimizing health system performance [45]. The articulated the goals remain appropriate today and require collaborative practice, namely, improving the experience of care (quality and satisfaction), improving the health of populations, and reducing healthcare costs. The IHI website has resources available for organizations and communities to facilitate their quest to achieve the interdependent goals.

## 28.8 Conclusion

Ideally, IPE would start early in health profession curriculums, then be practiced and emphasized during clinical experiences, and continue into the practice setting as a means of professional development. Done in this way, the desired outcomes of the Triple Aim could be realized. This chapter provides foundational resources needed to develop, implement, and evaluate educational efforts to foster the development of effective interprofessional collaborative practice involving nurses, radiologists, and radiologic technologists to transform the delivery of healthcare. Finally, future avenues for research and practice are shared.

## References

1. World Health Organization. Framework for action on interprofessional education and collaborative practice. Geneva: World Health Organization; 2010.
2. Institute of Medicine. Measuring the impact of interprofessional education (IPE) on collaborative practice and patient outcomes. Washington, DC: National Academies Press; 2015.
3. Brandt BF. Rethinking health professions education through the lens of interprofessional practice and education. New Dir Adult Cont Educ. 2018;157:65–76. https://doi.org/10.1002/ace.20269.
4. Potter TM. Partnership-imaging a new model in healthcare. JRadiolNurs. 2015;34:5–62. https://doi.org/10.1016/j.jradnu.2015.04.002.
5. Slanetz PJ, Mullins ME. Radiology education in the era of population-based medicine in the United States. AcadRadiol. 2016;23:894–7. https://doi.org/10.1016/j.acra.2016.01.017.
6. Interprofessional Education Collaborative Expert Panel. Core competencies for interprofessioanl

collaborative practice: report of an expert panel. Washington, DC: Interprofessional Education Collaborative; 2011.
7. Cronenwett L, Sherwood G, Barnsteiner J, Disch J, Johnson J, Mitchell P, et al. Quality and safety education for nurses. Nurs Outlook. 2007;55(3):122–31.
8. American Association of Colleges of Nursing. The essentials of baccalaureate education for professional nursing practice. Washington, DC: Author; 2008.
9. American Association of Colleges of Nursing. The essentials of master's education for advanced practice nursing education. Washington, DC: Author; 2008.
10. American Association of Colleges of Nursing. The essentials of doctoral education for advanced nursing practice. Washington, DC: Author; 2006.
11. National Organization of Nurse Practitioner Faculties. Domains and competencies of nurse practitioner practice. Washington, DC: Author; 2000.
12. American Association of Nurse Anesthetists (AANA). Standards for nurse anesthesia practice. 2019.https://www.aana.com/docs/default-source/practice-aana-com-web-documents-(all)/standards-for-nurse-anesthesia-practice.pdf?sfvrsn=e00049b1_2. Accessed 24 Feb2019.
13. Association for Radiologic and Imaging Nursing. Practice guidelines and position statements. Association for Radiologic and Imaging Nursing Position Statements; 2018 (Updated Nov2018). Available from https://www.arinursing.org/resources/practice-guidelines/. Accessed 18 Dec2018.
14. American Nurses Credentialing Center. Journey to magnet excellence.2015. Available from http://www.nursecredentialing.org/MagnetJourney. Accessed 24 Feb2019.
15. Kent F, Nankervis K, Johnson C, Hodgkinson M, Baulch J, Haines T. Considerations in the establishment of interprofessional education programs in the workplace. J Interprof Care. 2018;32:89–94. https://doi.org/10.1080/13561820.2017.1381076.
16. EngN. Focus your lectures with the 'One-Sentence Lesson Plan'. Faculty Focus.2018.https://www.facultyfocus.com/articles/teaching-and-learning/focus-your-lectures-with-the-one-sentence-lesson-plan/. Accessed 15 Feb2019.
17. United States Department of Health and Human Services, Agency for Healthcare Research and Quality. TeamSTEPPS course management guide. Available from https://www.ahrq.gov/teamstepps/index.html. Accessed 8 Jan 2019.
18. The Joint Commission. Hospital National Patient Safety Goals. 2019. https://www.jointcommision.org. Accessed 1 Mar2019.
19. Association for American Radiological and Imaging Nursing. ARIN position statement: nurse staffing in interventional radiology.2018.https://www.arinursing.org/ARIN/assets/File/public/practice-guidelines/2018_10_28_Staffing_Paper_Position_Statement.pdf. Accessed 20 Feb2019.
20. Knowles MS. The modern practice of adult education: From pedagogy to andragogy. 2nd ed. New York: Cambridge Books; 1980.
21. Reeves S, Fletcher S, Barr H, Birch I, Boet S, Davies N, et al. A BEME systematic review of the effects of interprofessional education: BEME Guide No. 39. MedTeach. 2016;38:656–68. https://doi.org/10.3109/0142159X.2016.1173663.
22. Gómez-Urquiza JL, Gómez-Salgado J, Albendín-García L, Correa-Rodríguez M, González-Jiménez E, Cañadas-De la Fuente GA. The impact on nursing students' opinions and motivation of using a "Nursing Escape Room" as a teaching game: a descriptive study. Nurse Educ Today. 2019;72:73–6. https://doi.org/10.1016/j.nedt.2018.10.018.
23. Adams V, Burger S, Crawford K, Setter R. Can you escape? Creating an escape room to facilitate active learning. J Nurses Prof Dev. 2018;34:E1–5. https://doi.org/10.1097/NND.0000000000000433.
24. Friedrich C, Teaford H, Taubenheim A, Boland P, Sick B. Escaping the professional silo: an escape room implemented in an interprofessional education curriculum. J Interprof Care. 2019;33:573–5. https://doi.org/10.1080/13561820.2018.1538941.
25. Strang Zook S, Hulton LJ, Dudding CC, Stewart AL, Graham AC. Scaffolding interprofessional education: unfolding case studies, virtual world simulations, and patient-centered care. Nurse Educ. 2018;43(2):87–91. https://doi.org/10.1097/NNE.0000000000000430.
26. Sandal S, Iannuzzi MC, Knohl SJ. Can we make grand rounds "grand" again? J Grad Med Educ. 2013;5:560–3. https://doi.org/10.4300/JGME-D-12-003551.
27. Matamoros L, Cook M. A nurse-led innovation in education: implementing a collaborative multidisciplinary grand rounds. J Contin Educ Nurs. 2017;48:353–7. https://doi.org/10.3928/00220124-20170712-06.
28. Poore JA, Stephenson E, Jerolimov D, Scott PJ. Development of an interprofessioanl teaching grand rounds. Nurse Educ. 2017;42:164–7. https://doi.org/10.1097/NNE.0000000000000351.
29. Bacon CT, Trent P, McCoy TP. Enhancing systems thinking for undergraduate nursing students using Friday Night at the ER. J Nurs Educ. 2018;57:687–9. https://doi.org/10.3928/01484834-20181022-11.
30. Young JK. Using a role-play simulation game to promote systems thinking. J Contin Educ Nurs. 2018;49:10–1. https://doi.org/10.3928/00220124-20180102-04.
31. Chetlen AL, Mendiratta-Lala M, Probyn L, Auffermann WF, DeBenedectis CM, Marko J, et al. Conventional medical education and the history of simulation in radiology. AcadRadiol. 2015;22:1252–67. https://doi.org/10.1016/j.acra.2015.07.003.
32. Kolb DA, Boyatzis RE, Mainemelis C. Experiential learning theory: previous research and new directions. Perspectives on thinking, learning, and cognitive styles. Mahwah, NJ: Lawrence Erlbaum Associates; 2001. p. 227–47.
33. Leithead J, Garbee DD, Yu Q, Rusnak VV, Kiselov VJ, Zhu L, et al. Examining interprofessional learn-

ing perceptions among students in a simulation-based operating room team training experience. J Interprof Care. 2019;33:26–31. https://doi.org/10.1080/13561820.2018.1513464.
34. Wang CL, Chinnugounder S, Hippe DS, Zaidi S, O'Malley RB, Bhargava P, Bush WH. Comparative effectiveness of hands-on versus computer simulation-based training for contrast media reactions and teamwork skills. J Am Coll Radiol. 2017;14:103–10. https://doi.org/10.1016/j.jacr.2016.07.013.
35. Niell BL, Kattapuram T, Halpern EF, Salazar GM, Penzias A, Bonk SS, et al. Prospective analysis of an interprofessional team training program using high-fidelity simulation of contrast reactions. Am J Roentgenol. 2015;204:W670–6. https://doi.org/10.2214/AJR.14.13778.
36. Ciro C, Randall K, Robinson C, Loving G, Shortridge A. Telehealth and interprofessional education. OT Pract. 2015;20:7–10.
37. Freeth D, Hammick M, Koppel I, Reeves S. A critical review of evaluations of interprofessional education. A review commissioned by the Learning and Teaching Support Network Health Sciences and Practice from the Interprofessional Education Joint Evaluation Team. 2002. Available at https://www.caipe.org/resources/publications/archived-publications/freeth-d-hammick-m-koppel-i-reeves-s-barr-h-al-2002-a-critical-review-of-evaluations-of-interprofessional-education-hea-health-sciences-and-practice-occasional-paper-2-2. Accessed 15 Mar 2019.
38. Kirkpatrick JD, Kirkpatrick WK. Kirkpatrick's four levels of training evaluation. Alexandria, VA: ATD Press; 2016.
39. Blue AV, Chesluk BJ, Conforti LN, Holmboe ES. Assessment and evaluation in interprofessional education. J Allied Health. 2015;44:73–82.
40. Rogers GD, Thistlethwaite JE, Anderson ES, Abrandt Dahlgren M, Grymonpre RE, Moran M, et al. International consensus statement on the assessment of interprofessional learning outcomes. MedTeach. 2017;39:347–59. https://doi.org/10.1080/0142159X.2017.1270441.
41. Curran V, Hollett A, Casimiro LM, Mccarthy P, Banfield V, Hall P, et al. Development and validation of the interprofessional collaborator assessment rubric (ICAR). J Interprof Care. 2011;25:339–44. https://doi.org/10.3109/13561820.2011.589542.
42. Thistlethwaite J, Dallest K, Moran M, Dunston R, Roberts C, Eley D, et al. Introducing the individual Teamwork Observation and Feedback Tool (iTOFT): development and description of a new interprofessional teamwork measure. J Interprof Care. 2016;30:526–8. https://doi.org/10.3109/13561820.2016.1169262.
43. Lockeman KS, Dow AW, DiazGranados D, McNeilly DP, Nickol D, Koehn ML, et al. Refinement of the IPEC competency self-assessment survey: results from a multi-institutional study. J Interprof Care. 2016;30:726–31. https://doi.org/10.1080/13561820.2016.1220928.
44. Dow AW, DiazGranados D, Mazmanian PE, Retchin SM. An exploratory study of an assessment tool derived from the competencies of the interprofessional education collaborative. J Interprof Care. 2014;28(4):299–304. https://doi.org/10.3109/13561820.2014.891573.
45. Berwick DM, Nolan TW, Whittington J. The triple aim: care, health, and cost. Health Aff. 2008;27(3):759–69. http://search.ebscohost.com.ezp.scranton.edu/login.aspx?direct=true&db=c8h&AN=105703563&site=ehost-live. Accessed October 28, 2019.

# Social Media

**Saad A. Ranginwala**

## 29.1 Introduction

Communication worldwide has been rapidly changing over the past 20–30 years. With the widespread adoption of email, the first step towards acceptance of digital correspondence was set. Particularly within the last 15 years, social media has become an integral part of the communication landscape.

Social media is a form of digital communication allowing for direct interaction between users. It differs from many other previous forms of communication in that there is, by design, often no intermediary between users, allowing for more direct communication. The sharing and consumption of content is governed by the unique features and rules inherent to each social media platform, which informs the best uses of each of these services.

Social media has become a required mode of communication in the business world. For businesses, the ability to reach and deliver content to consumers directly, large user bases, low start-up and maintenance costs, and ability to receive unadulterated feedback from consumers has proven to have great utility. While social media has clearly been embraced by the general public and businesses, medicine has relatively lagged behind in adoption of this mode of communication [1–3].

Currently, many in the medical world are beginning to use social media on a wider scale. While the level of adoption varies widely by institution and individual, social media has become a tool worth considering and employing on both a personal and institutional level.

## 29.2 Participation

Participation in social media can be performed on both a personal and institutional level. Each has different goals and purposes that should be properly utilized by the user account.

On the personal level, most institutions do not place restrictions on their employees creating accounts. However, care must be taken to share content responsibly. If there are restrictions per your employer on what types of content can be posted, these guidelines should be considered when posting on social media. Potential specific uses on different networks will be discussed later.

On the institutional level, it is very important to understand your organization's marketing and social media policies. Many institutions may require explicit approval from legal or marketing departments to participate in social media apart from restrictions on types of content allowed to be posted.

S. A. Ranginwala, MD (✉)
Department of Medical Imaging, Ann and Robert H. Lurie Children's Hospital of Chicago, Chicago, IL, USA

There are a few reasons for these types of restrictions by organizations, particularly in regard to the number of groups allowed to participate individually under the umbrella of an organization. First, organizations generally prefer a focused message to consumers and patients. The participation of multiple groups under the same organization can lead to garbling and dilution of the organizational message. Second, multiple groups raise the possibility of public blunders. Many organizations have made mistakes on social media requiring apologies after posting inappropriate content to their social media accounts. Last, regularly updated content is important to continue to stay relevant. Organizations aim to avoid orphaned accounts as they can demonstrate a lack of attention by the organization or even pose as a security risk due to targeting by hackers [4, 5].

Once an individual or group has decided to use social media, it's worthwhile to ask a few questions to guide their potential use. Who is the target audience? Which platform should be used? How often will content be propagated? Who will be in charge of both creating and managing content? What will content look like?

It's also very important to define how you or your organization will measure success. While each platform has its own specific metrics, some terms are important to know across platforms. For example, followers refer to individuals who have subscribed to your channel. Impressions measure the number of individuals who have seen your post. Engagement is a measure of how many people have interacted with a specific post. Many other metrics may be present which are more specific to a given platform.

## 29.3 Types of Platforms

In order to get a better understanding of how to use social media, it is beneficial to discuss some of the most popular platforms, their specific characteristics, and best uses.

### 29.3.1 Twitter

Twitter is a text and image-based social media platform based around interactions between users and followers via interactions called tweets (Fig. 29.1). As of February 2019, Twitter reported 321 million active monthly users [6]. Tweets are comprised of up to 240 characters with the ability to include embedded images, videos, and links. While these messages are brief, they can be posted in succession to form threads which can elicit deeper discussions. In addition, direct messages (DM) can be used to directly and privately communicate with individuals. Each user has a "handle," which is composed of a user name preceded by the "@" symbol. The main interactions on Twitter consist of tweets, replies to tweets, retweets (RT; reposting of another user's tweet), likes, and tags. Hashtags are words or phrases

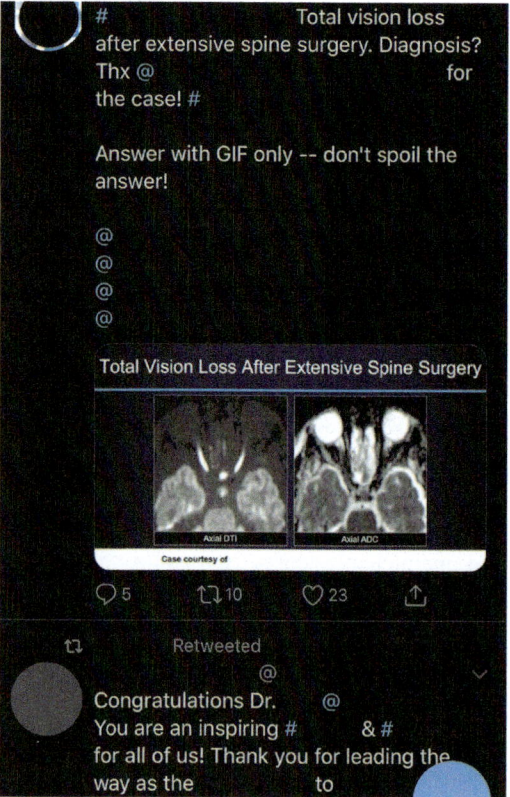

**Fig. 29.1** The feed on Twitter allows users to receive public posts from other users that they follow. Note the icons (message bubble, circular arrows, and heart) below the post which allow users to reply, retweet, and like, respectively

preceded by the "#" symbol which are used to emphasize a thought or categorize the tweet by a topic or trending discussion. For example, medical conferences often utilize hashtags to link tweets between attendees, such as #RSNA18 for the Radiological Society of North America 2018 Annual Meeting [7]. Anecdotally, Twitter is the most widely used social media platform for interactions between medical professionals in the United States.

On a personal level, Twitter can be used as a personal profile for interaction with others in your field online. An individual can share personal knowledge, accomplishments, events, and have discussions with colleagues. It can serve as a springboard for forming relationships with individuals that you may otherwise never have a chance to interact with. This can often serve as a bridge to in person interactions and new, beneficial professional relationships.

At the organizational level, Twitter can serve multiple purposes. First, it can serve as an organizational message board. Notable accomplishments, presentations, publications, profiles, and other items from members in the organization can be shared [8]. Interactions with other users on Twitter can also serve to establish the credibility of the organization with knowledgeable interactions with other credible individuals and organizations. It's important to determine the goals of your interaction and base your presence and voice around achieving those goals.

Metrics on Twitter are robust. Basic metrics include aforementioned universal metrics such as followers and impressions. In addition, platform-specific metrics include number of retweets, replies, and likes. Twitter provides access to these metrics and more advanced metrics within its analytics package [9].

### 29.3.2 Facebook

Facebook is a social media platform with the largest user base in the world, consisting of 2.38 billion monthly active users as of March 31, 2019 (Fig. 29.2) [10]. Facebook is a predominantly text and link-based platform with the ability to embed many different types of media within posts. It was among the first platforms to incorporate a specific platform for businesses rather than just individuals with analytics geared towards optimizing businesses.

On a personal level, the use of Facebook is somewhat limited in the medical space. Personal accounts generally remain geared towards family and friends rather than patients or customers.

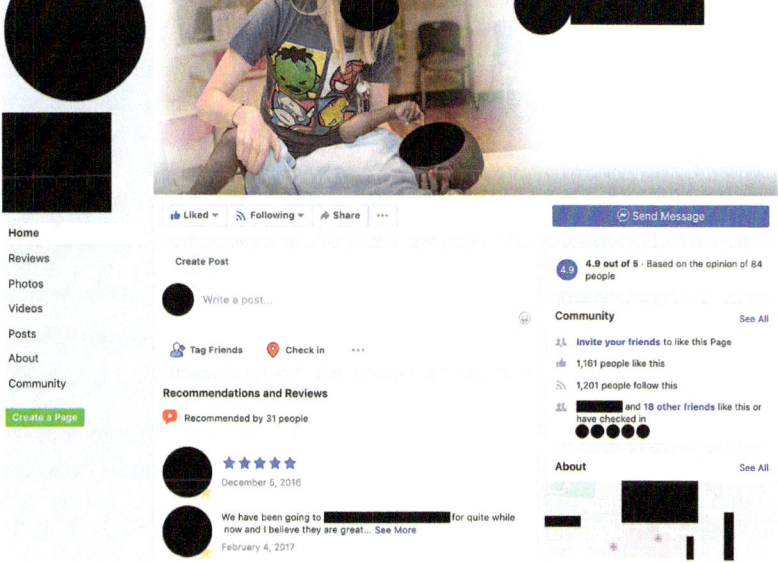

**Fig. 29.2** Business page on Facebook. Organizations can include any relevant information for their business and provide direct contact for customers, patients, and their families. Note that the public can also leave reviews and comments

On an organizational level, because of Facebook's large user base numbering in the billions, a presence is virtually necessary, if for no other reason than to serve as a landing page in such a widely used "directory." Business pages differ from personal pages in a number of ways, including organization, content, and how users subscribe to content. Unlike how personal accounts generally work through the "friend" concept requiring mutual agreement for content sharing, business accounts can be liked by users without explicit approval from the business, allowing the user to then receive content the business posts. General information such as location, hours of operation, addresses, phone numbers, and emails can also be included. Users are also able to "check-in" to let others in their network know that they have visited.

As platforms, Facebook and Twitter differ in a few ways. First, Facebook does not enforce a small character limit like Twitter, allowing for much longer and more detailed posts. Often, these posts are accompanied by links or other media, in order to better capture users' attention. Second, the manner in which content is distributed differs. Facebook offers differing levels of privacy for posts, while Twitter content is available either publicly or specifically only for followers [11].

Examples of uses for Facebook include making announcements, sharing content from other social media channels, and responding to user feedback and complaints.

Metrics on Facebook are among the most robust available on social media platforms. While basic metrics such as followers, likes, impressions, and engagement are available, advanced analytics through the Insights platform are also available.

### 29.3.3 Instagram

Instagram is an image-based social media platform with over 1 billion active monthly users (Fig. 29.3) [12]. The Instagram app is designed to be used exclusively on a mobile platform. It allows users to perform a variety of functions including editing images with filters and creating

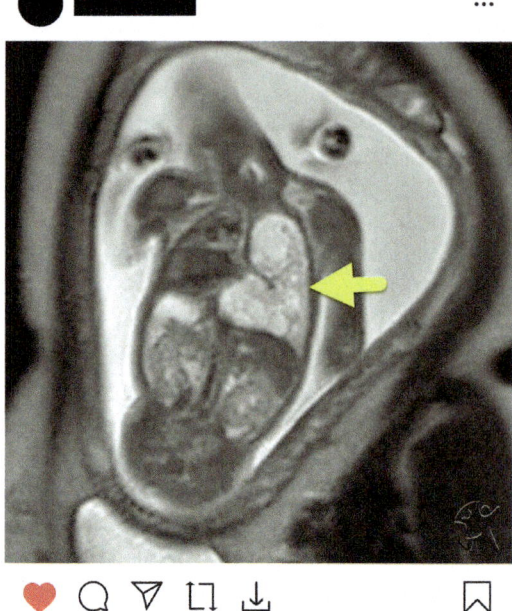

**Fig. 29.3** Instagram post. Note the image with releant caption below the image. The icons (heart, message bubble, paper airplane) allow users to like, reply to, and send the post to another user, respectively

descriptive captions with hashtags. While Instagram initially gained rapid popularity due to unique features such as square aspect ratio for images, filters, and mobile experience, Instagram has continually expanded its features and now allows posting in several forms. Traditional posts are viewed within the feed and consist of a mix of images and/or videos in each post with an accompanying caption. A newer feature called "Stories" allows users to post temporary images/videos which disappear after 24 h. One of the newest features, "IG TV," allows users to post videos of lengths greater than 1 min. The proliferation of these new features has anecdotally substantially changed the manner in which users have interacted, but generally interactions continue to occur mainly between users and their followers with additional interactions occurring secondary to categorization via hashtags [13–16].

Wilson, B. (2014). The Nerdy Nurse's Guide to Technology. Sigma Theta Tau International.

Indianapolis, Indiana.

Siegmund, L. A. (2019). "Like Us on Facebook®": Nursing in a World of Social Media. Journal of

Radiology Nursing, 38(30), 183-187.

**Fig. 29.4** Additional resources on social media and nursing

While the reliance on the mobile experience works well for personal uses, it may be suboptimal for education, a large focus in the radiology community. The reasons for this are as follows. First, mobile image capture has traditionally been the focus of Instagram. However, in the realm of radiology education and with imaging contained within PACS on desktop workstations, mobile capture of images is likely not the most effective manner of obtaining high-quality images. There are methods to get around this important limitation. Specialized screen capture applications can be used to copy these images in high quality. However, even after obtaining a high-quality image, another limitation of Instagram is that there is no official way to upload these images from the desktop/web to Instagram. Images are required to be sent in some manner to a mobile device to be uploaded. This can be achieved via email, text, or other services such as Dropbox™. Last, there are limited options for scheduling content within the app, though online services are available which skirt around these restrictions.

Despite these multiple limitations, the image-based focus of Instagram is well suited for a visible field such as radiology, particularly for education. With the ability to create posts via a multitude of methods using both images and videos, Instagram offers a robust platform for radiology focused users. However, prior to sharing images, it's important to consider the legal and institutional policies in your organization. Avoiding using identifiers such as age, gender, and specific clinical or social information can help to protect patients whose images are shared for educational purposes. In addition, newsworthy cases should also generally be avoided.

Instagram metrics are relatively basic but have become more robust over time. Basic metrics such as number of followers and number of likes in a post are easily accessible. Other more advanced metrics such as impressions, unique views, and more can be obtained by using a business account.

## 29.4 Conclusion

Social media has grown to become one of the most powerful media of communication. With its ability to reach large audiences directly using a number of different platforms with varying strengths, weaknesses, and demographics, individuals or organizations can connect with audiences within the radiology community (medical professionals) or outside of it (patients and families.) While the use of social media for and within medicine is in its relative infancy [17], the power of this form of communication is apparent and use will only continue to grow over time. See Fig. 29.4 for additional resources on social media and nursing.

## References

1. Glover M, Choy G, Boland GW, et al. Radiology and social media: are private practice radiology groups more social than academic radiology departments? J Am Coll Radiol. 2015;12:513–8.
2. Ranginwala S, Towbin AJ. The power of promotion: using social media to promote a radiology department. Acad Radiol. 2017;24(4):488–96.
3. Griner D. DiGiorno is really, really sorry about its tweet accidentally making light of domestic violence. Adweek. Available at: http://www.adweek.com/adfreak/digiorno-really-really-sorry-about-its-tweet-accidentally-making-light-domestic-violence-159998. Accessed 26 Jan 2016.
4. Moss C. US airways tweeted an extreme pornographic image and left it up for a long time. Business

Insider. Available at: http://www.businessinsider.com/us-airways-pornographic-tweet-2014-4. Accessed 26 Jan 2016.
5. Allen J. University of Michigan football's Facebook page hacked overnight. Mlive. Available at: http://www.mlive.com/news/ann-arbor/index.ssf/2015/08/university_of_michigan_footbal_3.html. Accessed 26 Jan 2019.
6. Twitter. About. Available at: https://about.twitter.com/company. Accessed 26 Jan 2019.
7. Hawkins C, Duszak R, Rawson J. Social media in radiology: early trends in Twitter microblogging at radiology's largest international meeting. J Am Coll Radiol. 2014;11:387–90.
8. Fitzgerald R, Radmanesh A. Social media and research visibility. AJNR Am J Neuroradiol. 2014;36:637.
9. Twitter. Twitter Analytics. Available at: https://analytics.twitter.com. Accessed 26 Jan 2016.
10. Facebook. Company Info | Facebook Newsroom. Available at: http://newsroom.fb.com/company-info/. Accessed 26 Jan 2015.
11. Aleo C, Hark L, Leiby B, et al. Ophthalmic patients' utilization of technology and social media: an assessment to improve quality of care. Telemed J E Health. 2014;20:887–92.
12. Instagram.com. Instagram. Available at: http://instagram.com/press/. Accessed 26 Jan 2016.
13. Mandviwalla M, Schuff D, Chacko M, et al. Is that all there is? Taking education to new levels in the social-media era. Change. 2013;45:51–8.
14. Bahner D, Adkins E, Patel N, et al. How we use social media to supplement a novel curriculum in medical education. Med Teach. 2012;34:439–44.
15. George D, Dreibelbis T, Aumiller B. How we used two social media tools to enhance aspects of active learning during lectures. Med Teach. 2013;35:985–8.
16. Karimkhani C, Connett J, Boyers L, et al. Dermatology on Instagram. Dermatol Online J. 2014;20
17. Glover M, Khalilzadeh O, Choy G, et al. Hospital evaluations by social media: a comparative analysis of Facebook ratings among performance outliers. J Gen Intern Med. 2015;30:1440–6.

# Response to Violence

**30**

Jeffrey Strickler

## 30.1 Introduction

Violence against healthcare workers is a widespread problem impacting care providers across the globe. This violence is coming from patients, family members, visitors, and even interpersonal violence from other employees. Such episodes of violence require health workers to be ever mindful of their risk and to develop new skill sets enabling them to better manage these incidents. In turn, it is requiring healthcare organizations to better prepare both staff and their facilities in ways to mitigate this violence. This chapter will look into the incidence of violence, describe how to assess for the factors putting individuals and organizations at higher risk, and most importantly prepare themselves and their organizations so that they can respond in a stronger and more proactive fashion to these threats.

## 30.2 Epidemiology

Hospitalization is stressful for all involved and navigating medical care can be frustrating for patient and family alike. As care providers, we need to understand that some individuals will respond to this stress and frustration with aggressive behavior. The challenge for healthcare workers is how to provide care to those under their watch while recognizing and responding to the cues of dissatisfaction and/or escalation so that a therapeutic relationship and environment can be maintained.

### 30.2.1 Incidence

The incidence of violence in a health setting is becoming more prevalent. A landmark study by the Emergency Nurses Association (ENA) in 2009 brought attention to this problem by showing that half of the emergency department (ED) nurses in their sample stated that they had been either verbally or physically assaulted in the previous 7 days with 12% suffering physical violence and 59% experiencing verbal abuse [1]. Further description revealed that 97% of this reported violence was perpetrated by patients and most nurses in the sample believed that the incidence of violence in their daily work had increased. This study revealed that incidences of violence had precipitated 25% of nurses to consider leaving the profession whereas 10% actually did leave. This study showed that greater than half did not feel safe or prepared to handle a violent encounter [2].

Although this example highlights that many incidents of violence are related to emergency

J. Strickler, DHA, RN, NEA-BC (✉)
UNC Health, University of North Carolina Health Care, Cary, NC, USA

care (80%), this problem is not unique to the ED. Other units such as the intensive care unit, psychiatric, pediatric, obstetric, and neonatal departments, as well as nursing homes or other long-term care facilities, are all shown to be at an increased risk for violence [3, 4]. According to the Occupational Safety and Health Administration (OSHA), 75% of the 25,000 annual workplace assaults occurred in the healthcare and social service setting and healthcare workers are four times more likely to be a victim of violence than workers in the private sector [5]. The National Crime Victimization Survey showed a 20% higher chance for healthcare workers to be a victim of violence compared to other workers [6]. A survey by the American Nurses Association (ANA) showed similar results to the ENA study with 21% of nurses reporting physical assault and 50% being verbally assaulted [7]. Further evidence of this increase, the Morbidity and Mortality Weekly reports showed that injuries from workplace violence doubled between 2012 and 2014 and workplace assaults averaged 24,000 incidents per year (2011–13) representing a 75% increase in workplace violence in healthcare [8]. Such statistics show that healthcare workers are now a common target for violence and our encounters with violence are unfortunately ubiquitous. Regardless of your practice setting, workplace violence is an increasing concern and one that all should be prepared to meet.

### 30.2.2 Definition

Workplace violence is considered to be any act of aggression, including any physical assault, emotional or verbal abuse directed toward persons at work or on duty [5]. These assaults or threats include physical, psychological, and verbal violence such as threats, verbal abuse, and harassment. Given this broader definition, it is clear that unfortunately many nurses have personal experiences with workplace violence.

### 30.2.3 Impact

These violent acts against healthcare workers have a profound impact on our profession. Hospitals have a direct cost for such acts for the treatment of any employees but also indirect cost for lost days from work. As a point of comparison, healthcare and social assistance have a greater than fourfold incidence of violent injuries resulting in days away from work as compared to other industries [5]. In addition to such financial indicators, the less visible but more impactful effect on nurses who encounter aggression in the workplace is that they often have feelings of anger, frustration, and hopelessness as well as more concerning issues with hyper-vigilance, post-traumatic stress disorder, depression, and anxiety all which may precipitate some to leave the profession. There are also other indicators such as resultant fatigue and stress leading to higher rates of medication errors and patient infections [5].

### 30.2.4 Causative Factors

The cause for this epidemic in violence directed toward healthcare workers is multifactorial. Some precipitating issues could be increased ED wait times, the unrestricted movement of the public in hospitals, decreased mental health funding and the resulting number of beds, increased patient acuity, increased use of hospital by law enforcement for those detained, and a general decrease in resources. Also, economic reasons such as the reduction in funding for mental health and substance abuse leading to drug seeking behavior or ED crowding with patients under the influence could be another factor [9]. Similarly, state reductions in mental health funding has put more such patients in emergency departments where staff are often unprepared to deal with violent outbursts [10]. Such closures have caused the number of mental health or substance abuse cases seen in EDs to climb from 1.6 million in 2005 to over 2 million in 2008 [11]. It is also important to consider some of the underlying social determinants of health such as unemployment, poverty, and homelessness. These all lead to feelings of hopelessness compounded by societal changes leading to decreased family and community support fractured families and fragmented services [12].

## 30.3 Assessment

There are several risk factors which increase the likelihood of an act of workplace violence with a prior history of assaultive behavior being deemed especially predictive. Other causes are age <40, clinical conditions with paranoia or poor impulse control, and a lifestyle with little or no social contact [13]. The DANGEROUS Behavior Screening Guide (Table 30.1) and the STAMP Nursing Assessment framework (Table 30.2) are valuable tools in highlighting these indicators.

The first warning sign of a possible violent encounter is agitation. Agitation is an acute behavioral emergency requiring immediate intervention. Agitation is further defined as anxiety leading to a private, chronic reaction to unmet emotional needs and stress resulting from experiencing life as a series of unpleasant events. Some of the warning signs for an agitated or anxious individual are exaggerated physical demonstrations such as pacing, finger tapping, loud and boisterous behavior; yet, it is important to note that others may be quiet and withdrawn. Eventually, the person may begin to lose rationality and the ability to think clearly. The second warning sign of an agitated person is defensiveness. The defensive patient exhibits irrational behavior such as challenging questions, verbally acting out, and attempting to intimidate staff with threatening behavior. Nursing staff should begin intervening when these signs are demonstrated. The final warning sign can be exhibited through violent behavior. Unfortunately, there are no diagnostic measures to determine violence, yet a history of violence is the best predictor of future violence, so a prompt recognition of patients with history of violence as soon as they present is imperative (see Table 30.3) [14].

When a patient becomes aggressive, the staff should ***take the threat of violence seriously***. Staff should isolate the patient by moving other individuals out of the area and removing all extraneous furniture and equipment. When approaching a violent and agitated person, one should approach with caution with a non-intimating and non-threatening appearance [14]. In such situations, it is important to maintain one's own behavior to diffuse anger and know in advance the steps to help to assist in diffusing a situation. One method for recalling these de-escalation

**Table 30.1** DANGEROUS behavior screening guide for higher risk of violent behavior

D—deviant thinking
A—alienation
N—negative home environment
G—gang affiliation
E—exposure to or history of violence
R—rebellion and poor socialization skills
O—obsession with violence
U—underachievement
S—substance abuse

Source: Adapted from [15, 30]

**Table 30.2** STAMP nursing assessment framework for potential violent behavior

Staring
Tone of voice
Anxiety
Mumbling
Pacing

Source: Adapted from [31, 32]

**Table 30.3** Signs of impending violence

- Flushed face
- Hand-waving and finger-pointing
- Direct, prolonged eye contact
- Encroachment into your personal space (closer than 3 ft but varies due to cultural norms) rapid, deep breathing
- Clenched teeth or hands
- Lack of response to verbal commands
- Defensive/offensive stance (lowering of center of balance, hands moving up and out)
- Searching for an exit or object to use as a weapon
- Brandishing of a weapon (e.g., firearm, knife, or any other item)

Source: Adapted from [28]

**Table 30.4** Responding to escalation

L = listening to what they are saying,
E = empathizing with their point of view,
A = asking reflective questions,
P = paraphrasing what you heard,
S = summarizing what your expectations of behavior

Source: Adapted from [28]

**Table 30.5** Strategies to de-escalate situations

- Let the individual vent
- Be assertive in your verbal communication
- Use a person's name frequently when addressing him or her
- Remain composed, use a firm but even-toned voice; set and enforce reasonable limits
- Redirect a person's anger by using the substitution technique (e.g., "I can't solve this problem, but let me check with Mr. Jones"); your subsequent call to "Mr. Jones" can actually be a call for assistance

Source: Adapted from [28]

techniques is the LEAPS acronym (listening, empathizing, asking, paraphrasing, summarizing) (see Tables 30.4 and 30.5) [15].

### 30.3.1 Physical Plant Considerations

Physical space can also be a consideration leading to increased risk for violent encounters. Space that is poorly designed with blind spaces out of view may put one at an increased risk. Other poorly light spaces such as parking lots are also concerning [16]. However, it is important to remind that many studies showed that in the majority of cases patients and relatives were the perpetrators of these violent incidences and as such the patient's room is the general site of these violent occurrences [2].

It is also important to consider administrative decisions in the context of the physical plant. Understaffing may lead to increased violent occurrences with an increased occurrence during times of increased unit activity such as meal times or visiting hours. A related risk factor is a staff member working alone or in isolation as the presence of a coworker was considered a potential deterrent. Similarly, timing of the day is also a consideration in that periods of peak census such as shift change inversely can lead to isolation in a room putting one at greater risk [13].

### 30.3.2 Personal Considerations

As to specific actions, it is critical that healthcare workers develop a greater awareness of the risk and potential for violence. One's personal behavior may also put one at a higher risk. Interpersonal interactions which are directly confrontational only increases the risk of a violent encounter. When communication is effective, mutual respect is maintained and the ability to openly talk ensures more effective interactions. Specific techniques that facilitate teamwork and communication include maintaining situational awareness, providing mutual support, and having a shared mental model. Situational awareness enables one to be aware of the surroundings and not be so focused on tasks that one loses sight of the patient and circumstances. Providing mutual support ensures that the entire team is providing backup and has the resources to complete the task at hand. Having a shared mental model assures that the entire team is on same page and sharing necessary knowledge and facts in order to complete the task [17].

## 30.4 Interventions

Such statistics are compelling but even more so when it is considered that such violence often goes under-reported by as much as 70% [8]. Furthermore, the ENA study showed that 72% of the staff did not feel safe nor prepared to handle such a situation [2]. Other surveys have shown that up to 74% of employers had no protocol for responding to such workplace violence [18]. In this same survey, 74% of the participants unfortunately relayed that there was no response by their employer after episodes of workplace violence and in 44.9% of the cases no action was ever taken against the perpetrator of the violent act. These points are particularly concerning since the ENA study showed that hospitals without such policies had an 18.1% physical violence rate as compared to only 8.4% for those institutions with a zero-tolerance position on workplace violence [13].

Such unpreparedness leads to significant personal costs in lost time, productivity, and turnover [8]. The ENA study looked at the reasons for this lack of reporting and identified five barriers to this reporting. These barriers are a fear of retaliation, the fact that there was no physical injury sustained, or that it was inconvenient to report. More surprisingly was the concern that reporting would adversely affect their customer service scores, or the acceptance that it was just a part of the job [2]. This issue with no action and a lack of reporting speaks to the significant part of the problem which is the apparent acceptance of this behavior from patients and families. Changing this paradigm is a major step for resolving this issue.

Many regulatory agencies in the United States have made positions statements related to workplace violence. The ANA adopted a Bill of Rights [19] where it noted that nurses have a right to work in an environment safe for themselves and their patients. Both NIOSH (National Institute for Occupational Safety and Health) and OSHA (Occupational Safety and Health Administration) developed national mandates where healthcare organizations have a duty to provide safe work environments [20]. The Joint Commission also has a leadership standard stating that institutions must "create and implement a process for managing disruptive and inappropriate behavior" [21]. It is therefore important that institutional leadership and other professional organizations adopt a policy where it is no longer acceptable to be assaulted while at work.

### 30.4.1 Organizational Plan

It is critically important that hospital leaders both develop the awareness of this problem and also adopt a zero-tolerance policy to this problem (violence-free culture) [22]. Frontline employee involvement on committees and in developing polices that create a safe workplace is equally critical. This involvement creates greater awareness of the issue and allows for change in the culture of acceptance around these instances while also enabling management to better understand the workplace environment and the particular threats encountered by their staff. A worksite analysis is a critical step in evaluating an institution's particular risks as such an analysis leads to both hazard prevention and control.

**Table 30.6** Summary of recommendations

1. Perform workplace analysis
2. Create comprehensive organizational violence prevention program
3. Adopt "zero tolerance" policy
4. Report violent events through organizational documentation system
5. Develop violence response plan
6. Perform post event reviews
7. Monitor key metrics
8. Provide de-escalation training for staff
9. Develop behavioral response team

A comprehensive organizational violence prevention program (see Table 30.6) has three necessary components. First, a reporting and documentation system must be in place to capture and trend data on violent incidents. Secondly, policy should note specific strategies to institute in the event of an incident. Finally, and perhaps most importantly, are post event incidence management and the necessary support for the staff impacted by the violent event. Other needed items are an employee identification system, improved access control, redesign for better security and management [23]. A family advocate program can provide specially trained staff that can intervene in crisis situations when hospital staff must focus on the care of the patient. Units should have standardized team huddles to increase staff's awareness of potentially violent patients [9]. Additional items in an organization response plan are the ability to flag dangers on electronic health records so that others may have proper situational awareness [12].

### 30.4.2 Training

Adequate training and education are of critical importance to improve the recognition and ability to safely respond to these situations. This training is focused on improving skills in communication and de-escalation techniques while also relaying important skills for self-protection if an encounter should turn violent. Such training should emphasize that anticipation is the most effective strategy as aggression rarely occurs without warning signs.

Detection and early intervention are essential to achieve desirable outcomes. Staff must be able to intervene appropriately when a patient or family member's behavior reflect anxiety or frustration. If staff members don't respond properly during the initial stages, then an agitated person may act on their emotions. A patient who progresses to acting on his or her emotions is an indication that staff have not responded during the initial stages [14]. During such a situation, the practitioner has three objectives: ensure safety of all, help the person become aware of their emotions so that they may re-gain control, and facilitate collaboration of patients and staff so that they may participate in the treatment plan at the direction of the healthcare team [14]. As mentioned, behaviors which point to an increased potential for violence are a patient exhibiting tension or anxiety through increased physical activity, such as pacing being particularly concerning. Skills such as active listening, a willingness to apologize and empathize, and utilizing distraction or deflection can be useful to prevent such a situation from escalating.

Verbal de-escalation requires staff to focus not only on what the patient is saying but also on nonverbal cues. Responses should be simple and direct as agitated individuals are less likely to understand complex responses. Staff should also respect physical boundaries. To establish verbal contact, only one staff member should interact with the individual to prevent unwarranted escalation. The staff member should speak calmly and concisely using simple words and short sentences, so the patient has time to process what has been said. The staff should expect to use repetition while speaking to an agitated person. A fourth area of de-escalation involves listening to what is said and identifying the needs as well as the wants of the individual. One should expect to exercise empathy while setting clear limits. The person should be told in clear simple language what is acceptable and unacceptable behavior. The staff should emulate respectful behavior while setting these limits. The final and most important consideration is debriefing after any involuntary intervention. It is the responsibility of the clinician to restore the therapeutic relationship as any coercive intervention is traumatic in nature and will aid in decreasing the risk of additional violence [14].

When working with an agitated patient the nursing staff should know that physical techniques are available for self-protection and control; however, such interventions should be considered a last resort. Healthcare workers should always focus first to ensure that basic needs are being met and that updates on the plan of care is provided; however, staff must also be able to use enhanced verbal and physical skills to successful deal with keeping patient and staff safe. Such physical techniques are best employed by a well-trained team for the safety of patient and staff alike and basic self-defense classes are not adequate or appropriate for such a response. Specific recommended interventions are that organizations should have an identified response team with skills in verbal de-escalation and non-coercive medication administration [14].

Other key points are to remember include wearing appropriate clothing that minimizes grabbing and choking hazards. In interactions, always maintain the appropriate positioning by maintaining a safe distance and use of a supportive stance when dealing with agitated person (see Fig. 30.1). Any situation in which a patient or family member feels helpless or trapped is cause for heightened awareness. In these situations, allow a safe distance between yourself and the individual of 4–6 ft, or at least farther than two steps or arm distance between yourself and the other person. The supportive stance places one at an angle from the patient and avoids face-to-face contact. Staff should keep their hands where the patient can see them at all times [14, 24]. Perhaps the best individual protective strategy to simply instruct the person to stop being violent is effective [25].

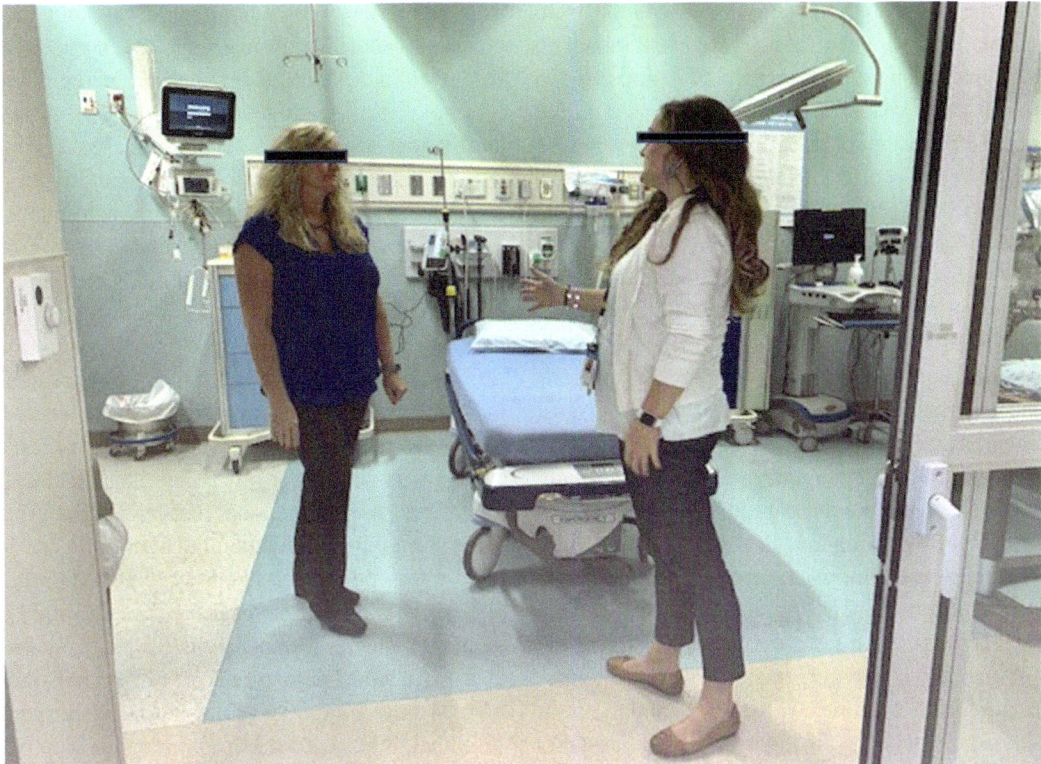

**Fig. 30.1** Supportive stance

## 30.4.3 Plant Improvements

In addition to awareness and de-escalation, the physical plant can be improved to lessen or mitigate incidents of violence. Recommended actions would be access control to clinical areas, in particular high-risk units such as the ED, intensive care units, psychiatry, obstetrics, etc. Metal screening at high-risk entry points such as the ED can also be a useful deterrent. Given the influx of behavioral patients in areas not historically designed for such patients such as the ED, the inclusion of behavioral health rooms into the design can enable staff to be more effective and safer. Inpatient units can be rearranged so that the environment can minimize risk of injury by better lighting and visibility. The IAHSS Security Design Guidelines (available at https://www.iahss.org/page/guidelines) are a useful guide for hospital design considerations [24].

## 30.5 Active Shooter Incidents

Increasingly, there are episodes of active shooter situations noted in the media. These multiple casualty events often capture the attention of the nation. As a large public venue, events impacting a hospital or other healthcare site have the potential for being an increasingly considered target. An active shooter incident is a situation in which "an individual [is] actively engaged in killing or attempting to kill people in a confined and populated area" [26, 27]. In the United States the Federal Bureau of Investigation (FBI) has identified 160 discrete incidents between 2000 and 2013 with 486 people killed and an additional 557 wounded. In the first half of that period, there were an average of 6.4 active-shooter incidents per year in the United States (US), but in the latter half of that period the number more than doubled to 16.4. Recently released FBI data reveal that the rate increased again in 2014 and 2015 to 20 incidents per year. Another study examined all US hospital shootings between 2000 and 2011 in which there was at least one injured victim and noted 154 incidents in 40 states causing death or injury to 235 people [26]. More specific to healthcare, the U.S. Bureau of Labor Statistics showed that the healthcare industry had a total of 19 homicides in 2015 with 16 due to gun violence representing a 46% increase from 2014 [27] (Table 30.7).

Although such events occurring in hospitals are still rare compared with other shooting sites, occurrences have increased in healthcare facilities with the emergency department being reported as the most common site for shootings followed by parking lot and patient rooms. These shootings were more common in larger (>400 beds) hospitals [27]. It should be noted that healthcare institutions present unique challenges for an active shooter event. Some challenges relate to the potential with large populations of vulnerable patients, 24-h-per-day operations, and reduced staff during off hours. These situations are also complicated by patients or staff who are unable to evacuate because of age, illness, or an ongoing medical procedure, and staff who may believe that they cannot leave patients or that they should respond to the injured [28]. Because most shootings have concluded before the police arrive, it is imperative that hospital staff be prepared to respond. One of the first keys for lessening such occurrences or mitigating the damage and lives lost is through hardening of the campus.

**Table 30.7** Best practices in an active shooter event

- If you are in an office, stay in place and secure the door by barricading with furniture or office equipment.
- If you are in a hallway, get into a room and secure the door. Silence cell phones or any other devices that might reveal your location. Close all blinds and curtains, turn off the lights, and move away from the door. Remain quiet.
- Remember, there is a difference between cover and concealment. Cover, such as a heavy desk, provides some protection from bullets such as a heavy desk, while concealment simply hides you from the shooter's direct line of sight.

Source: Adapted from [28]

The same activities mentioned throughout this chapter to address physical violence can be used to prevent access or movement of a perpetrator. Examples are identification (ID) badges, closed card reader access to units, and metal screening at high-risk locations such as ED. Similarly, discussing and securing a patient's belongings, which might include a handgun, lessen the risk of inadvertent discharge of a firearm. One of the facility challenges is that most hospitals are designed vertically with heavy reliance on elevators for transportation. Such design leaves small, narrow stairwells as alternative escape routes, which can become crowded choke points [26]. Also, unlike schools or office buildings, the treatment areas of hospitals have open designs with large common areas containing very little furniture, intersecting walls, or equipment to hide behind. For these reasons, safe rooms should be identified which include a door that can be locked or barricaded. These rooms should ideally not include any windows. If a window is present, staff should either cover this window or hide out of view of such windows. Staff should remain sheltered in place until area is safely secured and they are directed by police to exit. Under facility emergency plans should be a notification system that will allow personnel at the point of initial contact to trigger an alert that is immediately disseminated to the entire facility. The alert should be a simple, clear message that uses redundant pathways such as overhead speaker, paging, and texting systems [26].

Training is another important aspect as staff should know how to respond in the event of an active shooter situation. Staff should be taught to shelter in place unless evacuation can be easily and safely accomplished for both staff and patients. In such situations, they need to know how to secure their work area to protect patients and staff. A three-tier training program is recommended for hospitals and similar healthcare facilities. The first tier is general awareness training that presents the fact of the challenges presented by healthcare facilities. Staff should be trained to take note of the two nearest exits in any facility you visit or work in. The second tier is training regarding strategies for handling verbal aggression and intimidation. Tier three training is for staff in high-risk areas such as emergency departments and behavioral health units and encompasses more detailed skill and case-based training [27]. The above training should explain that healthcare workers should *not* attempt to disarm a subject if a weapon is seen or suspected [28].

The *"run, hide, fight"* directive [26] should be followed by any healthcare professionals, hospital workers, patients, and visitors who are able to comply with it; however, hiding can be problematic in the hospital setting as staff are responsible to care for patients who cannot run, hide, or fight owing to their medical condition. For this reason, a different set of responses should be considered—*"secure, preserve, fight"* [26]. This strategy includes the following actions—secure the location immediately, preserve the life of the patient and oneself, and fight only if necessary. The *"secure"* step would entail immediately securing patient care areas where essential life-sustaining treatment is being provided; deploying electronic or mechanical devices designed to barricade entrances into those areas so as to secure all access points from the inside; dimming or turning off all nonessential lights; and silencing telephones and pagers. In the *"preserve"* step, healthcare personnel should stay away from windows and doors and move patients into a sheltered area if possible, and provide only the essential medical care required to preserve life [26]. A wide range of inexpensive and easy-to-use products are available for installation on all types of doors. Similar to *"run, hide, fight"* strategy, fighting is a last resort effort in the *"secure, preserve, fight"* strategy and is reserved in the setting of contact with the perpetrator. This fighting is focused on incapacitating the individual and creating time and distance for escape. This defense uses any available items to use as a weapon and should be focused on particular vulnerable and disabling areas such as the eyes, throat, or groin.

Post-event mitigation can be improved by **Stop the Bleed** kits (see https://cms.bleedingcontrol.org/class/search). These kits should be considered similar to automatic external defibrillators and as such be available in all public areas. These kits contain essential supplies for hemorrhage control (a major cause of loss of life in such incidents) and contain gauze, gloves, and most importantly a medical grade tourniquet [26]. Facilities will also need a recovery plan including the notification system notifying families of patient status; a plan for rapid recovery and discharge of patients undergoing outpatient procedures; and a plan for media notification. A critical and often overlooked is attending to the psychological first aid needs of the patients, family, visitors, and healthcare workers who were present [26].

## 30.6 Legislative Action

For too long, the legal profession has not aggressively pursued cases of assault on healthcare workers. To address this problem, many US nursing, physician, and hospital groups have worked to introduce legislation making such violent acts a felony. Although this strategy does not address the root causes, it does provide a deterrent and sends the message that healthcare's difficult task should not be compounded by being concerned about staff safety. As of 2019, only 7 states have laws directing workplace programs, but 34 states have felony laws for assaults on healthcare workers [1, 29].

## 30.7 Conclusion

It is important that as professional nurses we work to better prepare ourselves to be alert practitioners. It is more important that we advocate within our hospitals and professional groups to have policies and procedures to better equip staff to handle these issues. Personal strategies such as always carrying a telephone or other communication device is critical. Perhaps most important that society works to address the poverty, homelessness, hopelessness, educational, and employment opportunities that has led to escalating levels of violence in our hospitals [12].

**Acknowledgments** Thank you to Rachel Ward BSN, RN, CCRN who provided invaluable assistance in the preparing of this manuscript.

## References

1. Emergency Nurses Association and Institute for Emergency Nursing Research. Emergency Department Violence Surveillance Study. 2010. ena.org. Retrieved 22 Jun 19.
2. Gacki-Smith J, et al. Violence against nurses working in US Emergency Departments. J Nurs Adm. 2009;39(7–8):340–5.
3. Papa AM, Venella J. Workplace violence in healthcare: strategies for advocacy. Online J Issues Nurs. 2013;18:5.
4. The Joint Commission. Preventing violence in the healthcare setting. 2010. www.workplaceviolencenews.com/2010/06/08. Accessed 29 Jan 11.
5. Occupational Safety and Health Administration. Workplace violence in healthcare: understanding the challenge. 2015. https://www.osha.gov/Publications/OSHA3826.pdf. Retrieved 20 Jul 2019.
6. The Joint Commission. Physical and verbal violence against health care workers. Sentinel Event Alert, Issue 59. 17 Apr 2018. https://www.jointcommission.org/assets/1/18/SEA_59_Workplace_violence_4_13_18_FINAL.pdf. Retrieved 20 Jul 2019.
7. Chetwynd E. Workplace violence in healthcare. 2019. https://www.everbridge.com/blog/workplace-violence-in-healthcare/. Retrieved 20 Jul 2019.
8. Potera C. Violence against nurses in the workplace. Am J Nurses. 2016;116(6):20–1.
9. Martinez AJS. Managing workplace violence with evidence-based interventions: a literature review. J Psychosoc Nurs. 2016;54(9):31–6.
10. Campbell AF. Why violence against nurses has spiked in the last year. The Atlantic. 1 Dec 2016.
11. American Nurses Association. American Nurses Association Health Risk Appraisal (HRA): preliminary findings. Oct 2013–2014.
12. Stempniak M. Finding a hospital's role in curbing Chicago's violence. 2017. www.hhnmag.com. Accessed 7 Jul 17.
13. Strickler J. When it hurts to care: workplace violence in healthcare. Nursing. 2013;43:58–62.
14. Phillips J, Stinson K, Strickler J. Avoiding eruptions: de-escalating agitated patients. Nursing. 2014;44:60–3.
15. McEwan D, Dumpel H. Workplace violence: assessing occupational hazards and identifying strategies for prevention, part 2. National Nurse. Mar 2012.
16. Occupational Safety and Health Administration. Guidelines for preventing workplace violence for healthcare and social service workers. 2016. https://www.osha.gov/Publications/osha3148.pdf. Accessed 21 Jul 2019.
17. Strickler J, Haynes J. Improving communication in healthcare. Nursing. 2014;44(1):62–3.
18. Shea T, Sheehan C, Donohue R, Cooper B, De Cieri H. Occupational violence and aggression experienced by nursing and caring professionals. J Nurs Scholarship. 2017;49(2):236–43.
19. American Nurses Association. Bill of Rights FAQ. 2019. Available at https://www.nursingworld.org/practice-policy/work-environment/health-safety/bill-of-rights-faqs/. Accessed 24 Jul 2019.
20. McPhaul KM, Lipscomb J. Workplace violence in healthcare. 2004. www.nursingworld.orgon. Accessed 21 Jan 11.
21. Schyve PM. Leadership in healthcare organization: a guide to Joint Commission Standards. The Governance Institute; 2009. http://www.governanceinstittue.com/ResearchPublications/ResourceLibrary/tabid/185/CategoryID/15/List/Level/a/ProductID/827/Default.asp?
22. Thompson P. Addressing violence in healthcare workplace. 2015. www.hhnmag.com. Accessed 8 Jul 17.
23. Clements PT. Workplace violence and corporate policy for healthcare settings. Nurs Econ. 2005;23(3):119–24.
24. Strickler J. Staying safe: responding to violence against healthcare staff. Nursing. 2018;48(11):58–62.
25. Gillespie GL, Gates DM, Miller M, Howard PK. Workplace violence in healthcare settings: risk factors and protective strategies. Rehabil Nurs. 2010;35(5):177–84.
26. Inaba K, Eastman AL, Jacobs LM, Mattox K. Active shooter response at health care facility. NEJM. 2018;379:6.
27. Sanchez L, Young VB, Baker M. Active shooter training in the emergency department: a Safety initiative. J Emerg Nurs. 2018;44(6):598–604.
28. Warren B, Bosse M, Tornetta P. Workplace violence and active shooter considerations for health care workers. J Bone Joint Surg Am. 2017;99:e88, 1–5.
29. Docksai R. Lawmakers and hospitals take action to curb violence against nurses. 2015. Available at from https://www.nursinglicensure.org/articles/workplace-violence.html.
30. Muscari ME. How can I detect the warning signs of extreme violence in my patients? J Clin Nurs. 2010;19:479–88.
31. Weeks SK, et al. Responding to an active shooter and other threats of violence. Nursing. 2013;43:34–7.
32. Luck L, Jackson D, Usher K. STAMP: components of observable behavior that indicate potential for patient violence in Emergency Departments. J Adv Nurs. 2007;59(1):11–9.

# Current Trends in Radiology

## 31

Thomas Hough and Joseph Marion

## 31.1 Introduction

Nursing and radiology hold a very symbiotic relationship. For this reason, individuals who are learning about the many different facets of nursing should have some insight into how radiology is being driven by the changes from Information Technology. In this chapter a look at Artificial Intelligence (AI), Computerized Physician Order Entry (CPOE), Electronic Health Records (EHR), and Enterprise Imaging will be covered.

## 31.2 Demand for Radiology Nurses

Nurses should be present in all modalities to increase patient safety and to respond to emergencies.

While the majority of radiology nurses will work in hospital settings, new free-standing diagnostic and interventional outpatient centers are growing in numbers. Radiology nurses volunteer in underserved areas of the globe via RAD-AID International (https://rad-aid.org) bringing radiology nursing education to developing countries.

The need for radiology nurses will only grow due to patient acuity and types of procedures (including those involving sedation and analgesia), many of which are performed on an outpatient basis. Nurses should be supervised and evaluated for annual performance reports by nurses who understand the role of the nurse and scope of practice for their locality. The nurse needs to have a good understanding of his/her scope of practice, especially when functioning autonomously in radiology.

Nurses need to be included in all aspects of education within radiology. They are essential members of the radiology team and are leaders in quality and safety. Radiologist and management support for nursing in radiology is key. Recruitment and retention of radiology nurses is important as the learning curve for this specialty is steep and radiology nursing education is not currently part of school curriculums but learned on the job during orientation period under the guidance of a preceptor, when available. Quick turnover is not only expensive for the department but also not detrimental to team cohesion, nursing morale, and patient safety. Radiology nursing education and networking is available through the Association for Radiologic and Imaging Nursing (www.arinursing.org).

---

T. Hough, CMC (✉)
True North Consulting & Associates Inc., Mississauga, ON, Canada

J. Marion, MBA, BA
Healthcare Integration Strategies, LLC, Waukesha, WI, USA

## 31.2.1 The Expanding Role of the Radiology Nurse

Nurses are the key people who can assure patient safety. Within radiology there are numerous risks and hazards for the patient. Falling off the exam table, receiving the wrong exam, imaging the right side when it should be the left side or a drug reaction to contrast media injections are all examples of patient risks and hazards. These are just some examples where nurses are needed to assist physicians and X-ray technologists in the safe delivery of patient care.

On-call responsibilities of nurses working in procedure areas allow for round the clock emergency procedures. Radiology nurses should also be involved in leadership through hospital-wide committees, e.g., pharmacy committee, institutional review board, and ethics committee. Nurses can also play a key role in renovation committees for radiology and on committees working on the EHR or forms/order sets.

## 31.3 Cybersecurity

Cybersecurity issues are increasing in all aspects of business and healthcare. Ransomeware incidents are on the rise and patient's healthcare data and care are at greater risk. Chapter 26 will discuss this growing threat.

## 31.4 Artificial Intelligence: What Is It, and Why It Is Relevant to Radiology

### 31.4.1 What Is It?

Artificial intelligence (AI) is the newest disruptive technology which will be written into history as an event equal to the introduction of personal computers (PCs) and propagation of the internet. Simply, AI is the ability to perform machine learned analytics on data sets in new or unique ways to seek answers to specific questions which have previously been held as a mystery contained in the large volumes of data. AI can be an application for analyzing stock market trends in order to predict future stock trends to recognizing lung cancer patterns in CT exams containing 20,000 images. AI is a technology platform which can be applied to just about any need in the world where there is an ability to collect data and perform analytics to find data patterns, outliers, or common denominators. Radiology is just one discipline where AI applications can be developed to improve productivity, accuracy, and patient outcomes.

*As each calendar day passes, a new volume of AI knowledge is written. This explosion of knowledge is proof of the interest and hype on the potential AI has. Due to limits in this chapter and volume of AI knowledge this chapter will focus on the challenges AI will face in radiology in the near term.*

AI is a platform permitting an application to be developed such as lung cancer detection via computed tomography (CT) chest exams. The application requires the validation of data using a huge data set to confirm what lung cancers looks like in CT exams. Simply, the computer needs to learn all the possible patterns, shapes, densities, and forms of lung cancer can show up as. It takes this information and creates an algorithm it can use to find CT exam lung cancer. The validation of all the variables of what lung cancer can look like is the machine learning. Each of these patterns need to be validated thousands of times by individuals who can recognize lung cancer in CT images before it can be considered to be validated. The validation process is analogous to teaching your computer to recognize family and friend's faces. The computer selects a number of photos of people and asks you—"Is this Aunt Jane?"; you reply to 10 or 15 requests from the computer, "This is Aunt Jane." This is the validation process. Once completed, the computer then goes through your photos and says—here, are all of Aunt Janes photos I can find. On your local computer, from time to time your computer will slip in your neighbor "Mary" as an "Aunt Jane." We know when sorting photos, making a mistake for "Mary" vs. "Aunt Jane" is not a life-or-death issue; however, when detecting a lung carcinoma, this is unacceptable. This is why verification

## 31.4.2 AI: Hype or Reality

process needs to execute 10,000 or more times to be valid.

Here is the challenge for AI in radiology. This process of validation needs to be repeated for every disease or pathology that can be diagnosed using radiology exams. Who is capable to do this validation? Radiologists need to execute the validation process which is time consuming and with the number of diseases and various forms they can take in radiology, this means it will take many years to have wide-enough applications (AKA Use Case) of algorithms (AKA applications) for it to be useful across the radiology spectrum. The long-term benefit is once fully validated, radiology-based AI Applications will be available 24/7 worldwide to aid in highly accurate diagnosis made by the imperfect observers we currently call radiologists.

Gartner, the world's leading research and advisory company (https://www.gartner.com), has developed a report called the *Hype Cycle for Emerging Technologies*, which has published every year since 2007. According to Gartner, the "Gartner Hype Cycles provide a graphic representation of the maturity and adoption of technologies and applications, and how they are potentially relevant to solving real business problems and exploiting new opportunities" [1].

At the peak of the *Hype Cycle for Emerging Technologies, 2018* [2], Deep Neural Nets (Deep Learning) are located in the Peak of Inflated Expectations (see Fig. 31.1 below), and are starting the downward descent into the Trough of Disillusionment, which phase is defined as

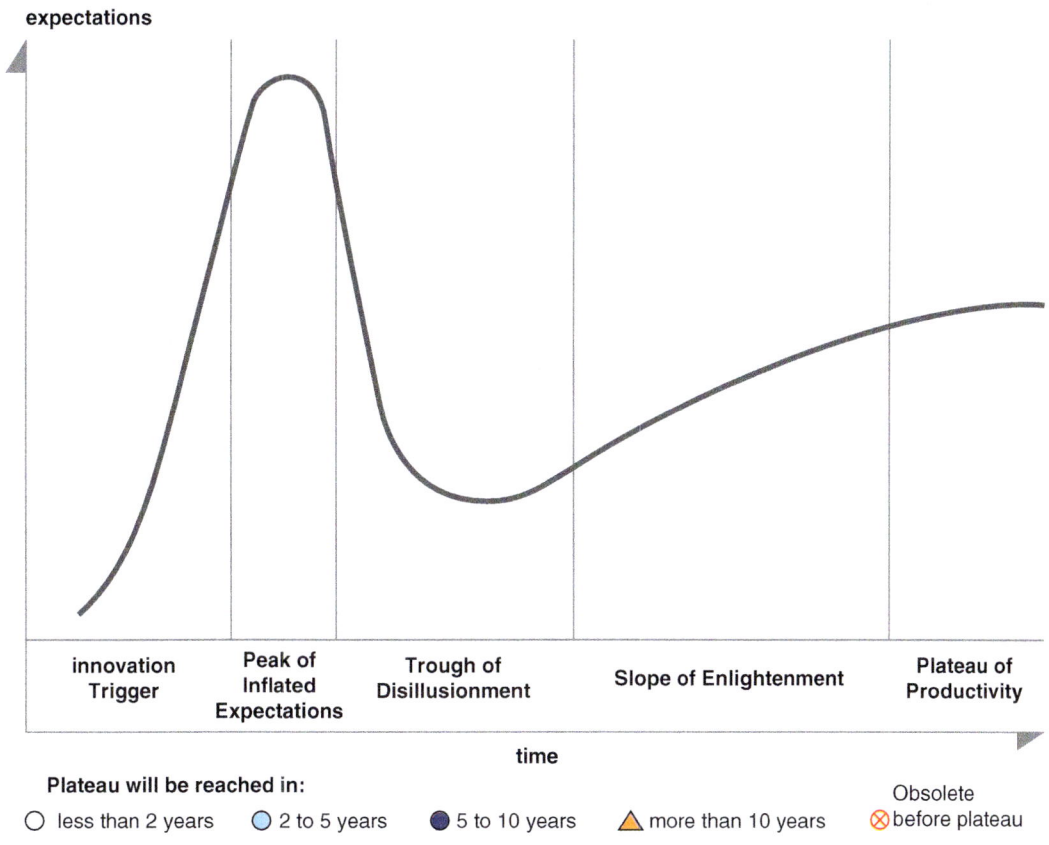

**Fig. 31.1** Gartner Hype Cycle, Gartner Inc., 2017. Reprinted with permission of Gartner

"Interest wanes as experiments and implementations fail to deliver. Producers of the technology shake out or fail. Investments continue only if the surviving providers improve their products to the satisfaction of early adopters" [1]. In diagnostic imaging, the chapter authors believe this is seen as the process required to validate useful use cases (applications) where AI can be used with enough efficacy for the diagnosis of patient's pathology. Accordingly, disillusionment comes from the amount of work required to develop these use case applications for each and every disease and how long it is going to take to develop a large enough library of applications to be developed for widespread use.

For the past few years there has been much hype in healthcare identifying how AI will revolutionize the delivery and costs within healthcare. The chapter authors believe radiology clearly has inflated expectations of how AI is going to revolutionize radiology with some going as far as saying the radiologist will be a profession of the past in 5–10 years.

Through our research we found that another significant challenge for AI is the timeline for technology adoption. Numerous companies and applications are coming to market in the 2018–2022 era. With the realization now, the validation of each disease needs to be completed before AI can take on the variety of diagnostics currently done every day, and so comes the downhill of the Trough of Disillusionment on how long it is going to take to have all applications ready for daily diagnostic imaging use. In other words, having a few AI applications to find lung cancer or brain hematomas does not facilitate a radiologist with primary diagnosis. It will likely take over a decade for enough AI applications to be developed before AI can take on a workload of exams where the radiologists can oversee the exam reports produced.

This Trough of Disillusionment is followed by the Slope of Enlightenment. As vendors and healthcare providers will learn during the Trough of Disillusionment phase, the authors believe the lessons needed to maximize benefits of AI will come when an orchestrated workflow is implemented. In passing through these phases, healthcare IT needs to ensure their IT enterprise-wide environments are ready to deploy AI. Once completed, the authors feel the Plateau of Productivity will then be achievable permitting the realization of the return on investment (ROI) required for healthcare.

Currently there are many companies and academic centers entering into AI application development and validation. With this influx of enthusiasm and capital, it is not known who will be successful and who will fail. Additionally, market consolidation has not occurred (where large companies acquire one or more winning smaller firms to broaden their market offering and to speed their go-to-market and sales efforts). The quality of applications will start to present itself and certain applications will rise to be industry leaders to set standards of care in AI. Due to the industry evolution as described by Gartner above, the authors believe it could be considered premature at this time to spend money on AI purchases while looking for a clear predictable ROI in AI.

### 31.4.3 Race Cars Need Fuel and Roads—Fuel

Healthcare enterprises would be better hedging their bets on AI at this time and should be doing other work in preparation for AI deployment. Credit needs to be directed to Paul Chang, MD, FSIIM Professor of Radiology, Enterprise Imaging at the University of Chicago Pritzker School of Medicine. In February 2019, Dr. Chang presented a webinar to the Society for Imaging Informatics in Medicine (www.SIIM.org). The following analogies, theories, and ideas for this presentation have come from his presentation [3].

The analogy focuses on two areas. Let's consider AI as a race car, but without "Drilling for Fuel" and "Building Roads" there is no point in having a race car.

The race car is AI's Machine Learning Algorithm (AKA the Use Case or Application)—once validated for an application such as CT lung cancer there may be no better nor faster method for diagnosis of lung cancer. However, what does a race car run on—fuel; in this case the fuel is data. Once fueled-up the race car needs to run on roads; in this case the roads are workflow integration. Currently in today's world the current workflow integrations are not a part of a capable IT infrastructure.

In reality, can anyone in healthcare IT say: (1) The desired data required for AI is accessible and, in the scale, required in real time; (2) Can the data be trusted to be accurate and in the right format(s); and (3) Can the data be reliably correlated with reliable outcome measures at scale?

Most of the integration of workflow between patient EHR, PACS, RIS, and pathology is done by humans with the exception of the IHE (Integrating the Healthcare Enterprise) [3] Integration Profiles (IPs) which facilitate interoperability. Real workflow integration requires much more integration than what is currently available to facilitate the productivity of key clinical people. The ability to access the different relevant clinical data stored in any one of the different applications or access this from a centralized data repository in an organized and rapid fashion is what is required.

## 31.4.4 Service-Oriented Architecture

The movement to a service-oriented architecture (SOA) is key to ensure data is prepared for access in rapid real-time format for event processing such as required in AI. Migration to SOA requires data to be extracted from the format it is native to, such as DICOM, HL-7, or FHIR, and to be transferred and loaded into a web service such as XML, for use by other rapid applications like AI (Fig. 31.2).

The SOA business layer function takes relevant data from other file platforms and formats regardless of source and extracts, transfers, loads (ELT) into xml to store the data—this then goes into an enterprise service bus which hands this off to continuous event processing. This process is a Middle "Business Logic" Layer where data can be found in agents, ORBs, or web services and accessed much more rapidly than other methods. Moving to a SOA can be considered as preparing the IT environment to be an advanced IT environment as required for AI.

The image below illustrates the current level of integration and interoperability achieved by many vendors today using IHE integration profiles. This is integrated workflow where the movement of

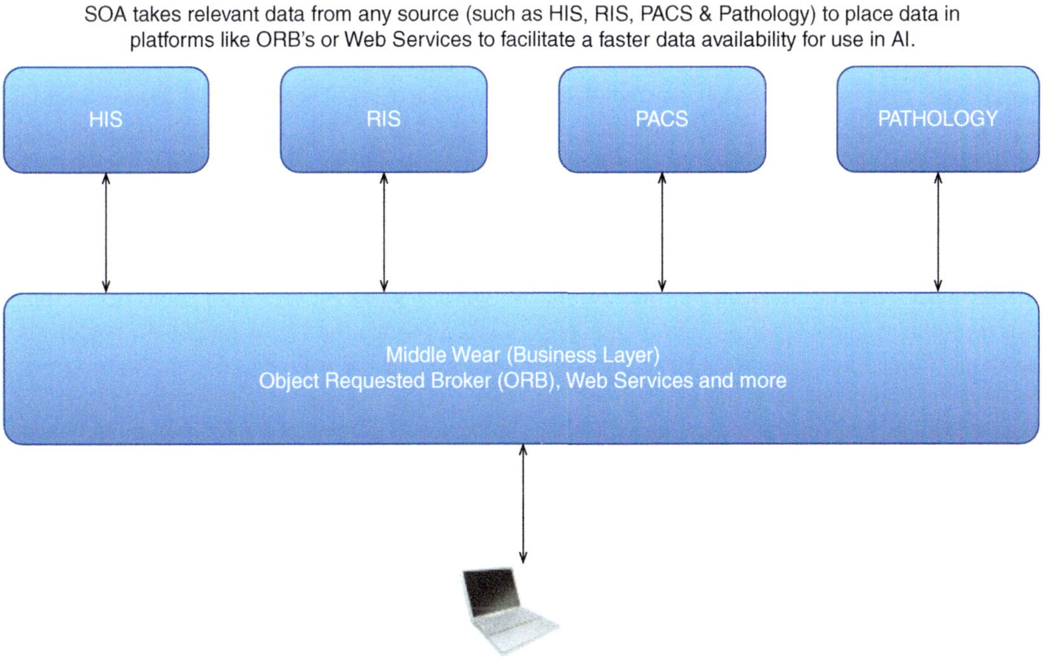

**Fig. 31.2** Enterprise integration model for service-oriented architecture

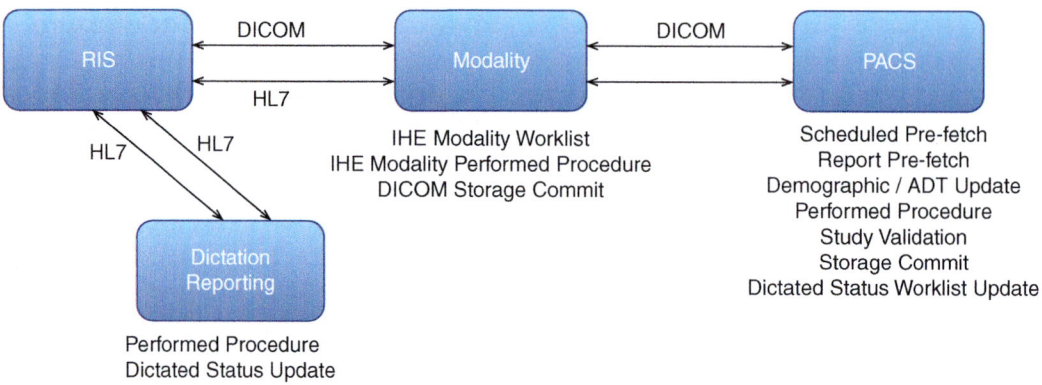

When integrating, the use of IHE Integration Profiles, DICOM and HL-7 Provide a level of integration resulting in workflows. These standards and protocols do not go far enough to achieve workflow orchestration which provides users with the information they require to make a lot of decisions required during the diagnosis of the patient.

**Fig. 31.3** IHE, DICOM, and HL7 integrated workflow

data triggers and confirms specific data transfer which can enable workflow (Fig. 31.3).

Advanced IT requires IT middleware solutions to collect relevant data from different data sources to assemble relevant information such as the patient has endured a recent Crohn's flare-up. When orders are placed through computerized physician order entry (CPOE) software that do not share relevant patient information like recent Crohn's flare-up to assist the radiologist in making a better diagnosis this leaves the radiologist handicapped when making the best possible diagnosis. Employing a SOA will collect this relevant information and share it at an appropriate time in the diagnosis process to facilitate the radiologist to be more productive and accurate with the diagnosis. Sharing relevant information like this is workflow orchestration—information presented at a time to enhance where and when it is most useful in the diagnosis and treatment of the patient. This is the fuel which is required for the race car (AI) to deliver advanced productivities.

### 31.4.5 Race Cars Need Fuel and Roads—Roads

An IT Big data and deep learning hedge strategy needs to be deployed. This hedging strategy is designed to ensure optimal workflow integration is completed as preparation for workflow orchestration. This level of advanced IT preparation is required for applications optimization of AI and the productivity of those who use AI. The IT infrastructure needs to be able to feed near future advanced decision-making support agents, such as AI and analytics which are often cloud-based applications. Currently, deep learning applications are driven by data availability—not by a use case. There are use cases which are "nice to have's" and "not must have" at this stage of AI deployment. The Catch 22 in this evolution is a lack of clinically relevant and vetted datasets for training for the computers. As stated before, there are not enough relevant validated use case algorithms (where use case is defined as a diagnostic application for diagnosis of lung cancer) to assist in the training of computers across a wide array use cases at this time. The current focus of AI is image centric when it really needs to evolve to collection of data from many sources as identified so all relevant information is considered when formulating a diagnosis. The current state is validation via images to identify the pathology. AI needs to have SOA to have relevant data shared with the radiologist, so they can become more productive and accurate by going through the diagnostic interpretation process.

Clinicians need to be told the patient had a recent flare-up of Crohn's disease and has cancer based on information collected from other sources such as lab work, other test and clinical encounter reports, pathology, biopsies, etc. in order for the system to be considered "poly-capable." Without most recent clinical information, the radiologist who gets a requisition stating unexplained pain in chest and abdomen is left to diagnose cancer and Crohn's disease each time a new exam is presented for this patient. Currently, vendors can be considered to be missing the use case sweet spot with how they are developing and deploying AI. Solutions are attempting to go from hard wired, rules based algorithmic solutions and jump directly to deep knowledge and primary diagnosis.

What is needed is a non-threatening process for the radiologist that takes away menial tasks such as hanging protocols and pathology measurements and augments the process with useful and pertinent information such as "patient has had a recent Crohn's flare-up."

Workflow integration needs to move toward a level of machine intelligence which is real time and knows where the clinician is in any process to provide relevant clinical information to enable a more productive clinician who delivers better quality diagnosis as a result of the workflow orchestration.

Workflow orchestration is achieved when clinical context information is searched out by the machine intelligence. The content is presented in an intelligent format and at a time and location when needed to support the work of the diagnostician.

### 31.4.6 Conclusion: Is AI Ready for "Prime Time"?

AI conclusion: Now is too early to be "picking a winner" as there is not enough information available on the reality of AI and its application within radiology. Therefore, selecting a "hedge strategy" is much more reasonable. The hedge strategy needs to prepare IT infrastructure for advanced IT applications (to be the FUEL) for AI. Diagnostic imaging IT needs to set goals for "Deep Integration" with workflow by having data-driven optimized workflow orchestration (the Roads).

## 31.5 Electronic Health Record—EHR

Electronic Health Records (EHR), frequently referred to as electronic medical records (EMR) originated as a means to automate much of the clinical records documentation previously done by hand. The primary benefit of EHR systems is to reduce errors and make more patient information available to the clinician to better manage the patient in the achievement of the desired patient outcome.

### 31.5.1 Background of an EHR

In the United States EHR implementation was greatly impacted by changes in healthcare policy, namely the American Recovery and Reinvestment Act (ARRA) passed in 2009 [4]. Part of the ARRA includes the Health Information for Technology and Clinical Health (HITECH) that specifically addressed an incentive program for use of an EHR. This was to be implemented in several phases, known as stages, with increasing incentive payments to eligible physicians (EP) or eligible hospitals (EH) for meeting certain electronic reporting criteria objectives (Clinical Quality Measurement, or CQM).

To qualify for payments, EHR systems needed to be certified for each stage, as each stage contained a progressive number of CQMs. Over the course of implementation of the first two stages, experience demonstrated that inventive payments were helpful in fostering use, but that physicians were spending more time entering information into the EHR and less time with patients! Consequently, changes are being made to shift emphasis of the regulations from *compliance measurement* to an emphasis on *interoperability* of EHRs with other systems to help improve the health of patient populations.

## 31.5.2 EHR Interoperability with Imaging

The spreading use of EHRs has implications for imaging, which affect the operational workflow and the importance of interoperability of EHRs with imaging systems.

### 31.5.2.1 Study Identification

Picture archive and communications systems (PACS) originally relied on themselves for identification of the study, which meant there could be discrepancies with other systems in terms of patient identification. Subsequent iterations relied on interoperability with a radiology information system (RIS) for patient identification for consistency and interoperability.

EHRs are gradually taking over many of the patient management functions of a RIS, and consequently require interoperability with PACS for patient identification. A key component in terms of PACS' ability to manage patient identification of studies performed by modalities such as computed tomography (CT) and ultrasound (US) was the definition encompassed in the Digital Imaging Communications in Medicine (DICOM) Standard, known as modality worklist. By use of this standard, PACS is able to pass the patient demographic and study information to the imaging device, avoiding duplication at the imaging device and subsequent errors.

The growing use of portable devices such as portable ultrasound in other clinical areas, as well as within radiology, presents a conundrum in terms of accurately identifying the patient and study information for inclusion in the PACS, as such devices typically do not support the DICOM modality worklist, or they do not encompass a means for patient/study identification. In these instances, vendors are developing ways of capturing this information from the EHR and associating it with the portable study so that it can be correctly identified within a PACS.

### 31.5.2.2 Imaging Integration

One of the objectives of an EHR is the consolidation of patient health information such as lab test results, patient history and notes, and radiology results. Because PACS were in place prior to the implementation of EHRs, imaging was not considered a part of an EHR, and imaging associated with radiology results were not included in an EHR.

EHR and PACS vendors have worked to address this deficiency by means of application program interfaces (API) between an EHR and PACS. These APIs enable an EHR to embed a "placeholder" that links to a specific patient study in the PACS. These are oftentimes referred to as "hyperlinks" that enable the ability to launch an image viewer application by selecting the link in the EHR. This capability has been important to insuring that EHRs can directly present relevant imaging information in association with the EHR.

### 31.5.2.3 Workflow Considerations

Accessing imaging studies within PACS has classically been accomplished by selecting the correct patient study from a "worklist" of presented studies. The next iteration of PACS utilized the information from a RIS worklist to first select the study, including additional information such as the reason for the study and prior study reports that resided in the RIS.

As EHRs replace RIS, PACS workflow has been modified to rely on the EHR for the "worklist" to select a specific patient study and then launch the images from the PACS. As with the RIS, the EHR can present the radiologist with additional patient information, including study results from other clinical services such as cardiology, patient history, and lab results. Experience is finding this additional information can potentially impact the radiologist's perception of what they see in the images. As suggested previously, the radiologist may initially expect liver discrepancies to be cysts, whereas with the additional patient history and lab results, it might alter the diagnosis to be cancer.

## 31.6 Computerized Provider Order Entry—CPOE, and Clinical Decision Support—CDS

According to the Agency for Healthcare Quality and Research (AHRQ) [4] "Computerized provider order entry (CPOE) is an application that allows healthcare providers to use a computer to directly enter medical orders electronically in inpatient and ambulatory settings, replacing the more traditional order methods of paper, verbal, telephone, and fax." With the advent of the American Recovery and Reinvestment Act of 2009 (ARRA) and the push to increase the use of EHRs, CPOE is a natural extension of automation and improving healthcare delivery.

### 31.6.1 Why CPOE?

According to the Office of the National Coordinator for Health Information Technology (ONC), Clinical Decision Support (CDS) "is a sophisticated health IT component. It requires computable biomedical knowledge, person-specific data, and a reasoning or inferencing mechanism that combines knowledge and data to generate and present helpful information to clinicians as care is being delivered" [5]. In conjunction with CPOE, CDS can provide a more structured and consistent means for radiology study orders.

### 31.6.2 How Do CPOE and CDS Relate to Radiology?

Signed into law on April 1, 2014, the Protecting Access to Medicare Act of 2014 (PAMA) includes the most extensive reform of the Medicare Clinical Laboratory Fee Schedule (CLFS) since it was established in 1984. It requires clinical decision support systems to confirm appropriate use criteria (AUCs) on ambulatory (outpatient), non-emergent advanced imaging studies such as MRI, CT, and PET scans. Following several delays, enactment is now set for January 1, 2020.

One of the more active initiatives to apply CDS in radiology has been the American College of Radiology (ACR) ACR Select®, a digital representation of the ACR Appropriateness Criteria® for diagnostic imaging. The ACR licensed ACR Select® to the National Decision Support Company (NDSC), now part of Change Healthcare [6]. The NDSC licenses the ACR Select® criteria to EHR companies for incorporation in their CPOE and CDS products.

The major impact of CPOE and CDS will be to substantially automate the ordering process of radiological studies, and to provide greater standardization and less ambiguity in radiology orders. This should free up radiology staff from the time spent verifying and correcting orders which can be as high as 35% of all exam orders.

### 31.6.3 CPOE and CDS Benefits

The use of CPOE and CDS will result in multiple benefits to care delivery organizations. First and foremost is the potential cost savings by reducing episodic costs, lowering the total cost of care, and lowering the cost to the patient.

In a definitive study of the effects of CDS, the Institute for Clinical Systems Improvement (ICSI) conducted a study of high technology diagnostic imaging (HTDI) exams involving 4500 providers ordering the top 90% of HTDI studies using appropriateness criteria [7]. The results demonstrated a savings of approximately $150 million attributed to the use of decision support criteria.

Another benefit is in the reduction in low utility ordering, or in other words the ordering of exams that have little utility in the overall diagnosis. Conversely, CPOE and CDS can result in an improvement in diagnostic efficiency by selecting the appropriate exam for the criteria presented.

### 31.6.4 Challenges

CPOE and CDS are not without their challenges. CPOE relies on physician acceptance and utilization. There may be physician resistance to CPOE utilization, as it represents another electronic task to be performed by the physician. In many instances, a physician may rely on his staff to actually place the order, in which case appropriate use criteria may not be addressed by the physician.

Appropriate use criteria may be based either on similar demographics and symptoms or on iterative questions. The iterative approach can be more intrusive to the physician, but they can also be more precise in terms of appropriateness. The more CPOE and CDS can be integrated into the physician's normal workflow, the more likely they are to use it.

Another challenge is insuring that the radiologists become the "gatekeeper" for appropriateness criteria. CDS is not static and it must keep up with changing imaging procedures. Since radiologists are most informed on what constitutes an appropriate exam, they need to take a leadership position in continuing efforts to refine appropriateness criteria.

## 31.7 Enterprise Imaging: Digital Imaging Across a Large Enterprise and Geography

Radiology has been the classical service line for imaging, but that doesn't mean other service lines don't utilize imaging. Somewhat related to radiology is cardiology imaging, which probably represents the second-most imaging-intensive service. There are a number of other areas, which utilize imaging that are not classically addressed within image management applications.

Areas such as ophthalmology, dermatology, urology, and pathology to mention a few of the "ologies" all create images of some sort. Historically, individual service lines have managed their own images in some form or another. For example, dermatology may produce images with digital cameras or smart phones. These images may be off-loaded to some storage media such as a hard disk drive, or they may be retained on the capture device for some indeterminant period.

A key factor in terms of considering these other areas is the audience for the images. Typically, it may be strictly for the physicians treating the patient, or for referral physicians. There have been no standards associated with how these images are managed or communicated.

With the advent of EHRs, a key intent is to provide a single source of access to all patient information. The EHR can track imaging content and launch an appropriate viewer to an image. This would be referred to as an image-enabled EHR. The EHR itself doesn't have to manage the images. It only has to provide a linkage, better known as an application program interface (API) to the PACS.

### 31.7.1 Enterprise Imaging

Why it matters without a common image application, the EHR would need to manage multiple application interfaces, and the physician would need to know how to manage multiple viewing applications. Such a scenario would have negative implications for the acceptance of such a solution. An approach that consolidates all image content into a single system application would be more widely accepted and represents the best scenario for image—enabling the EHR on an enterprise-wide basis.

### 31.7.2 How Does It Impact PACS? Enterprise Archive and Viewing

As stated above, a singular solution for enterprise-wide image access via the EHR is more clinically viable. To achieve this, images need to be centrally managed and accessed via a common viewer. The central management of images suggests an enterprise-wide archive that can manage image content from multiple sources in a patient-centric manner.

Since content might be in multiple formats, an enterprise archive needs to be able to accommodate multiple data formats. Standard radiology and cardiology images might be handled via a standard created for that—Digital Imaging and Communications in Medicine Standard (DICOM). The DICOM standard encompasses a way to handle the identification information regarding the images (metadata), as well as a format for storing the actual image content.

Other imaging services may produce image content in other standard formats, such as Joint Photographic Experts Group (JPEG). This format is widely used for photographic purposes. Given that it is a widely accepted format, it would be redundant to convert it to another format such as DICOM. Therefore, an enterprise archive should be able to manage multiple formats in their native format.

Similarly, a viewing device associated with the enterprise archive would need to be able to display images from multiple file formats such as PDF, JPEG, and DOCX. These so-called "universal viewers" can present images from multiple formats, simplifying how clinicians can view images from multiple service lines.

PACS has embraced both image archive and image viewing technologies, but they are optimized for the service line addressed. For example, in the case of radiology, since most image content is handled via DICOM, the archive and viewing devices are structured around the DICOM standard. With the advent of an enterprise archive and viewing application, some of this capability is redundant within PACS. Therefore, the PACS capability for long-term image archive and clinical display can be replaced by an enterprise application. Figure 31.4 illustrates the impact that Enterprise Image Management (EIM) can have on a PACS.

Note in the first case of PACS, all the functionality including the archive and clinical viewing is part of the PACS. In the second case, the PACS focuses on image acquisition and diagnostic viewing, and the EIM assumes responsibility for image archive and clinical viewing. This primarily differentiates a PACS in an EIM environment.

## 31.8 Health Insurance Portability and Accountability Act

The Health Insurance Portability and Accountability Act (HIPAA) was enacted by the United States Congress in 1996. The HIPAA act recognizes the importance of securely managing patient information by what is referred to as Protected Health Information, or PHI. According to the Health and Human Services (HHS), "HIPAA Privacy Rule provides federal protections for personal health information held by covered entities and gives patients an array of rights with respect to that information. At the same time, the Privacy Rule is balanced so it permits the disclosure of personal health information needed for patient care and other important purposes" [8].

### 31.8.1 Safety and Security Involving Imaging Equipment and PACS

Image content from imaging equipment as stored within a PACS is considered to be protected health information (PHI). Such content must be managed in a manner consistent with the law. Image content must be managed securely and breeches or failure to comply with HIPAA means the entity managing the image content may be subject to fines if not corrected within 30 days.

### 31.8.2 Importance of Archive Policy and Testing

Hard copy material may be easier to manage than digital content, as it can only be in one physical place at a time, unless copied. Digital content can be harder to manage as it may be in multiple places at the same time. For example, a CT exam may reside on a scanner, however, it may also be archived to PACS. To be HIPAA-compliant, there needs to be rules and means for handling digital content.

In terms of the example above, a CT exam can be managed within the capabilities of DICOM, whereas once the image has been transferred to PACS and verified, the CT scanner is free to delete the study; the PACS is now the "owner" of the data (Modality Performed Procedure Step, or MPPS).

Managing imaging data in an archive in a HIPAA-compliant manner means there needs to be a policy for handling availability of data, as well as periodic testing of the policy. If data is

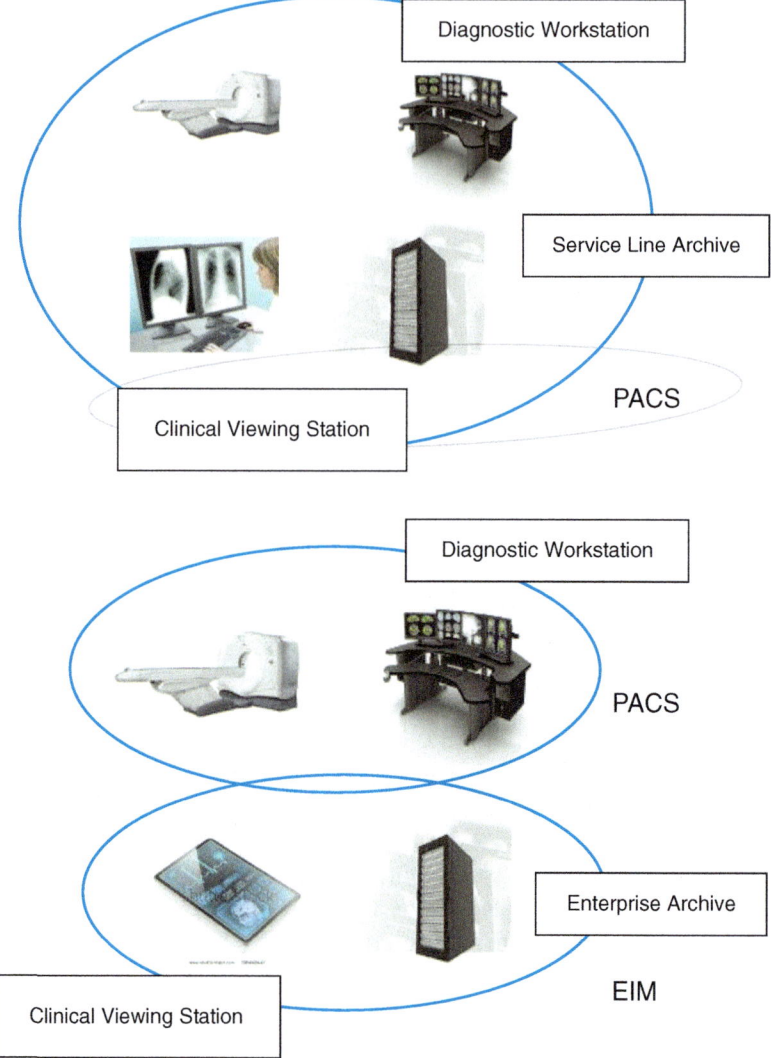

**Fig. 31.4** Impact of enterprise image management on PACs

Note in the first case of PACS, all the functionality including the archive and clinical viewing is part of the PACS. In the second case, the PACS focuses on image acquisition and diagnostic viewing, and the EIM assumes responsibility for image archive and clinical viewing. This primarily differentiates a PACS in an EIM environment.

stored in multiple levels of an archive, if for some reason an exam is deleted, the policy determines how the data can be restored. The policy needs to include a mechanism for testing the ability to restore data. When the archive incorporates a "backup" capability where there is a backup instance of the data, the policy must define both the process and the ability to restore the data from the backup to the primary archive. Failure to do so could mean the archive is not HIPAA-compliant.

## 31.9 Conclusion

Nurses and radiology should go together like bread and butter. Unfortunately, there are not enough nurses for this to occur. Individuals who volunteer to become a much-needed asset in radiology will be rewarded with an interesting and compelling career of helping patients when they need it the most. The technical information shared in this chapter is a small part of what makes diagnostic imaging an interesting discipline within nursing. Individuals who are wanting to see huge changes in healthcare should choose diagnostic imaging as AI will impact radiology and play a huge role in the EMR evolution that will affect patient outcomes in a very positive way.

## References

1. Gartner Methodologies, Gartner Hype Cycle. Available at https://www.gartner.com/en/research/methodologies/gartner-hype-cycle.
2. Gartner Hype Cycle for Emerging Technologies, 2018, Mike Walker, 6 Aug 2018.
3. Machine learning and artificial intelligence in radiology: a "gentle" introduction. Available at https://siim.org/page/19w_ml_ai_introduction?&hhsearchterms=%22webinar+and+february+and+2019%22.
4. Health Information Technology Archive. Computerized provider order entry. Available at https://healthit.ahrq.gov/key-topics/computerized-provider-order-entry.
5. Health IT.gov. Clinical decision support. Available at https://www.healthit.gov/topic/safety/clinical-decision-support.
6. CareSelect®. Available at http://nationaldecisionsupport.com/.
7. Institute for Clinical Systems Improvement. Clinical decision support. Available at https://icsi.org/_asset/0g594t/htdi-Decision-Support-Overview.pdf.
8. United States Department of Health and Human Services summary of the HIPPA privacy rule. Available at www.HHS.gov.

# Correction to: Advanced Practice Providers

Randi L. Collinson

---

**Correction to: K. A. Gross (ed.), *Advanced Practice and Leadership in Radiology Nursing*, https://doi.org/10.1007/978-3-030-32679-1**

There were two misspellings in Fig. 1.1 in the original version of the book in Chap. 1. The spelling errors have now been corrected.

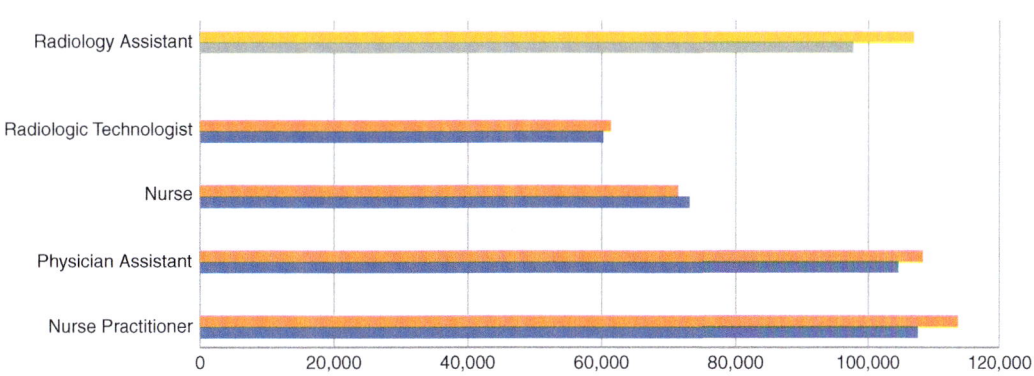

|  |  | Nurse Practitioner | Physician Assistant | Nurse | Radiologic Technologist | Radiology Assistant |
|---|---|---|---|---|---|---|
| ■ | 2016 Mean Wages |  |  |  |  | 106,777 |
| ■ | 2008 Mean Wages |  |  |  |  | 97,891 |
| ■ | 2018 Mean Wages | 113,930 | 108,430 | 71,730 | 61,540 |  |
| ■ | 2017 Mean Wages | 107,480 | 104,760 | 73,550 | 60,320 |  |

**Fig. 1.1** Medical professionals in the United States. (Source: From refs. [42–44])

---

The updated online version of this chapter can be found at
https://doi.org/10.1007/978-3-030-32679-1_1

The manufacturer's authorised representative in the EU is Springer Nature Customer Service Centre GmbH, Europaplatz 3, 69115 Heidelberg, Germany. If you have any concerns regarding our products, please contact ProductSafety@springernature.com

Printed and bound by CPI Group (UK) Ltd, Croydon, CR0 4YY
23/03/2026
02076660-0001